D1119997

Home Health and Rehabilitation

Concepts of Care

Home Health and Rehabilitation

Concepts of Care

Bella J. May, EdD, PT, FAPTA
Professor
Department of Physical Therapy
School of Allied Health Sciences
Medical College of Georgia
and
Co-Director
PhysioTherapy International, PC
Augusta, Georgia

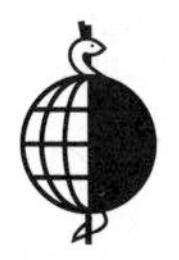

F.A. DAVIS COMPANY • Philadelphia

Printed in the United States of America

Last digit indicates print number: 10 9 8 7 6 5 4 3 2 1

Senior Allied Health Editor: Jean-François Vilain
Senior Allied Health Developmental Editor: Ralph Zickgraf
Production Editor: Crystal S. McNichol
Cover design by: Steven R. Morrone

As new scientific information becomes available through basic and clinical research, recommended treatments and drug therapies undergo changes. The author(s) and publisher have done everything possible to make this book accurate, up to date, and in accord with accepted standards at the time of publication. The authors, editors, and publisher are not responsible for errors or omissions or for consequences from application of the book and make no warranty, expressed or implied, in regard to the contents of the book. Any practice described in this book should be applied by the reader in accordance with professional standards of care used in regard to the unique circumstances that may apply in each situation. The reader is advised always to check product information (package inserts) for changes and new information regarding dose and contraindications before administering any drug. Caution is especially urged when using new or infrequently ordered drugs.

Library of Congress Cataloging-in-Publication Data

Home health and rehabilitation : concepts of care / [edited by] Bella J. May.
p. cm.
Includes bibliographical references and index.
ISBN 0-8036-5939-3 (hardback : alk. paper)
1. Home care services. 2. Home care services—United States.
3. Sick—Home care. 4. Handicapped—Home care. I. May, Bella J. [DNLM: 1. Decision Making. 2. Home Care Services.
3. Rehabilitation. 4. Reimbursement Mehanisms. WB 320 H765]
RA645.3.H6467 1992
362. 1′4—dc20
DNLM/DLC
for Library of Congress

92-49433
CIP

PREFACE

Several years ago, a colleague and I presented a workshop on decision making in home health care. After the workshop, one of the participants thanked us and voiced a concern over the dearth of written materials and workshops for the therapist working in home health. A survey of the literature supported her premise and led to the birth of this book. Several occupational and physical therapists reviewed the original chapter outlines and made content suggestions. The book reflects topics of greatest interest to most reviewers. It is not meant to be an encyclopedia of home health and rehabilitation care, and there are areas that have not been included, such as the special needs of the ventilator-dependent individual, because of the need to balance size, cost, and number of chapters.

Home health is a unique practice arena. Home health therapists may travel many miles in the course of a day. They visit rural and urban homes, enter affluent and inner city neighborhoods, and work with clients of all ages and varied socioeconomic status. Home health therapists have no medical charts to review, no colleagues close at hand, and no readily available medical support services. Their equipment is limited to what they can carry in their cars. They generally work in isolation, although they function as part of a team. There are a number of similarities and differences between home health and rehabilitation care. Both are concerned with functional outcomes and both work with clients with multiple problems. Several therapists working in rehabilitation facilities reviewed the chapter outlines and indicated interest in the content. Thus, the book was designed for occupational and physical therapists working either in home health or in rehabilitation. Future practitioners will also find many topics of interest, and we recommend *Home Health Care and Rehabilitation* to faculty as a reference or text for entry-level and advanced graduate students.

Each author is an experienced practitioner either now or recently involved in clinical practice in home health or rehabilitation. Each chapter is a blend of theoretical and practical information and is designed to help the practitioner or future practitioner design programs for total client care. Many chapters use a case-based approach, providing examples of major concepts; a reference list is included for the reader seeking a more in-depth approach to the topic.

The book is divided into four sections. The first section provides an overview of home health care: Chapter 1 describes the history and dynamic growth of home health; Chapter 2 introduces the major players and investigates problems created by the isolation of home care. Chapter 3 focuses on decision-making, and while the examples used in this chapter are drawn from home health, the process is equally applicable to any client decision.

The second section includes chapters on specific therapeutic interventions. Functional assessment is the focus of Chapter 4, which includes examples of different types of forms used to document client status. Chapter 5 considers the application of therapeutic exercises in the home setting. It focuses on ways to adapt exercises and is not intended to be a compendium of therapeutic exercises or to provide complete illustrations of home exercises for sharing with clients. Other publications fill that role admirably. The most commonly seen disabilities and frequently used exercises were selected. The illustrations were designed as a guide to the practitioner. Chapter 6 provides a motor control approach to mobility and, again, will be valuable to therapists in any setting who are concerned with helping clients regain mobility capabilities. Functional independence happens in the home and community; therapists working in rehabilitation settings and those involved in home health are responsible for assessing the home environment and making recommendations for change. Chapter 7 presents home environment assessments. Therapists also recommend special or adapted equipment, the topic of Chapter 8. Chapter 9 discusses medications and provides clear descriptions of major pharmacologic concepts, including problems of substance abuse, found as often among the elderly as among younger clients. The appendix outlines major drugs and their effects, providing an excellent reference guide for practicing therapists and students.

We function in a multicultural society (Chapter 10), interact with many individuals with cognitive and motivational problems (Chapter 11), and work with caregivers as well as clients themselves (Chapter 12). The third section of the book is designed to provide the reader with a greater understanding of these important areas. Chapter 13 outlines the many roles and functions of the medical social worker, a resource person we often look to for help.

The fourth section focuses on independent topics. Chapter 14 presents the complex issues related to documentation and reimbursement clearly and concisely. Chapter 15 explores pediatric home health care, a specialty in itself. For the many therapists who find themselves working with the terminally ill client, Chapter 16 provides a greater understanding of the hospice movement and the special needs of the terminally ill.

The book is primarily designed as a resource and guide for practitioners and students. I believe it will be a good companion in anyone's home health kit or departmental or personal library.

Bella J. May

ACKNOWLEDGMENTS

From conception to birth, preparing a book is not a solitary job. Many people contribute to its creation. I would like to thank the chapter authors, who tolerated my nagging and deadlines, who wrote and rewrote, and who willingly shared their expertise. Special thanks go to the two authors who cheerfully took on additional work to help out at difficult times. Reviewing manuscripts is a critical but often unappreciated task. Thank you, Lynn Colby, MA, PT, Ohio State University; Christine M. Crivello, PT, NovaCare, Milwaukee; Debra Feingold-Stern, MSM, PT, Sunrise Rehabilitation Hospital, Fort Lauderdale; Laura Gitlin, PhD, OT, Thomas Jefferson University, Philadelphia; Robert G. Ingrisano, MS, PT, National Therapeutic Systems, Westchester, Illinois; Maureen K. Kavalar, PT, NovaCare, Milwaukee; JoAnn Niccum-Johnson, PT, Visiting Nurse Association, St. Louis, Missouri; Susan Parker, OTR/L, Austill's Rehabilitation Services, Exton, Pennsylvania; and Phyllis Plotnick, PT, Gulfport, Florida; you helped each of us write more relevant and readable chapters. I would also like to thank some special people whose names do not otherwise appear in the book: Marlene Kay Goodman of MKG Graphics in Mt. Prospect, Illinois, for the drawings in Chapter 5 and for her willingness to redraw figures for a picky editor; Cecelia King, Administrative Coordinator in our department, for dependably completing so many onerous duties; and Jean-François Vilain and Ralph Zickgraf, Senior Editors for F.A. Davis, for providing a listening ear and solutions to seemingly overwhelming problems. Finally, my thanks to all my clients who, over the years, have taught me humility, patience, and the rewards of being a therapist.

BELLA J. MAY

CONTRIBUTORS

Rebecca Austill-Clausen, MS, OTR/L, FAOTA
President
Austill's Rehabilitation Services, Inc.
Exton, Pennsylvania

Lynn Allen Colby, MS, PT
Assistant Professor
The Ohio State University
School of Allied Health Medical Professions
Physical Therapy Division
Columbus, Ohio

Jancis K. Dennis, M.App.Sci.(Phy), PT
Associate Professor
Department of Physical Therapy
School of Allied Health Sciences
Medical College of Georgia
and
Codirector
PhysioTherapy International, PC
Augusta, Georgia

Margaret E. Strolle Gossens, PT
Physical Therapist
Addison County Home Health Care Agency
Middlebury, Vermont

Marianne Hart, MSW, LCSW, BCD
Individual, Family, and Child Therapy Medical Social Service Consultant
and
Adjunct Professor
Department of Physical Therapy Education
College of Osteopathic Medicine of the Pacific
Pomona, California

Bette Horstman, MEd, PT, LNHA
President and CEO
Allied Health Service, Ltd.
Des Plaines, Illinois

Barbara Nowell Jackson, MPH, MS, OTR/L
Private Practitioner and Consultant
Raleigh, North Carolina

Donald E. Jackson, MS, PT
Executive Vice President
National Easter Seal Society
Chicago, Illinois

Maureen K. Kavalar, BS, PT
Administrator
NovaCare, Inc.
Milwaukee, Wisconsin

Bella J. May, EdD, PT, FAPTA
Professor
Department of Physical Therapy
School of Allied Health Sciences
Medical College of Georgia
and
Codirector
PhysioTherapy International, PC
Augusta, Georgia

D. Michael McKeough, EdD, PT
Associate Professor of Physical Therapy
School of Allied Health Sciences
Department of Physical Therapy
Medical College of Georgia
Augusta, Georgia

Elsa L. Ramsden, EdD, PT
Associate Professor
Office of the Provost
University of Pennsylvania
and
Adjunct Associate Professor
Temple University and Beaver College
Philadelphia, Pennsylvania

Rick Reuss, PT
Director
Department of Rehabilitation
King's Daughter's Hospital
Madison, Indiana

Carol Schunk, PsyD, PT
Regional Director
Medicare and Rehabilitation Specialists
Portland, Oregon

Maredith Spector, MS, PT
Geriatric Consultant
Physical Therapy and Sports Medicine Center, Inc.
Ridgefield, Connecticut

Betty J. Williams, PhD
Professor of Pharmacology
Department of Pharmacology
University of Texas Medical Branch—Galveston
Galveston, Texas

Barbara W.K. Yee, PhD
Associate Professor
School of Allied Health Sciences
University of Texas Medical Branch—Galveston
Galveston, Texas

CONTENTS

Chapter 1

Home Health Past and Present

BARBARA NOWELL JACKSON

HISTORY OF HOME HEALTH CARE

The care of sick persons in their homes is not a new idea in America. Its beginnings go back as far as 1796, when the Boston Dispensary created the first hospital-based home care program provided by lay persons or training physicians. It would be almost a century later, however (1877), before the New York City Mission sent trained graduate nurses to minister to the sick in their homes. The first voluntary (nongovernmental) agency specifically organized to provide home nursing services was founded in Buffalo, New York, in 1885. Stewart[1] noted that the Visiting Nurse Associations, started in 1896 in Boston and Philadelphia, were to become the prototypes for early home care, especially in the northeastern United States. In other regions of the country, the nursing functions were usually supplied by the local health departments, such as the Los Angeles County Health Department, which in 1898 hired graduate nurses to provide home care to sick persons.

Early Beginnings

Home care expanded slowly, largely due to the lack of funding. Early programs depended on philanthropy or private funds to care for the poor in their homes. However, some life insurance companies saw the benefits of home nursing care. In 1909, Metropolitan Life Insurance Company was the first to offer such services to its policyholders. Other insurance carriers, such as John Hancock, emphasized health promotion as much as curing the sick.

The use of antibiotics and immunizations and the many wounded World War II veterans who wanted treatment in their local communities became the impetus for expanding home health care. Crowded hospitals looked to community health programs where they could send their discharged patients for further treatment. Home health agencies (HHAs) slowly began to include physical therapy, social services, and nutrition in their programs. Later, such programs included speech therapy, occupational therapy, and homemaker and home health aide services.

Modern home care is often thought to have begun with the "hospital without walls" program of the Montefiore Hospital in New York City in 1947. Hospital staff provided medical, nursing, and social services to the chronically ill in their homes. Pegels[2] states that this program was unique at this time in treating all kinds of patients, not just the poor or elderly, and in expanding the scope of its providers to include vocational rehabilitation, occupational therapy, laboratory, and x-ray services.

Social Security Act of 1965

By far the most important piece of legislation to affect the use of home care services was the passage in 1965 of Title XVIII of the Social Security Act, known as Medicare. It provided for reimbursement of certain health care services delivered in the home under specific guidelines to a specific population group. Medicare reimbursement of home health services is made only to a beneficiary who is at least 65 years of age and who has paid into the Social Security or Railroad Retirement system. People less than 65 years of age are entitled to Medicare benefits if they have been disabled for at least 24 months or have end-stage renal disease. Spouses of beneficiaries more than 65 and dependent children of those entitled because of disability or end-stage renal disease may also be eligible for Medicare benefits.[3] Medicare states that the beneficiary must be homebound, under the care of a physician, and in need of intermittent part-time skilled nursing, physical therapy, or speech therapy. If these conditions are met, then occupational therapy, social work, medical supplies and equipment, and home health aide services are also eligible. Until July 1, 1981, home health visits were limited to 100 visits in a benefit period; the client had to have been hospitalized at least 3 days prior to receiving home care services. The Omnibus Reconciliation Act of 1980 removed these limitations and added occupational therapy as a primary service qualifying for benefits. This law was in effect from July 1, 1981, to December 1, 1981. It was replaced by the Omnibus Budget Reconciliation Act of 1981, which stated that occupational therapy was not a primary service but could continue even after the primary service of nursing, speech, or physical therapy had stopped. This was important in qualifying the beneficiary to continue to receive home health aide or social services as long as the client received occupational therapy. For the services to be reimbursed, the home health agency must be certified by Medicare (Table 1 – 1). (See Chapters 13 and 14 for more information on Medicare.)

Medicare has two parts, both of which cover home health care. Part A (Medicare Hospital Insurance) automatically covers an unspecified number of home care visits by a Medicare-certified HHA, as long as the three qualifying conditions are met. Although Part A states that these services are covered, certain official and unofficial guidelines have been developed by the fiscal intermediary who pays the bills that determines which services will be reimbursed. An appeal process can be initiated by the home health agency to challenge these denials. In *Dugan vs. Boen* (1989), the National Association of Homecare made one such appeal over the definitions of "homebound" and "intermittent," which resulted in a more liberalized interpretation of these terms.

Title XIX, or Medicaid, was created by the Social Security Act of 1965. Medicaid finances health care services to the indigent in many settings, one of which is the home.[4] Medicaid is less restrictive than Medicare in that the client does not need to receive skilled care to be eligible for any service. Medicaid is a joint federal and state program. Benefits for such programs vary from state to state. Medicaid requires that states provide home care nursing, equipment and appliances, medical supplies, and home health aide services, but it has the option of providing physical, occupational, and speech thera-

TABLE 1–1

Sources of Reimbursement for Home Health Care

Source	Eligibility	Requirements	Coverage	Limitations (Not Covered)
Medicare (Title XVIII of the Social Security Act)	1. Over 65 and payment into the Social Security or Railroad Retirement system 2. Disabled at least 24 months 3. End-stage renal disease 4. Spouse of 1, 2, and 3	1. Homebound 2. In need of skilled care on an intermittent basis 3. Treatment plan established by a physician	• Skilled nursing care • Physical therapy • Speech therapy If at least one of the above is needed, coverage may also be provided for • Home health aide • Occupational therapy • Medical social work • Medical supplies and equipment	1. Custodial care 2. Homemaker/chore services
Medicaid (Title XIX of the Social Security Act)	Meeting categorical and income requirements	1. In need of medically necessary care on an intermittent basis 2. Treatment plan established by a physician	Federal mandates: • Nursing care • Home health aide • Medical supplies and equipment At state's option: • Physical therapy • Occupational therapy • Speech therapy	Medical social work services
Older Americans Act (Titles III and VII)	Over age 60—special emphasis on those with low incomes	—	• Senior centers • Home-delivered meals • Transportation • Home repair • Information and referral	N/A
Social Services Act (Title XX of the Social Security Act)	Primarily based on financial need; exact criteria vary from state to state	—	Homemaker/chore service workers	N/A
Private insurance	Paid insurance policy with home health benefits	Generally, in lieu of hospitalization	Varies greatly	Depends on policy
Veterans Administration (VA)	Service-connected disability	Prior hospitalization at a VA facility	Usually the same as Medicare	Available only for service-connected disability; occasional coverage for veterans with no other funding source

Source: Reprinted from Home Health Care Nursing by S. Stuart-Siddall, p. 28, with permission of Aspen Publishers, Inc., © 1986.

pies. States can determine the scope, duration, and amount of services they will provide; therefore, many of their clients have chronic conditions that would not conform to the "intermittent" part-time service requirements of Medicare.

Title XX was added by the Social Security Act of 1975 and provides a broad range of social services to persons who meet eligibility requirements, such as homemaker and chore worker service, personal care, and home-delivered meals. Homemaker and chore worker services funded by Title XX monies provide ancillary, in-home support services; home health aides are HHA employees who provide personal care services under the supervision of a registered nurse or professional rehabilitation specialist as part of the physician's plan of treatment.[3]

Medicaid waiver programs have been developed to address persons who are at risk for institutionalization. Wagner[5] describes the New York State Long Term Care Program, which was established in 1978 to fund in-home services up to 75 percent of the average cost of residential care. It addressed the total mental, social, and health needs of the client that could be delivered in the home.

Social Security Amendment of 1983

The most recent health legislation that affected the development of the home care movement was the Social Security Amendment of 1983. Pegels[2] explains that this law established a prospective payment system, based on 468 diagnostic-related groups (DRGs), for all US hospitals reimbursed by Medicare, with the exception of rehabilitation or mental health hospitals. Hospitals were paid a specific amount per diagnosis no matter how long the client stayed in the hospital or how many tests or procedures were done. Discharging the client from the hospital as soon as possible became financially beneficial, and HHAs began to see much more seriously impaired clients than previously. This change in home health case mix, which could now include high-risk premature babies or hospice clients, paved the way for new high-technology manpower.

COMPONENTS OF HOME HEALTH CARE

Definitions

There has never been a definitive definition for home health care; rather, a concept has evolved. In 1974, the Council of Home Health Agencies defined home health services as comprising "an array of health care services provided to individuals and families in their places of residence or in ambulatory care settings for purposes of preventing disease and promoting, maintaining, or restoring health or minimizing the effects of illness and disability" (ref. 2, p. 94). Pegels goes on to describe these services as "appropriate to the needs of the individual as planned, coordinated, and made available by an organized health agency through the use of agency employed staff, contractual arrangements, or a combination of administrative patterns. Medical services are primarily provided by the individual's private or clinic physician" (ref. 2, p. 96). This general definition, however, would not be acceptable under current Medicare regulations, which restrict reimbursement to short-term, skilled, restorative services.

In 1988, Hankwitz defined home health care as "that component of a continuum of comprehensive health care whereby health services are provided to individuals and families in their places of residence for the purpose of promoting, or restoring health, or maximizing the level of independence, while minimizing the effects of disability, and illness, including terminal illness" (ref. 6, p. 294). By including services to the dying, this definition is more inclusive than the World Health Organization definition of health "as a state of complete physical, mental, and social well-being, and not merely the absence of disease or infirmity" (ref. 7, p. 29). At the 1989 annual meeting of the American Medical Association, the Council on Scientific Affairs gave a succinct definition of home care: "Home care can be defined as the provision of equipment and services to the patient in the home for the purpose of restoring and maintaining his or her maximal level of comfort, function, and health" (ref. 8, p. 1241).

Levels of Care

Within the current broad definition of home health care there are various levels. In 1988, Hankwitz described these levels as "High-Tech Acute Care, Long-term Care and Home Hospice" (ref. 6, p. 294). In 1986, J. Friedman separated these into "intensive, intermediate, and minimal care" (ref. 9, p. 32). Intensive care requires a variety of providers and equipment in the home at a high rate of use of services, similar to the care that would have been received in the hospital. Intermediate care includes both the restorative therapies and less skilled support services such as a choreworker or transportation. Minimal care includes those services that are not skilled but are necessary for a client to remain at home (Table 1–2). Hennessey and Gorenberg[10] suggest separating home care services into preventive, supportive, and therapeutic categories (Fig. 1–1).

Home Health Agency Categories

Medicaid law does not define "home health agency," but its regulators define it as a public or private agency or organization primarily engaged in providing skilled nursing or other therapeutic services.[4] The Health Care Financing Administration of the Department of Health and Human Services[11] has divided HHAs into five categories:

TABLE 1-2
Home Care Services Required At Various Impairment Levels

SERVICE	UNIMPAIRED	SLIGHTLY IMPAIRED	MILDLY IMPAIRED	MODERATELY IMPAIRED	GENERALLY IMPAIRED	EXTREMELY IMPAIRED
Transportation	X	X	X	X	X	X
Monitoring	X	X	X	X	X	X
Social/ recreational	X	X	X	X	X	X
Homemaker			X	X	X	X
Housing			X	X	X	X
Administrative/ legal				X	X	X
Meal preparation				X	X	X
Food, groceries				X	X	X
Personal care						X
Continuous supervision						X
Nursing care						X

Source: With permission of author and publisher. From Spiegel, AD: Home Healthcare. Baltimore, MD: National Health Publishing Co., 1983, p. 254.

1. Official (government): Administered by a state, county, city, or other local unit of government. Its major responsibilities are disease prevention and community education. It must offer nursing of the sick in the home.
2. Voluntary: Administered by a community-based board of directors and is usually financed by earnings and contributions. The function is care of the sick in the home. Some voluntary agencies are operated under church auspices.
3. Combined official and voluntary: Administered jointly by a voluntary and an official agency, supported by tax funds, earnings, and contributions, and providing nursing and therapeutic services.
4. Private not-for-profit: A privately developed and administered non-profit organization other than a visiting nurse association that provides care of the sick in the home. This agency must qualify as a tax-exempt organization under Title 26 USC 501(c) of the Internal Revenue Code.
5. Proprietary: Owned and operated by an individual or a business corporation. The organization may be a sole proprietorship, partnership (including limited partnership and joint stock company), or corporation.

A more definitive description by Stuart-Siddall states, "Home health agencies are classified further according to location and government struc-

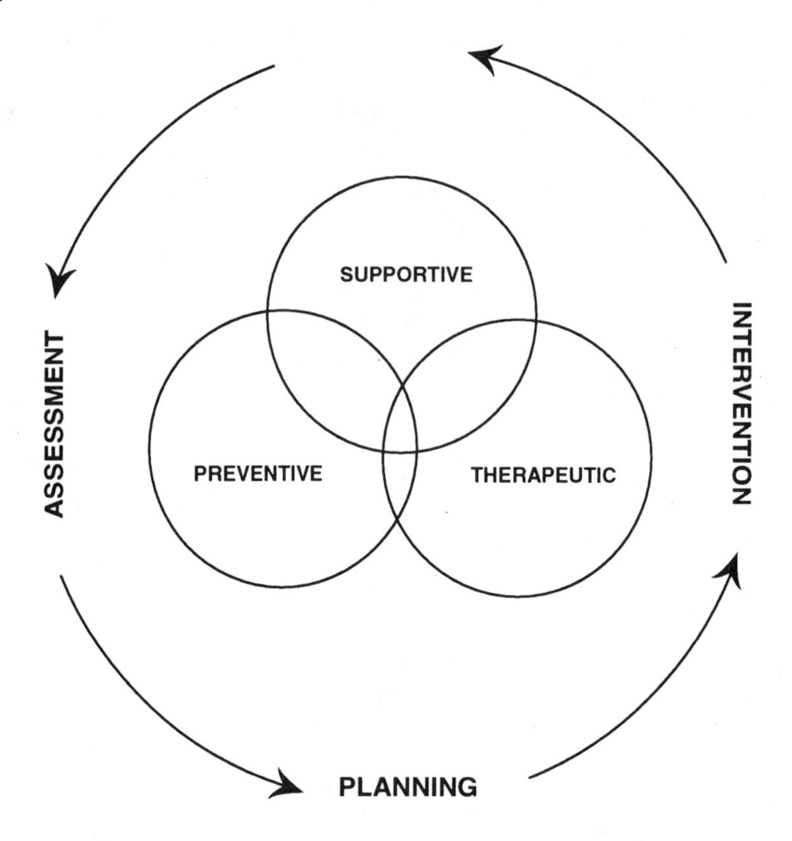

Preventive	*Supportive*	*Therapeutic*
Dental Care	Legal	Nursing
Health Education	Financial	Physical Therapy
Police Assistance	Home Help	Occupational Therapy
Outpatient Care	Nutrtion	Inhalation Therapy
Protective Services	Social	Dental Care
Home Safety	Religious	Mental Health Therapy
Recreation	Recreation	Medical
Peer Interaction	Transportation	Pharmaceutical Services
Employment	Shopping	Laboratory Services
Volunteer Work	Grooming	Family Respite Care
	Visitors	Night Sitters
	Handyman	Trustee Services
	Laundry	
	Information and Referral	

Figure 1–1. The three-way segmentation of home care services. (From Hennessey and Govenberg,[10] p. 357, with permission.)

ture. Those that are not housed within another type of service delivery system or institution are defined as freestanding. Conversely, agencies that are housed within another service delivery system are commonly grouped according to the type of provider. As a result, skilled nursing facility (SNF)-based and hospital-based agencies are common terms within the industry" (ref. 3, p. 24).

A Home Health Line summary of HHAs, certified as of December 10, 1990, gave the following totals[12]:

Veterans Administration	476
Combined Official	14
Official	941
Rehabilitation Hospital	9
Hospital	1537
Skilled Nursing Facility-based	105
Proprietary	1970
Private Nonprofit	701
Other	0

In addition, many prepaid health care systems, such as health maintenance organizations (HMOs) and preferred provider organizations (PPOs), have developed their own health programs or contracted with an HHA to provide care for their Medicare or Medicaid clients.

CLIENT POPULATION

In 1756, the population served were the elderly poor who wanted to be treated with dignity in their homes rather than in hospitals, which were considered repositories for the indigent or alms cases. After the establishment of the Visiting Nurses Association at the end of the 19th century other people, including children and individuals with chronic diseases, were seen. Titles XVIII and XIX of the Social Security Act of 1965 expanded funding for home health services to include the disabled, the elderly, and people with chronic illnesses. Medicaid also broadened the concept of home health care to include such nonskilled services as homemaking and home-delivered meals.

Between 1980 and 1990 home care expanded to new populations. Medical technology has made it possible for clients to receive intravenous chemotherapy, home renal dialysis, total parental and enteral nutrition, ventilator-dependent infusion services, defibrillators, intravenous therapies, and special cardiac monitoring in the home. These special treatment modalities require extensive monitoring, which, until recently, could only be accomplished in a hospital. They require highly trained providers who can educate caregivers regarding procedures and precautions. The legal and quality-assurance aspects of such high-technologic treatments have changed the image of home care from a "cottage" medical service to an extension of the hospital.

USE OF SERVICES

On the other end of home health care service delivery is the expanded need for the semiskilled or nonskilled services of homemakers, personal care attendants, and other supportive personnel. The largest financial outlay in

TABLE 1–3
Average and Median Ages of Postacute Care Clients
(All Medicare Hospital Discharges; Live Discharges Only)

DRG	No PAC Use	SNF	Home Health	Rehabilitation
Average Age				
14 Stroke	76.4	79.6	76.8	74.9
88 COPD	71.1	75.7	73.2	73.6
127 Heart failure	76.0	81.6	78.5	76.2
209 Major joint procedures	73.6	80.6	75.9	76.2
210 Hip and femur procedures	80.8	82.6	79.7	80.2
All DRGs	72.6	79.9	76.1	74.1
Median Age				
14 Stroke	76	80	77	75
88 COPD	71	77	73	73
127 Heart failure	76	82	79	75
209 Major joint procedures	73	81	76	77
210 Hip and femur procedures	82	83	80	81
All DRGs	73	80	76	75

DRG = diagnostic-related group; PAC = progress assessment chart; SNF = skilled nursing facility; COPD = chronic obstructive pulmonary disease.

Source: Adapted from Neu et al,[14] p. 12, with permission.

recent years has been Title XX funds that deliver nonskilled services to elderly and disabled clients in their homes. It is the inability to take care of dressing, feeding, and bathing, or the lack of a primary caregiver—not necessarily the type or severity of the disability—that most often puts a disabled person at risk for institutionalization (see Chapters 12 and 13).

Ginzberg and associates[13] divide home care use into various patient characteristics such as age, living arrangement, sex, diagnosis, and functional status. A 1989 Rand study showed that, although there is an increasing number of home care clients younger than 65 years of age, the principal age group of persons using those services in five primary DRG groups remains older than 65 (Tables 1–3 and 1–4).[14] It is a well-known epidemiologic fact that the population of the United States is getting older, with the fastest-growing group being more than 85 years of age[15] (Table 1–5). This age-related use is partially a reflection of the funding sources for Medicare and Medicaid, but other age groups are now being served by home health agencies through such insurance programs as HMOs, PPOs, Blue Cross–Blue Shield, or other private insurance companies whose case mix populations reflect working families with children.

Caregivers have changed in recent years: adult children and spouses are both employed, families move farther apart, and single parents are more prevalent. Yet only about 5 percent of the elderly population resides in nursing homes (see Chapter 12). Pegels states, "The majority of the older people, and especially the very old, are women. At the beginning of the 20th century,

TABLE 1-4

Tendencies of Clients to Use Postacute Care, By Age

(All Medicare Hospital Discharges; Live Discharges Only)

Age Group	SNF	Home Health	Rehabilitation
DRG 14: Stroke			
<65	6.9	24.3	7.8
65–69	8.4	25.7	9.6
70–74	11.1	28.2	8.7
75–79	14.9	28.4	7.6
80–84	18.4	28.9	6.5
>84	21.8	23.9	3.8
DRG 88: COPD			
<65	0.8	13.0	0.1
65–69	0.9	14.3	0.1
70–74	1.0	17.6	0.1
75–79	1.7	21.3	0.1
80–84	2.9	23.3	0.2
>84	4.3	22.3	0.2
DRG 127: Heart Failure and Shock			
<65	0.4	11.5	0.1
65–69	0.9	14.8	0.1
70–74	1.3	18.1	0.2
75–79	2.1	21.6	0.1
80–84	2.7	23.6	0.1
>84	4.2	24.8	0.1
DRG 209: Major Joint Procedures			
<65	3.6	28.6	2.1
65–69	5.3	27.4	1.6
70–74	8.9	34.3	1.9
75–79	15.0	38.6	2.7
80–84	23.5	40.6	2.6
>84	34.6	32.2	2.4
DRG 210: Hip or Femur Procedures			
<65	11.9	29.4	3.0
65–69	17.8	41.9	3.1
70–74	22.4	40.9	2.9
75–79	27.9	40.8	3.1
80–84	33.4	37.0	2.9
>84	36.9	26.5	2.4
All DRGs			
<65	0.8	9.0	0.4
65–69	1.2	10.1	0.5
70–74	2.0	13.5	0.5
75–79	3.3	16.9	0.6
80–84	5.0	19.6	0.6
>84	7.7	20.1	0.5

DRG = diagnostic-related group; SNF = skilled nursing facility; COPD = chronic obstructive pulmonary disease.

Source: Adapted from Neu et al,[14] p. 13, with permission.

TABLE 1 – 5

Actual and Projected Growth of the Elderly Population, 1900–2050 (In Thousands)

YEAR	TOTAL POPULATION ALL AGES	55 to 64 Years		65 to 74 Years		75 to 84 Years		85 Years and Over		65 Years and Over	
		NUMBER	PERCENT	NUMBER	PERCENT	NUMBER	PERCENT	NUMBER	PERCENT	NUMBER	PERCENT
1900	76,303	4,009	5.3	2,189	2.9	772	1.0	123	0.2	3,084	4.0
1910	91,972	5,054	5.5	2,793	3.0	989	1.1	167	0.2	3,950	4.3
1920	105,711	6,532	6.2	3,464	3.3	1,259	1.2	210	0.2	4,933	4.7
1930	122,775	8,397	6.8	4,721	3.8	1,641	1.3	272	0.2	6,634	5.4
1940	131,669	10,572	8.0	6,375	4.8	2,278	1.7	365	0.3	9,019	6.8
1950	150,967	13,295	8.8	8,415	5.6	3,278	2.2	577	0.4	12,270	8.1
1960	179,323	15,572	8.7	10,997	6.1	4,633	2.6	929	0.5	16,560	9.2
1970	203,302	18,608	9.2	12,447	6.1	6,124	3.0	1,409	0.7	19,980	9.8
1980	226,505	21,700	9.6	15,578	6.9	7,727	3.4	2,240	1.0	25,544	11.3
1990	249,657	21,051	8.4	18,035	7.2	10,349	4.1	3,313	1.3	31,697	12.7
2000	267,955	23,767	8.9	17,677	6.6	12,318	4.6	4,926	1.8	34,921	13.0
2010	283,238	34,848	12.3	20,318	7.2	12,326	4.4	6,551	2.3	39,195	13.8
2020	296,597	40,298	13.6	29,855	10.1	14,486	4.9	7,081	2.4	51,422	17.3
2030	304,807	34,025	11.2	34,535	11.3	21,434	7.0	8,612	2.8	64,581	21.2
2040	308,559	34,717	11.3	29,272	9.5	24,882	8.1	12,834	4.2	66,988	21.7
2050	309,488	37,327	12.1	30,114	9.7	21,263	6.9	16,034	5.2	67,411	21.8

Source: Reprinted with permission from *America's Aging: Health in an Older Society*, © 1985 by the National Academy of Sciences. Published by National Academy Press, Washington, D.C.

men actually outnumbered women. Improvements in health care have changed that statistic dramatically. In 1980, elderly women outnumbered men by 6 million and are projected to outnumber men by 12 million by the year 2036" (ref 2, p. 20). These data translate to higher use of home health services by women than by men (ref. 14, pp. 14 and 15) (Tables 1–6 and 1–7). Ginzberg and associates state, "The most prevalent diagnostic group that was treated at home was that comprising circulatory disorders, including stroke, followed by neoplasms. Other frequent primary diagnostic categories include endocrine diseases, musculoskeletal disorders and injuries" (ref. 13, p. 15).

The functional status of the client being treated in the home is probably a more accurate indicator of needs for services than the diagnosis. Kane and Kane[16] reviewed various types of physical assessment tools such as the Katz Activities of Daily Living (ADL), the modified ADL Scales, the Barthel Index of Performance, and the Rapid Disability Rating Scale. No single assessment tool can be used as a predictor of function in home care. However, studies have correlated the level of disability or dependence with the cost effectiveness of home care, indicating that home care may be more effective with people in need of rehabilitation services and individuals with chronic problems whose families were willing to provide care.[17, 18] Research also indicates that early home rehabilitation following geriatric assessment in chronic illness can forestall functional decline and may even re-establish functional independence.[18] (See Chapter 4 for a more detailed discussion of functional assessment.)

TABLE 1–6

Tendencies of Clients to Use Postacute Care, by Sex

(All Medicare Hospital Discharges; Live Discharges Only)

DRG	Sex	No PAC Use	SNF	Home Health	Rehabilitation
14 Stroke	Male	59.8	12.1	25.8	7.9
	Female	54.5	16.9	27.9	6.6
88 COPD	Male	83.3	1.2	15.6	0.1
	Female	77.7	1.8	20.7	0.1
127 Heart failure	Male	81.3	1.7	17.1	0.1
	Female	75.0	2.5	22.7	0.1
209 Major joint procedures	Male	65.4	10.1	26.1	1.7
	Female	49.5	17.5	37.6	2.5
210 Hip and femur procedures	Male	44.6	26.7	34.1	2.7
	Female	40.4	32.0	34.8	2.8
All DRGs	Male	85.6	2.3	12.2	0.5
	Female	80.1	3.8	16.6	0.5

Note: Row totals may exceed 100 percent because some patients use postacute care in more than one setting.
DRG = diagnostic-related group; PAC = progress assessment chart; SNF = skilled nursing facility; COPD = chronic obstructive pulmonary disease.

Source: Adapted from Neu et al,[14] p. 14, with permission.

TABLE 1–7

Tendencies of Clients to Use Postacute Care, by Age and Sex

(All Live Medicare Discharges; In Percent)

		Age Group					
	Sex	**<65**	**65–69**	**70–74**	**75–79**	**80–84**	**>84**
SNF	Male	0.8	1.0	1.7	2.7	4.0	6.1
	Female	0.9	1.4	2.3	3.7	5.6	8.4
Home health	Male	7.6	8.3	11.3	14.6	17.8	19.5
	Female	10.9	11.7	15.5	18.6	20.7	20.3
Rehabilitation	Male	0.4	0.5	0.5	0.6	0.6	0.4
	Female	0.4	0.5	0.5	0.6	0.6	0.5

SNF = skilled nursing facility.

Source: Adapted from Neu et al,[14] p. 15, with permission.

Occupational and Physical Therapy

In 1986, the American Occupational Therapy Association[15] surveyed 281 occupational therapists known to be practicing in home health. The most frequent number of visits per diagnoses were, in order, cerebral vascular accidents, burns, spinal cord injuries, head injuries, and cerebral palsy. Occupational therapists spent most of their treatment time on ADL, assessment, and muscle re-education. Analyzing expenditures in 1986 and 1987, the National Association for Home Care indicated that more than 17,000 therapists provided services in 1986 and more than half a million clients received services in 1987 (Tables 1–8 and 1–9). Table 1–10 depicts the increase in the number of occupational therapists and assistants working primarily in home health since 1973; Figure 1–2 depicts the geographic distribution of occupational therapists. The 1990 Active Membership Profile Report of the American Physical Therapy Association[19] also indicates the increasing numbers of therapists involved in home health care since 1978

TABLE 1–8

Number of Clients, by Type of Provider, In-Home Care, 1987

TYPE OF PROVIDER	CLIENTS
Homemaker–home health aides	2,643,000
Nurses	2,143,000
Doctors	969,000
Therapists	633,000
Other (medical)	1,512,000
Total	5,878,000*

*The numbers do not add up because some individuals receive services from more than one type of provider.

Source: Reproduced by permission of The National Association for Home Care, from *Basic Statistics About Home Care —1991*.

TABLE 1-9

Number of Providers, by Type, Working in Medicare-Certified Home Care Agencies, 1986

PROVIDERS	SALARIED	CONTRACT*	TOTAL
RN	39,552	1,680	41,232
LPN	3,827	163	3,990
Physical therapists	6,234	7,902	14,136
Occupational therapists	1,997	1,807	3,804
Speech therapists	3,113	6,215	9,328
Homemaker–home health aides	26,324	7,302	33,626
Other	23,991	521	24,512
Total	105,038	25,590	130,628

*Estimated.

RN = registered nurse; LPN = licensed practical nurse.

Source: Reproduced by permission of The National Association for Home Care, from *Basic Statistics About Home Care —1991*.

(Table 1–11). The percentage drop from 8.29 percent in 1983 to 7 percent in 1990 probably reflects the change in status of many providers from staff physical therapists to contract physical therapists. The Health Care Financing Administration data indicate that Medicare-certified agencies more than doubled in number since 1967. With Medicare providing the greatest percentage of reimbursement for home health care clients, the major increase in agencies providing occupational therapy services reflects the acceptance of occupational therapy for reimbursement in Medicare regulations (Tables 1–12 through 1–14). The North Carolina Association for Home Care surveyed its members in 1990 and reported both the number of visits made by each discipline and the percentage of services received by each client (Table 1–15; Fig. 1–3). The growth and current use of therapy in the scope of total home health services is clearly illustrated in these data.

TABLE 1-10

OTRs and COTAs Working Primarily in Home Health Settings (1973–1988)

	OTRs		COTAs	
	%	NO.	%	NO.
1973	0.9	77	0.2	4
1977	2.2	300	0.4	13
1982	3.8	853	0.8	43
1986	4.6	1317	1.2	79
1988	5*	1413	1.5*	118

*Estimate.

OTR = registered occupational therapist; COTA = certified occupational therapy assistant.

Source: From *Occupational Therapy News*, March 1989, with permission of The American Occupational Therapy Association.

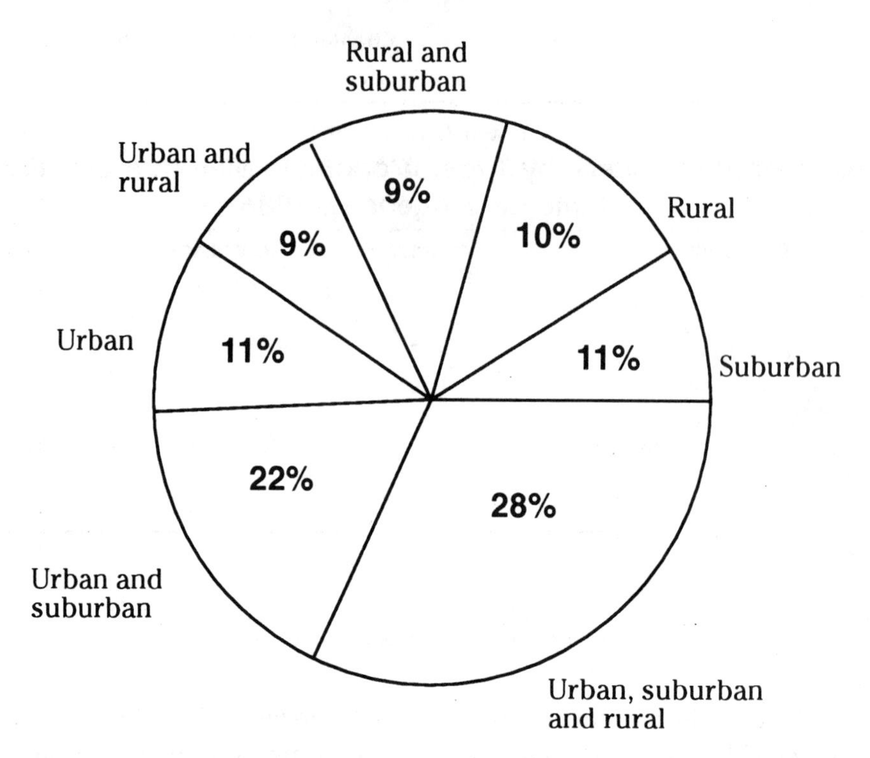

Figure 1–2. Geographic areas served by home health agencies. (From *Occupational Therapy News*, September, 1986, with permission of the American Occupational Therapy Association.)

TABLE 1–11

Types of Facility or Institution in Which (or for Which) Respondents Practice

FACILITY/INSTITUTION	1978	1982	1983	1990
Hospital	47.11	42.71	41.39	29.6
Private office	9.92			
Private physical therapy office		11.01	14.66	24.9
Physician's office		3.01	2.75	2.2
Rehabilitation center, with or without beds	9.24	8.46	9.15	10.8
Extended care facility/nursing home	8.20	7.50	6.00	5.5
Home health agency	5.88	8.26	8.29	7.00
Public or nonpublic school	5.65	6.78	4.68	5.1
Academic institution	5.20	4.23	4.25	4.0
Specialty clinic	1.67	1.19	1.93	N/A
Residential care facility	1.53	1.46	1.13	N/A
Governmental department or agency	1.44	1.12	0.98	N/A
Voluntary health agency	0.41	0.30	0.15	N/A
Prepaid health care organization	0.39	0.76	0.92	1.2
Research center	0.19	0.36	0.22	0.2
Industry	0.11	0.17	0.31	N/A
Other/missing	3.06	2.68	2.69	9.5

Source: From American Physical Therapy Association 1990 Active Membership Profile Report, with permission.

TABLE 1-12

Number and Percent of Home Health Agencies Providing Occupational Therapy Services, 1975–1986

	1975	1976	1982	1984	1986
All agencies	2254	2185	3415	4271	5900
Agencies providing OT services:					
Number	533	590	1360*	2104	3510
Percent	23.6	27.0	40.0*	49.3	59.5

*Estimate.

Source: From the Health Care Financing Administration, US Department of Health and Human Services, with permission.

TABLE 1-13

Revenue Sources of Home Health Care (1987) (%)

78	Medicare
7	Medicaid
4	Blue Cross/Blue Shield
5	Commercial insurance
3	Self-pay
1	HMO
1	Philanthropy
1	Other

Source: Adapted from the Health Care Financing Administration, US Department of Health and Human Services, with permission.

TABLE 1-14

Clients Receiving Each Service (%)

Nursing	77
Occupational Therapy	5
Physical Therapy	32
Speech Therapy	7
Medical Social Service	10
Home Health Aide	28

Source: Adapted from North Carolina Association for Home Care: A Summary of the 1990 Home Health Data. Raleigh, NC, 1991, with permission.

TABLE 1-15

Number of Medicare-Certified Home Health Agencies in Selected Years

1967	1809
1977	2496
1981	3178
1983	4258
1985	5983
1986	5898
1987	5785

Source: From the Health Care Financing Administration, US Department of Health and Human Services, with permission.

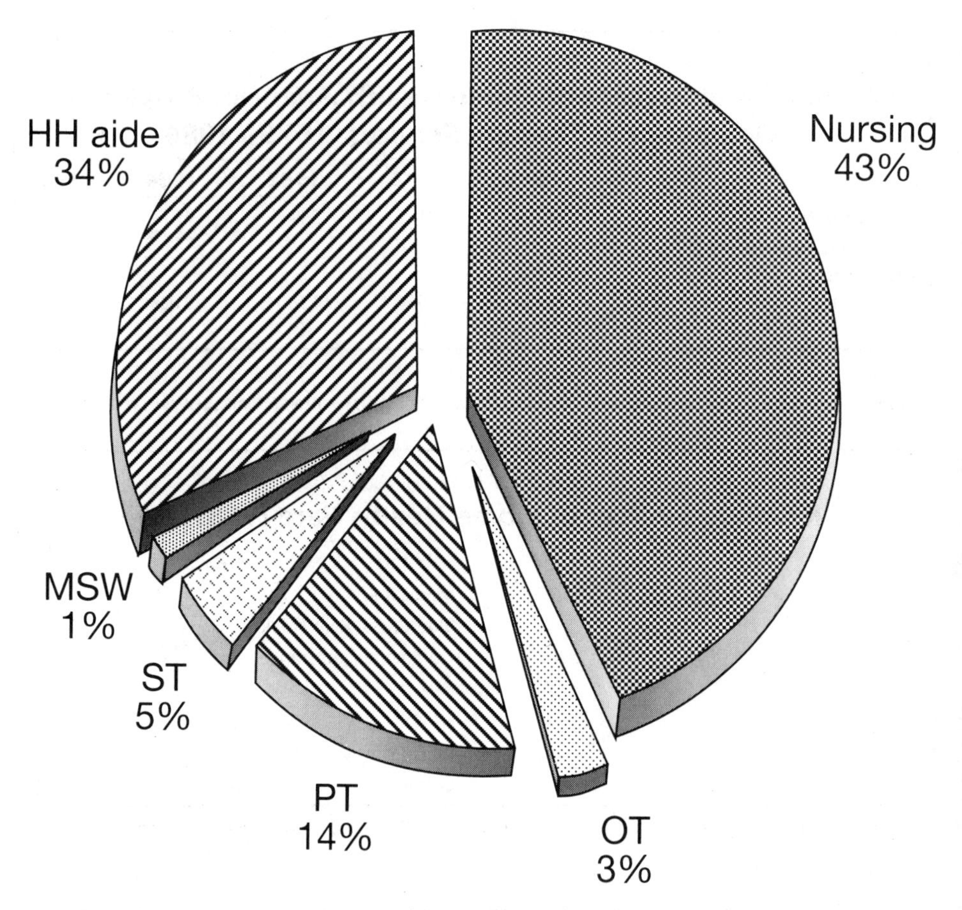

Figure 1–3. Percent of visits by discipline. (From North Carolina Association for Home Care: A Summary of the 1990 Home Health Data. Raleigh, NC, 1991, with permission.)

HOME CARE IN THE TOTAL HEALTH CARE DELIVERY SYSTEM

Home health care, as a part of the continuum of health services, is a rapidly growing system for a variety of reasons. Home care (1) can prevent or delay hospitalization and residential placement, (2) can be cost effective in comparison with institutional care if the level of skilled care necessary is contained, (3) is the preferred alternative for most people, (4) addresses the needs of various age groups, not just the ill elderly, (5) can be delivered in a variety of settings depending on the restrictions and eligibility criteria of funding sources, and (6) gives financial advantage to hospital systems using DRGs to discharge clients to a community setting. The advantages and disadvantages of home health care are depicted in Table 1–16 (ref. 6, p. 298).

Public policy questions have arisen about the availability, accessibility, and quality of home care services. The need for skilled and unskilled per-

TABLE 1-16
Advantages and Disadvantages of Home Health Care

Advantages	Disadvantages
Provides more efficient use of physician's time by expanding use of the team approach.	Gives physicians heavy and often unreimbursed management responsibilities (a significant intrusion on physician time with supervisory demands, paperwork, and lengthy phone calls).
Expands physician's patient base through coordinated home care programs because physician can order all ancillary care easily through one coordinator.	May require physician to see patient at home rather than in the office.
Gives physician comprehensive perspective of patient and family.	Requires deep involvement of family members and may disrupt family functioning at the same time that it permits the family to remain technically intact.
Provides educational opportunity for house staff physicians and medical students.	Indirect costs may be high when cost of family members' or caregivers' time and out-of-pocket expenses are considered.
Continues health care.	May be lack of coordination and communication between physician, home health agency, family, and patient.
Identifies day-to-day problems early; reduces emergency situations.	Quality of care delivered in the home is not easily measured, monitored, or documented.
Permits earlier discharge from hospital and other health care institutions.	Third-party payers may not cover costs of identical home care supplies and services that are covered when provided in an institutional setting.
Reduces institutional readmissions.	
Enhances recovery and emotional well-being, freedom, and personal dignity in the company of the client's family in a more comfortable and cheerful atmosphere.	
Does not expose clients to institution induced illness.	
Client's own food tastes can be met.	
Long-term and terminal illnesses may better be cared for at home.	
Family is part of care team.	
Improves progress in activities of daily living with less deterioration in indices of socioeconomic functioning.	
Visiting home care personnel provide support and understanding.	
Reduces costs to client and third-party payer when compared with costs of institutional care.	
Reduces unnecessary capital construction costs for inpatient facilities.	
Provides educational benefits to clients and their families, with the home being a more effective site for learning and motivational activities with achievement of a relatively independent status.	

Source: Adapted from Portnow, J (ed): Home health care and rehabilitation. In Physical Medicine and Rehabilitation: State of the Art Reviews, 2(3), 1988, p 298, with permission.

sonnel continues to increase beyond available resources. There is a need to expand services to the rural population, inner city clients, and socioethnic minorities. Monies are often available for institutional care, but not for community-based home care. Access issues include the fragmentation and non-coordination of services due to various criteria for eligibility and funding sources; knowledge of what services are available; the cost involved; and whether a caregiver is available to assist and augment the home health plan.

Home care must also be acceptable to the client, the physician and other gatekeepers to services, and the caregiver. Increasingly, HHAs are conducting "exit satisfaction surveys" with clients and their caregivers. Educational programs are being targeted toward physicians and discharge planners regarding the scope and diversity of services offered in the home.

Two of the most critical aspects of home care center around the issue of accountability — the lack of definitive research in the area of home care and quality assurance. Research has been restricted by the numerous factors that are not easily measurable — for example, the total cost of keeping a client at home; the amount of care now given without financial remuneration; and lack of control studies on caregiver stress. Wagner[5] suggests that the rising costs of Medicare and Medicaid in the 1970s led to a demand from third-party payers and the government for professional accountability of health care providers. The American Nurses Association (ANA) developed a model of quality assurance that included structure, process, and outcome criteria to assess the quality of care for professional performance, patient care, and organizational settings. This ANA model, adapted for the home care setting, led to the 10 Step Model of Quality Assurance of the Joint Commission on Accreditation of Healthcare Organizations and that organization's recent implementation of a voluntary accreditation for HHAs. The *Quality Assurance Primer* (1988) of the North Carolina Association for Home Care[20] and the "Quality Assurance in Home Health" model for occupational therapists developed by the American Occupational Therapy Association,[21] address the need to assess the quality of care. In both models, quality is measured through internal and external review. The internal review is generated and administered by the agency and includes the audit and advisory committees, whereas the external review refers to compliance with state licensing practice or to fiscal intermediators.

Barhydt-Wezenaar[22] characterizes the 1960s as the decade of hospital expansion, the 1970s as the decade of nursing home expansion, and the 1980s and 1990s as the decades of home care expansion. She notes:

> Until the early 1980s, home care was considered to be a stepchild in the health care delivery system. This attitude was held by government, legislators, regulators, and even within the professional health care community. As a result, there was a pervasive perception within the community that home care is often chosen as a last resort (ref. 22, p. 252).

Home health care is expanding at an accelerating rate. The fact that it is often cheaper and preferred by the client enhances this trend. The major detriment to expansion is limited funding sources. Home care in the 1990s is an old idea in an old setting, with new populations and new providers. If the present political situation continues, consumer demands will dictate that a financial health package, including home care, be developed by the federal, state, local, or the private sector during this decade.

SUMMARY

The history of home health care since 1796 has changed a small, charity-financed or personal payment system of lay persons, treating the poor and sick in their homes, to a system of various services financed by government, state, or private insurance under defined agreements to specific populations. The populations served have been primarily the elderly, the chronically ill, or the disabled but recently have expanded to include infants, ventilator-dependent clients, enteral feeding clients, and the terminally ill. The services rendered primarily by nurses are now augmented by a variety of rehabilitation specialists, ventilator and respiratory personnel, and highly trained technicians. Delivery of home care services has broadened from primarily visiting nurse associations and health departments to skilled nursing homes, adult day care centers, hospital-based agencies, and agencies located in the community, nursing homes, or other places of residence. The future of home health care in the United States continues to expand at an explosive rate within the confines of reimbursement parameters and federal, state, and local requirements.

REFERENCES

1. Stewart, JE: Home Health Care. CV Mosby, St Louis, 1979, p. 20.
2. Pegels, CC: Health Care and the Older Citizen: Economic, Demographic, and Financial Aspects. Aspen, Rockville, 1988, p 73.
3. Stuart-Siddall, S: Home Health Care Nursing. Aspen, Rockville, 1986, p 27.
4. Spiegel, AD: Home Healthcare: Home Birthing to Hospice Care. National Health Publishing, Owings Mills, 1983, p 10.
5. Wagner, DM: Managing for Quality in Home Health Care. Aspen, Rockville, 1988, p 2.
6. Hankwitz, PE: The Role of the Physician in Home Care. In Portnow, J (ed): Physical Medicine and Rehabilitation: State of the Art Reviews, 1988.
7. World Health Organization: The Constitution of the World Health Organization. World Health Organization Chronicle. Geneva, 1944, p 29.
8. Council on Scientific Affairs: Home Care in the 1990s. JAMA 263: 1241, 1990.
9. Friedman, J: Home Health Care. WW Norton, New York, 1986, p 32.
10. Hennessey, MJ and Govenberg, B: The significance and impact of the home care of an older adult. Nursing Clinics of North America, 14(2): 357, 1980.
11. Health Care Financing Administration: Provider Reimbursement Manual. Part 2, Section 402.1, Subsection 9402A, Part 1. Commerce Clearing House, Chicago, 1986.
12. Home Health Line: Personal communication, March, 1991.
13. Ginzberg, E, Balinsky, W, and Ostow, M: Home Health Care: Its Role in the

Changing Health Services Market. Rowman and Allanheld, New York, 1984, p 12.

14. Neu, CR, Harrison, SC, and Heilbrunn, JZ: Medicare Patients and Postacute Care: Who Goes Where? Rand, Santa Monica, 1989, p 11.
15. American Occupational Therapy Association: Guidelines for Occupational Therapy Services in Home Health. Author, Rockville, 1987, p 5.
16. Kane, RA and Kane, RL: Assessing the Elderly: A Practical Guide to Measurement. Lexington Books, Lexington, KY, 1981, p 39.
17. Sager, A: Planning Home Care with the Elderly. Ballinger, Cambridge, UK, 1983, p 134.
18. Keenan, JM: In-Home geriatric rehabilitation. In Kemp, D, Brummel-Smith, K, and Ramsdell, J (eds): Geriatric Rehabilitation. Little, Brown & Co, Boston, 1990, p 361.
19. American Physical Therapy Association: 1990 Active Membership Profile Report. Author, Alexandria, VA, 1990, p 23.
20. North Carolina Association for Home Care: Quality Assurance Primer (1988). Author, Raleigh, 1988.
21. American Occupational Therapy Association: Quality Assurance in Occupational Therapy: A Practitioner's Guide to Setting Up a QA System Using Three Models. Author, Rockville, 1991.
22. Barhydt-Wezenaar, N: Home Care and Hospice. In Jones, S (ed): Health Care Delivery in the United States, ed 3. Springer-Verlag, New York, 1986, p 252.

BIBLIOGRAPHY

Brickner, PW: Home Health Care for the Aged: How to Help Older People Stay in Their Own Homes and out of Institutions. Appleton-Century-Crofts, New York, 1978.

Cromwell, FS (ed): The Roles of Occupational Therapists in Continuity of Care. Occupational Therapy and Health Care 2:1, 1985.

Crystal, S, et al: The Management of Home Care Services. Springer-Verlag, New York, 1987.

Dunlop, BD (ed): New Federalism and Long-Term Health Care of the Elderly. Center for Health Affairs, Project HOPE, Millwood, 1985.

Gaitz, CM and Samorajski, T: Aging 2000: Our Health Care Destiny. Springer-Verlag, New York, 1985.

Gallo, JJ, Reichel, W, and Andersen, L (eds): Handbook of Geriatric Assessment. Aspen, Rockville, 1988.

Greenberg, W and Southby, RMcKF: Health Care Institutions in Flux. Information Resources Press, Arlington, 1984.

Haddad, AM: High Tech Home Care: A Practical Guide. Aspen, Rockville, 1987.

Hiatt, HH: America's Health in the Balance: Choice or Chance. Harper & Row, New York, 1987.

Holt, SW: Securing the Future Through Innovation: New Dimensions in Home Health Care. Caring, 8:35, 1989.

Jonas, S: Health Care Delivery in the United States, ed 3. Springer-Verlag, New York, 1986.

Kane, NM: The Home Care Crisis of the Nineties. The Gerontologist 29:24, 1989.

Keenam, JM and Fanale, J: Home Care: Past and Present, Problems and Potential. J Am Geriatr Soc 37:1076, 1989.

Liebig, PS and Lammers, WW (eds): California Policy Choices for Long-Term Care. Ethel Percy Andrus Gerontology Center, University of Southern California, Los Angeles, 1990.

Martinson, IM and Widmer, A: Home Health Care Nursing. WB Saunders, Philadelphia, 1989.

Mundinger, MO'N: Home Care Controversy: Too Little, Too Late, Too Costly. Aspen, Rockville, 1983.

Parker, M: How to Succeed in the Home Care Business in the 1990s. Caring 9:8, 1990.

Pegels, CC: Health Care and the Elderly. Aspen, Rockville, 1980.

Pelham, AO and Clark, WF (eds): Managing Home Care for the Elderly: Lessons from Community-Based Agencies. Springer-Verlag, New York, 1986.

Polich, C, et al: The Provision of Home Health Care Services through Health Maintenance Organizations: Conflicting Roles for HMOs. Home Health Care Quarterly 11:47, 1990.

Rowland, D: Measuring the Elderly's Need for Home Care. Project HOPE 8:39, 1989.

Somers, AR and Fabian, DR: The Geriatric Imperative: An Introduction to Gerontology and Clinical Geriatrics. Appleton-Century-Crofts, New York, 1981.

Zola, IK: Aging, Disability and the Home-Care Revolution. Arch Phys Med Rehabil 71:93, 1990.

Chapter 2

Health Care Providers: Functions and Issues

BARBARA NOWELL JACKSON

Geraldine Tifton, 78 years old, has had severe osteoarthritis of the upper and lower extremities for many years. She also has a history of diabetes, hypertension, and chronic heart failure. She underwent a total replacement for the left hip 9 days ago and is being referred to the home health department at the time of discharge from the hospital. The referral requests nursing services, a home health aide, and physical therapy. Ms. Tifton lives with her husband Kenneth, 82 years old, who has hypertension and sustained a mild cerebral vascular accident about 6 years ago. The Tiftons live in a double-width trailer in a local trailer park. They have no relatives in the town; a son and daughter-in-law and three grandchildren live in the next town about 70 miles away.

The Tiftons represent a fairly typical home health care referral. Ms. Tifton was referred by the orthopedic surgeon but has been under the care of an internist for many years. Mr. Tifton is under the care of the same internist but has been treated by a neurologist as well. While in the hospital, Ms. Tifton had a urinary tract infection and was treated by a urologist. On discharge she had a number of different medications, a walker, and an appointment to see the orthopedic surgeon in 3 weeks. While Ms. Tifton was in the hospital, communications about her, if any were desired, took place through the medical chart notes and personal contact between health care providers.

If Ms. Tifton were being discharged to a rehabilitation center rather than to her home, she would be automatically evaluated by all the services on admission, a physician would review her medical status making contact with her community physicians as needed, and the health professionals would meet on a regular basis to plan her care and discuss her progress. If questions arose between team meetings, all the health professionals would be on the premises and in relatively close contact. Occupational and physical therapists may work in adjacent areas; health professionals may see each other in the hall or meet in dining areas and are generally available by telephone. Casual as well as formal communications are enhanced by the close proximity.

Contrast the scenario above with the situation in home health care. Ms. Tifton's referral is faxed to the home health agency, where a patient coordinator, usually a nurse, assigns it to one of the intake nurses, notifies the home health aide coordinator, and either sends the referral to the therapy coordinator or assigns it directly to a physical therapist. Each person receiving the referral works independently. On receiving the initial referral, each person may or may not know the names of the other people involved; providers function relatively independently, rendering services at different times and on different days. Providers may not even meet in the home health office because each person follows an independent schedule. The potential for fragmented rather than coordinated care is great unless each person treating Ms.

TABLE 2–1
Health Care Providers

PHYSICIAN PERSONNEL	NURSING PERSONNEL	REHABILITATION PERSONNEL	SOCIAL SERVICE PERSONNEL
Referring Physician	Registered Nurse	Dietitian	Social Worker
Family or Specialty Physician	Licensed Practical Nurse	Medical Equipment Vendor	Social Worker Assistant
Consulting Physician	Home Health Aid	Occupational Therapist	
		Occupational Therapy Assistant	
		Physical Therapist	
		Physical Therapist Assistant	
		Respiratory Therapist	
		Speech Therapist	

Tifton makes a concerted effort to make necessary contact. Often it is left to the client and the family to coordinate care.

The concept of the team approach to health care is well known. As health care becomes increasingly complex, as clients require services from a greater variety of health care providers, and because independent practice and contractual working arrangements are frequent, the team approach may be no more than a concept. In home health care, as in a rehabilitation center, it is important for goals to be coordinated and treatment plans integrated. On initial referral, Ms. Tifton was to receive three services: nursing, a home health aide, and physical therapy. Depending on total needs, there may be many different people involved in the care of any one client (Table 2–1). This chapter presents a brief discussion of the role of primary home care providers followed by some of the issues faced in the rendering of such care. Because one of the concerns of all health professionals is high-quality care, quality assurance in home health care is also discussed.

KEY ROLES

Like most home health care clients, Ms. Tifton may use many general health services such as a medical laboratory or radiology. Services not provided in the home are not discussed in this chapter.

Physician

A physician generally acts as the gatekeeper for the delivery of home care. The orthopedic surgeon referred Ms. Tifton to home health care prior to discharge from the hospital. In other instances, the referring physician may be the client's primary physician. If the client has been treated in a rehabilitation center, the medical officer may make the referral. The referring physician receives the reports of care and must authorize the services given. Like Ms. Tifton, most clients may have several physicians providing care. The coordination of services, which may become an issue, is discussed later in the chapter.

Nurse

Ms. Tifton will most likely be seen first by a registered nurse (RN), who is responsible for gathering all intake information and completing all the paper work including medical and social history, medications, insurance data, caregiver status, consent for treatment, and emergency information. In addition, the nurse explains the new "Patient Advance Care Directives," which requires an agency to honor any living will or durable power of attorney the client may have. While talking to the Tiftons, the nurse notes the kind of personal care Ms. Tifton will need and completes the aide assignment sheet. The nurse also assesses Ms. Tifton's nursing needs such as learning proper care and monitoring of her diabetes. Ms. Tifton's incision is draining a little at one end; the nurse will teach the Tiftons how to change dressings, will provide the necessary supplies, and will supervise proper dressing care. The Tiftons are concerned with Ms. Tifton's difficulty in getting in and out of the bathroom, which has a narrow door. The nurse discusses the advantages and disadvantages of obtaining a bedside commode. If one is needed, the nurse will make the necessary referral to the durable medical equipment company.

The nurse is the primary liaison between the client and the physician, keeping the physician abreast of recent changes in the client's medical or social condition. A great deal of the nursing role is to educate the client and family in ways that enhance recovery or support the highest level of function. The nurse frequently makes referrals to other services such as occupational or physical therapy or social services. The nurse supervises other levels of nursing care, such as that given by a licensed practical or vocational nurse (LPN) and the home health aide.

Licensed Practical/Vocational Nurse

The terms "LPN" and "LVN" are used interchangeably, depending on the state or community; "LPN" will be used to refer to both care providers. LPNs are graduates of practical nursing schools and hold state licenses. In some states, they supervise home health aides, attendants, or orderlies as well as perform routine nursing care such as dressing and wound care. LPNs also participate in client education programs related to self-care and health care practices.

Home Health Aide

The home health aide (HHA) assigned to Ms. Tifton has been requested to provide personal care: helping Ms. Tifton bathe, brush her teeth, comb her hair and get dressed. She will also make the bed, change the linens, and clean the portable commode. She must be able to help Ms. Tifton move in and out of the bed safely and get to the bathroom or to the commode. In some circumstances, the HHA may help Ms. Tifton walk around the house and perform some of the exercises outlined by the occupational or physical therapist. The HHA is usually supervised by an RN or LPN but can be supervised by other team members such as a physical therapist (PT), occupational therapist (OT), or speech therapist (ST). Supervisory visits are usually made at least every 2 weeks, either through direct observation of the aide's performance or by questioning the client to determine if goals are being met. In some communities, the HHA might help the Tiftons prepare a meal, do the laundry, or shop for food. In other communities, such services are provided by homemaker aides.

In some communities the HHA is required to complete a number of continuing education hours, pass a test, and then work a designated length of time before being hired by a home health agency. Other communities, however, have few restrictions or eligibility criteria. Sometimes the role of the HHA and that of the homemaker are combined under the term "homemaker/home health aide." The homemaker alone gives service at a lower level of care, assisting mainly with household duties such as cooking, laundry, cleaning, and shopping. Homemaker aides are not supervised by nursing personnel and thus are not considered a part of the home care professional team, but they are often the vital link in being able to maintain a client in the home.

Rehabilitation Personnel

Dietitian

The registered dietitian (RD) holds an undergraduate or graduate degree in nutrition and has passed a national registry examination. Dietitians generally work in inpatient centers such as hospitals and rehabilitation centers but may be available for consultation with clients in home care. Ms. Tifton may need the services of a dietitian if she has difficulty with her diabetic diet. In some agencies, the RN may have some specialized nutrition training and function in that role.

Medical Supply Vendor

The medical supply vendors may work directly with nurses, respiratory, physical, and occupational therapists in providing durable medical equipment supplies, nutritional supplements, or assistive devices. A medical supply vendor would deliver a bedside commode to Ms. Tifton and set it up properly, showing the Tiftons how to take care of it. If anything was wrong with it, the vendor would return and service or exchange it (see Chapter 8).

Occupational Therapist

An OT is a graduate of a baccalaureate or master's degree curriculum approved by the American Occupational Therapy Association who has passed a national registry examination. In many states the OT is licensed by a state licensing board. On initial evaluation, the PT may note that Ms. Tifton has difficulty with self-care skills because of the osteoarthritis in her hands and may request an OT referral. The OT is concerned with functional deficits in activities of daily living (ADLs) and with physical barriers to accessibility and home safety. Following an assessment of Ms. Tifton's abilities and deficits, the OT would teach her adaptive dressing and housekeeping skills, possibly providing some equipment to aid in the task (e.g., reachers, magnifiers, and jar openers). The OT might help the Tiftons adapt the environment; for example, making kitchen modifications or rearranging bathroom equipment. With other clients, the OT might teach compensatory techniques for sensory loss, energy conservation techniques, and work simplification and might provide perceptual and ataxic training. If Ms. Tifton needs a splint for her hands, it will be designed and fabricated by the OT. The OT interacts with the PT on mobility issues and with the HHA to implement daily living skills training.

Occupational Therapy Assistant

The certified occupational therapy assistant (COTA) is a skilled technician who holds an associate degree in occupational therapy and has passed the national certification examination given by the American Occupational Therapy Association Certification Board. An individual can also become a COTA by having 2 years of experience as an occupational therapy assistant (OTA) and passing the proficiency examination approved or sponsored by the US Public Health Service before December 13, 1977. The COTA works under the supervision of a registered occupational therapist (OTR) to carry out the established plan of treatment. A COTA might actually work with Ms. Tifton, with the OT making supervisory visits as required by law. The COTA can perform most regular treatment functions but cannot evaluate, establish, or revise the plan of care.

Physical Therapist

A PT holds an undergraduate or graduate degree in physical therapy from a college or university program accredited by the American Physical Therapy Association (APTA) and is state licensed to practice after passing an examination. With Ms. Tifton, the goal of treatment is to regain strength and flexibility in the involved extremity, learn a home exercise program to maintain total function, and regain the ability to move around the house and take care of her needs. The PT would teach Ms. Tifton to get in and out of the bathroom and the trailer safely. Prevention of further deterioration of other affected areas would also be a concern. The PT might use such equipment as a transcutaneous electric nerve stimulation unit or ultrasound to relieve pain, as well as hot and cold packs, electricity, or traction. Client and family education is an integral part of PT function. Ms. Tifton's referral to the OT probably would come from the PT, who, on initial evaluation, would note deficits in dressing and self-care. PTs often work with OTs to maximize independence in ADLs, and with HHAs to teach transfer techniques or range of motion exercises. Some clients are referred to home health care for physical therapy only and do not require nursing interventions. In such instances, the PT may be expected to complete the intake interview and paperwork.

Physical Therapist Assistant

A physical therapist assistant (PTA) is a skilled technician who holds an associate degree in physical therapy from a college program accredited by the APTA and is licensed in many but not all states through examination. The PTA could well be the person providing regular PT services to Ms. Tifton, with the PT making supervisory visits at least once every 2 weeks. PTAs are educated to carry out most PT treatment activities, but they cannot evaluate, reevaluate, or determine the plan of care. The PTA will usually not treat a client whose physiological state is precarious and needs close monitoring or one requiring complex therapeutic interventions. PTAs write progress notes while working closely with PTs.

Respiratory Therapist

Respiratory therapists (RTs) and respiratory therapy technicians perform diagnostic tests and provide treatments to patients with respiratory problems. To become certified, the candidate must complete a 2-year training program accredited by the Committee in Allied Health Education and Accreditation and pass an examination to become a registered respiratory therapist (RRT). An RT technician receives 1 year of training and must take an entry-level examination to become certified. The technician is supervised by an RRT or by a physician. Both examinations are administered by the National Board of Respiratory Care. Although Ms. Tifton would not need respiratory services at this time, a client with chronic obstructive pulmonary disease might be using oxygen or a ventilator and require regular respiratory care. The RT is especially trained to assist clients in the use of ventilators, oxygen, supplies, pressure machines, and other breathing equipment. The RT teaches clients proper breathing exercises; for example, how to clear mucous from the lungs or how to increase functional lung capacity.

Speech Therapist

If Mr. Tifton had received home health services when he had his cerebral vascular accident several years ago, he might have received speech therapy. The speech therapist (ST) holds a master's degree in speech or audiology, has completed 1 year of field experience, and has passed a national examination to obtain the Certificate of Clinical Competence authorized by the American Speech and Hearing Association. Some states require licensing to practice. A speech evaluation includes speaking, hearing, reading, writing, understanding, and communicating with others. The ST treats articulation, fluency, and organization of spoken or heard language as well as dysphagia problems. The goal of treatment is to maximize speech and language recovery and facilitate communication to its highest functional level. The ST may work with the OT to correct swallowing problems, positioning, and cognitive processing deficits that relate to daily living skills; with the PT in areas of mobility; with the RN to determine medicine regimens; and with the HHA in carrying out the instructions of the home communication program.

Social Service Personnel

Social Worker

There are a number of ways in which social services might be involved with the Tiftons. They might need assistance in obtaining equipment or a referral to a social support group to obtain volunteer assistance for transportation. (Details of social work function can be found in Chapter 13). The social worker (MSW) has completed a master's degree from a school of social work accredited by the Council on Social Work Education, and 1 year of practical field work. Some states require licensing, whereas others require registration. Social workers are concerned with mental, social, economic, and emotional problems of home health care clients. They are also a referral source to a variety of community resources and services. They function as counselors, client advocates, and often as case managers. A social worker is an educator to the family and a consultant to the other members of the home health team for social or economic issues.

Social Work Assistant

A social work assistant is one who has completed an undergraduate degree in social work or a related field and has acquired at least 1 year's social work experience in a health care setting. The assistant may work in conjunction with an MSW or independently. Generally, the social work assistant performs functions similar to those of the MSW without the latter's specialized education and training.

Personnel Issues

One of the major issues of the 1990s in home care, as in health care in general, centers around the shortage of qualified personnel to support and staff the increasing number of programs. Ms. Tifton can expect to be seen by the RN within 48 hours of the time the referral is received by the agency. The PT is to make the initial visit within 5 days. If the agency is short of staff, such requirements can sometimes be difficult to fulfill. Personnel projections continue to predict shortages of professional staff. Projections are determined by the numbers and types of personnel needed to provide services to a

TABLE 2-2
Trends in North Carolina Health Care Needs

OCCUPATION	1987 Actual EMPLOYMENT	1989 ESTIMATED EMPLOYMENT	1991 PROJECTED EMPLOYMENT	ANNUAL AVERAGE OPENINGS
Dietetic technicians	502	544	586	48
Dietitians and Nutritionists	981	1035	1089	77
Electrocardiograph technicians	409	443	477	25
Electroencephalograph technologists and technicians	173	187	201	10
Emergency medical technicians, ambulance drivers and attendants	87	139	191	6
Health practitioner, technologists, technicians and related health occupations	715	715	715	25
Home health aides	1591	1673	28,183	105
Medical and clinical lab technicians	2071	2145	2219	74
Medical and clinical lab technologists	3293	3569	3845	202
Medical assistants	3208	3414	3621	208
Medical records technicans and technologists	898	974	1032	54
Medical scientists	204	212	220	7
Medical secretaries	5295	5914	6534	288
Medicine and health service managers	7005	7481	7957	272
Nurse, licensed practical	13,720	14,818	15,916	1152
Nurse, registered	32,435	35,225	38,015	2348
Nursing aides, orderlies, attendants	24,236	26,209	28,182	2582
Nursing instructors (postsecondary)	1361	1394	1426	77
Occupational therapists	347	419	491	21
Occupational therapy asssistants and aides	109	119	129	9
Opticians, dispensing and measuring	592	634	676	32
Pharmacists	4608	4830	5052	323
Pharmacy assistants	1810	1906	2002	106
Physical therapists	1198	1326	1454	86
Physical therapist assistants	706	776	846	60
Physicians and surgeons	11,298	11,996	12,694	1076
Physicians' assistants	829	887	945	53
Radiologic technicians	1450	1548	1646	62
Radiologic technologists	1308	1402	1497	59
Podiatrists	62	70	78	9
Recreational therapists	547	595	643	30
Respiratory therapists	1045	1141	1236	55
Speech pathologists and audiologists	774	804	834	26
Surgical technolgists and technicians	990	1072	1154	59

Source: Adapted from Trends in North Carolina Health Care Needs. Med Life 1:49, 1990. Copyright 1990, Medical Life Publishing Inc., with permission.

defined population over a given period. An example of such a projection, shown in Table 2-2, is derived from data compiled by the Employment Security Commission of North Carolina from an actual employment base.[1] Although projecting from 1985 data, the table depicts the types of personnel projections frequently publicized now. A 1991 publication indicates a continuing need for a large number of health care providers (Table 2-3).[2]

TABLE 2 – 3
Health Careers

OCCUPATION	WORK DESCRIPTION	EDUCATION NEEDED	SALARY	EXPECTED GROWTH
Biological Scientist	Study the growth and makeup of living organisms and the relationships of animals and plants to their environments. Use knowledge to help solve problems in medicine, industry, and agriculture.	Bachelors, Masters, Ph.D.	$37,000	Average
Clinical and Medical Lab Technician	Perform tests in labs to get information for doctors to use. Use chemicals, microscopes, and other technical equipment.	OJT, 2-year CC, Bachelors, Masters	$18,000	Average
Dentist	Examine, diagnose, and treat problems of teeth and gums.	Doctor of Dental Surgery (DDS)	$60,000	Average
Dietitian	Plan and direct how food will be prepared and served. Try to see to it that the food people eat meets their health needs.	2-Year CC, Bachelors	$25,000	Average
Emergency Medical Technician	Administer first aid treatment and transport sick or injured persons to medical facilities. Work as a member of an emergency medical team.	OJT, 1-year CC, 2-year CC	$19,000	Average
Licensed Practical Nurse	Take care of sick and injured people in hospitals, clinics, or other places. Work under supervision of a registered nurse or physician.	HS vocational ed., 1-year certificate/license, 1-year CC	$18,000	Above average
Medical Lab Technician	Perform routine tests in medical laboratories for use in the treatment and diagnosis of diseases.	OJT, 2-year CC, Bachelors, Masters	$18,000	Average
Medical Record Technician	Compile and maintain medical records of hospital clinical patients.	OJT, 2-year CC	$19,000	Above average

Occupational Therapist	Plan, organize, and conduct programs to facilitate rehabilitation of mentally, physically, or emotionally handicapped people.	Bachelors, Masters	$26,000	Above average
Optometrist	Provide care for eyes. Examine and test eyes for problems and diseases. May prescribe lenses and treatment.	Doctor of Optometry (OP)	$50,000	Above average
Pharmacist	Mix drugs and medicines as doctors prescribe.	Bachelors plus license, Masters, Ph.D.	$50,000	Average
Physical Therapist	Plan, organize, and administer treatment in order to restore mobility, prevent and relieve pain for those suffering from a disabling injury or disease.	Bachelors, Masters	$28,000	Above average
Physician	Diagnose and treat human diseases and injuries as well as practice preventive medicine.	Doctor of Medicine (MD)	$73,000+	Above average
Physician Assistant	Provide patient services under direct supervision of a doctor of medicine.	Trade, Bachelors, Masters	$23,000	Above average
Podiatrist	Diagnose and treat diseases and deformities of the human foot.	Doctor of Podiatry (DPM)	$63,000	Above average
Radiologic Technologist	Take x-rays to help doctors diagnose illness. Also use radioactive materials to treat patients.	2-Year CC	$21,000	Above average
Registered Nurse	Plan and supervise health programs and personnel, instruct people in health edcation and prevention of disease, and give nursing care.	2-Year CC, Bachelors, Masters	$26,000	Above average
Respiratory Therapist	Specialize in the evaluation, treatment, and care of patients with breathing disorders	2-Year CC, Bachelors	$23,000	Above average

OJT = on the job training; CC = community college.

Source: From Health Careers. Med Life 2:34, 1991. Copyright 1991, Medical Life Publishing, Inc, with permission.

The location and number of educational programs preparing health care providers is considered by many professionals to be related to personnel shortages. A telephone survey of representatives from three national health professional organizations was conducted by this author in October, 1991 to determine the current number of available education programs in key professions. The APTA representative stated that 123 institutions provide 130 entry-level professional PT programs, 112 PTA programs, 41 advanced master's degree programs, and 9 doctoral programs in the United States.[3] The American Occupational Therapy Association representative stated that 81 institutions provide 97 entry-level professional OT programs and 69 COTA programs, 31 advanced master's degree programs, and 3 doctoral programs.[4] The American Speech, Language and Hearing Association reported 195 accredited programs, 84 awarding only speech degrees, 2 awarding only audiology degrees, and 109 awarding both degrees.[5] Yet existing educational programs for rehabilitation professionals are not meeting current demands for graduates. In December, 1990, the North Carolina State Rehabilitation Task Report noted in part: "The shortage of these health professionals . . . is a multidimensional problem that should be jointly addressed by employers, health profession schools, funding resources and various departments of state government" (ref. 6, p. 38).

Health professionals working in home care need more than a basic professional degree. Because they often function independently, with little direct supervision or colleague support, they must be flexible in scheduling clients, must adapt to new and challenging situations, and must possess high levels of integrity and ingenuity. Most home health agencies require at least 1 year's professional experience in a health care setting following entry into the profession.

COMMUNICATION AND COORDINATION

The isolation of home health care providers raises special issues in communication and coordination and requires particular attention to this topic.

Communication among team members can be formal or informal, daily, weekly, monthly, or at the end of the 60-day Medicare certification period. With little face-to-face contact, team members often must rely on the telephone, answering machine, or written notes for exchanging information. Substantial interchange of ideas is often difficult, as is finding mutually satisfactory times for team meetings. Many home care professionals work part-time or on a contractual basis or work for more than one agency, having chosen home care because of the flexibility of work hours.

Updated information regarding clients and referrals should be furnished to the practitioner in the most expedient manner using the most modern communication technology. Agencies must develop specific procedures to ensure appropriate communications between care providers. Each health care provider also must be aware of communication difficulties and make every effort to share information with others on the team. Although each client has an individual chart, most providers do not have ready access to that chart, and notes may not be filed soon enough to make chart reading an effective agent for communications. If Ms. Tifton is to receive coordinated care, each health professional must assume responsibility for communicating with the others to achieve such coordination.

Meetings

The interchange of information and mutual goal sharing often stimulates personal and professional growth. Regular team meetings are the hallmark of the rehabilitation center but are more difficult to schedule in home health care. Most home health agencies will have regular case conference meetings attended by the full-time staff. Contractual and part-time staff are invited but usually not required to attend. Sometimes the scheduling of such meetings or the list of clients for discussion is not generally communicated. Informal meetings may occur when team members pass each other in the agency office or at social gatherings. On occasion, a case conference may be held between the client and the caregiver in the client's home. The issue of team meetings for joint planning and information sharing remains to be resolved.

Physicians

The number of physicians involved with any one client can also create problems for the health care providers. Ms. Tifton is being treated by the orthopedic surgeon and her general internist and may be asked to make a follow-up visit to the urologist. She also, of course, sees an ophthalmologist (for any vision problems) and a dentist. Any or all of these physicians may prescribe medication or make other recommendations that may impinge on the services provided in home health care. (See Chapter 8 for a discussion of medications.) Generally, providers report patient progress and discuss issues with the referring physician. However, it may be necessary to discuss medication with one physician and ambulation status with another. If nursing services are involved, the nurse may coordinate care; however, not all home care clients receive nursing services. In such instances, the OT or PT may provide the only skilled service involved and must function as care coordinator and client advisor.

Coordinators

One individual in an agency may function as a coordinator. This person is available to take and give messages and distribute information. This person may be a member of the office staff or may be a health professional, usually a nurse, who functions as team leader, coordinates the activities of the team members, and delegates certain functions to other persons. The team leader, or supervisor, is the link to the organization and communicates policies and procedures to the staff and caregivers. It is the duty of the team leader to ensure that appropriate services are provided in a timely manner and documented correctly.

Performance evaluation is an important part of home health care, as is the evaluation of the collective team and the agency as a whole. Functional evaluation forms documenting qualitative outcomes can objectively record the client's progress toward a specific goal. Quality assurance or quality management techniques are used successfully to address problems of high risk or high volume or problem-prone clients. Many agencies also evaluate staff members, addressing such aspects as quality of work, dependability, and timely and accurate documentation. (See Chapter 14 for information on documentation). Some agencies hire outside rating services such as the Joint Commission on Accreditation of Health Organization (JCAHO) or the National League of Nursing (NLN) to evaluate the efficiency and effectiveness of its program and recommend improvements.

Territoriality

Issues related to professional territory may be another problem not necessarily limited to home health care. Team members apply their own educational backgrounds and philosophies of health care as well as different cultural backgrounds or value systems. Team members may have different treatment approaches; the RN may believe a particular client could benefit from therapy and request an evaluation, whereas the therapist may not see the need for skilled treatment and not accept the client. If the same RN makes a number of referrals that are rejected by the therapist, negative attitudes may develop. Problems also may arise over logistic issues such as scheduling. Because home health care clients can tire easily, services must be scheduled over a wide range of time. However, individual practitioners may not think of sharing their schedules with others, and contract or part-time providers may not schedule a client at the same time for each visit. To reduce the potential for provider conflict, problems must be anticipated and procedures instituted for sharing relevant information.

Isolation from peers and from direct supervision can be a problem for health care providers who are accustomed to a structured, supervised hospital or institutional setting. Ongoing continuing education programs, professional meetings, and staff enrichment opportunities can help to alleviate such feelings of isolation. Overlapping professional task boundaries may induce stress. Staff meetings and social gatherings, recognition and awards, or written documents such as agency newsletters may be used to improve intercommunication.

Other Issues

Provider independence requires that the home health care agency be vigilant toward the abuse of provider privileges. Providers who are paid per visit may be tempted to provide minimal care to maximize the number of clients seen in one day. Supervisors must review client scheduling carefully to guard against this practice. Careful selection of employees, thorough and effective orientation to agency policies and procedures, accurate job descriptions, careful document review, and open communications help to reduce poor or inadequate client care.

One of the major problems noted by all team members is the amount of paperwork required to generate acceptable documents that enhance quick and timely reimbursement. Without staff support, each provider must complete all required paperwork, which can be very time-consuming. Computer technology may alleviate this problem in the future, but many agencies do not have the resources to hire staff to transcribe dictation or to purchase appropriate computers and software. Time taken to complete paperwork is time taken from client care.

As has been previously stated, most agencies require at least 1 year of professional experience before allowing employees to work in home health care. New graduates often lack the maturity, judgment, flexibility, and experience necessary to function effectively without supervision. However, persistent personnel shortages have led some agencies to hire less qualified personnel. This issue is expected to continue in the future. Effective quality management is one way to improve the delivery of care in the home.

QUALITY MANAGEMENT

Quality can be variously defined, depending on the individual, the setting, and the item being evaluated. For purposes of this discussion, quality is defined as "The degree of adherence to generally recognized standards of good practice and the achievement of anticipated outcomes for a particular service or procedure" (ref. 7, p. 5). If the Tiftons develop a positive rapport with each of their health care providers, and if Ms. Tifton is able to return to an improved level of independent function, they will believe that they received high-quality care. The clinical staff, on the other hand, may define quality in terms of technically correct care and procedures. The RN may document the wound healing, the PT, the ambulation distance and degree of assistance required, and the OT, independence in dressing. Medicare and other third-party payers may define quality in terms of number of services, visits, or days of home care provided.

Quality assurance (QA) is the sum of all agency activities that ensure that the client care delivered by the agency is necessary, appropriate, safe, and effective. The North Carolina Association for Home Care states:

> Quality assurance encompasses these major management functions. First, it ensures that the quality of client care provided by the agency meets norms of practice. Second, it assists with the reduction of potential risks to clients and staff, minimizes the agency's liability if incidents occur, and assures appropriate use of incident reports and response to incidents. Third, quality assurance ensures the suitability of a particular procedure, treatment, or service to clients and determines if the care provided was sufficient, yet not excessive, and provided in the setting best suited to the client's needs (ref. 7, p. 5).

QA is a comprehensive, cyclic program that evaluates an agency through the mechanisms of internal and external structure review, procedures, and outcomes of care. QA is both objective and systematic. The North Carolina Association of Home Care QA Primer states:

> Through this program an agency should:
>
> 1. Use a planned, systematic process to identify the strengths and weaknesses of the agency.
> 2. Provide an ongoing process rather than a series of random activities.
> 3. Monitor all major functions or service areas of the agency.
> 4. Use indicators that reflect current knowledge and clinical expertise.
> 5. Take action to correct identified problems.
> 6. Evaluate the effectiveness of all corrective actions.
> 7. Document findings and actions.
> 8. Evaluate annually the entire quality assurance program for effectiveness (ref. 7, p. 6).

Several regulatory bodies have been involved in QA over the last 50 years. Prior to 1965, "The emphasis was on supervision of nurses in the field, the annual evaluation of agency functioning, the collection of statistical data on patients and patient care to project future needs, and nursing education requirements" (ref. 8, p. 8). In 1965, Medicare was established and home care coverage became law, with certain eligibility restrictions. NLN has had an accreditation program for community nurses since 1967. In 1972, JCAHO developed accreditation criteria for nurses, and, in June, 1988, developed specific standards of practice for home care. As of December 1991, accreditation by JCAHO or NLN was voluntary, but both organizations petitioned the Health Care Finance Agency (HCFA) of the Department of Health and

Human Services for "deemed" status to review all home care agencies requesting Medicare certification.

Many home care agencies have adopted the generic 10-step Model of Quality Assurance summarized below:

1. Assign Responsibility: The ultimate responsible body is the governing board, which delegates authority to the administrator, who gives it to the QA Coordinator and then to the managers and staff.
2. Delineate Scope of Care: Which part of the agency's program should be addressed? Types of patients? Treatments and activities performed? Conditions or diagnoses? Types of providers? Types of treatments?
3. Identify Important Aspects of Care: Are these high volume, high risk, or problem prone?
4. Identify Indicators: An indicator is a measurable variable that represents the quality of care. A structural indicator examines the characteristics of the organization providing the care (numbers and qualifications of staff, resources, equipment, etc.). A process indicator evaluates the delivery of care or behavior of the caregiver (assessment, planning, education, etc.). An outcome indicator evaluates the result of the provider intervention or change in status of the client (client satisfaction, knowledge of a procedure, ADL status, etc.).
5. Establish Thresholds for Evaluation: Action will be taken at the pre-established level in the data analysis, or at a level indicating that a problem needs further review and evaluation. In most cases, it is recommended that neither 100 percent or 0 percent be used, to avoid further investigation when certain variables cannot be controlled.
6. Collect and Organize Data: Data are obtained for each indicator. The process should be systematic, coordinated, and integrated and can be concurrent or retrospective. A data collection sheet or a flow sheet helps to summarize data. It is valuable to get staff members involved in this process as much as possible.
7. Evaluation of Care: Cumulative data are analyzed to show whether professional practice and patient care compare with expected outcomes. The purpose is to improve care by educating staff in the area of specific deficits through continuing education, in-services, counseling, increased supervision, or a systems change in policies or procedures.
8. Take Action to Solve Identified Problems: The solution should be specific to the problem identified and its cause; should be realistic and achievable; and should identify who or what must change,

who is responsible for implementing action, what action is appropriate to the problem, cause, scope, and severity, and when change is expected to occur.

9. Assess Actions and Document Improvement: Actions are reassessed with the same indicator and data collection tool as before. If results remain the same, the problem, its cause, and the proposed action should be reassessed and resolved before additional data are collected.
10. Communicate Relevant Information to the Organization-Wide QA Program: The evaluation and monitoring information is communicated to the QA committee, managers, and staff as stated in the QA plan. This is usually done through a written report on a monthly or quarterly basis. All QA activities are protected and considered confidential.[9]

An agency establishes a quality assurance committee composed of representatives from the major disciplines. Each committee member then uses the 10-step JCAHO process to evaluate an aspect of care that is high volume, high risk, or problem prone. Examples of QA review forms for occupational care given to clients with cerebral vascular accidents are provided in Tables 2–4 through 2–9.[10] Tables 2–10 through 2–12[11] exemplify the use

TABLE 2-4

Quality Management

Aspect of care: Occupational therapy management of patients with the diagnosis of CVA in the home setting.

Indicator (outcome): Client and/or caregiver will correctly verbalize or demonstrate the following at time of discharge:

1. Verbalize effects of immobility (total or partial)
2. Demonstrate therapeutic exercises as ordered and taught
3. Demonstrate ability to safely and effectively use proper DME, splints, and adaptive equipment.
4. Demonstrate safe and appropriate positioning techniques for bed and/or chair
5. Demonstrate safe, effective, and appropriate techniques for bathing, dressing, feeding, writing, and personal care
6. Demonstrate effective, safe emergency skills for telephone use and ability to get outside

Sample size: 100%

Standard/Threshold: 95%–5%

Data source: Discharge Outcome Criteria Checklist

Methodology: All clients with diagnosis of CVA who receive occupational therapy services will complete a discharge checklist with the occupational therapist to determine whether goals were reached. A copy of the D/C Outcome Criteria checklist is given to the QM Coordinator. The QM Coordinator or a designee will tally results and submit cumulative data monthly to the QM Committee for evaluation, recommendations, and/or actions.

CVA = cerebral vascular accident; DME = durable medical equipment; D/C = discharge; QM = quality management.

Source: From Rex Home Services/Rex Home Care. Quality Management Committee. Raleigh, NC, 1991, with permission.

TABLE 2–5

Discharge Outcome Criteria

Diagnosis Specific CVA–Occupational Therapy

	P/C	YES/NO	N/A
1. Client/caregiver correctly verbalizes effects of immobility (total or partial)	____	____	____
2. Client/caregiver correctly demonstrates therapeutic exercises as ordered and taught	____	____	____
3. Client/caregiver correctly demonstrates safe and proper use of			
DME	____	____	____
Splints	____	____	____
Adaptive Equipment	____	____	____
4. Client/caregiver correctly demonstrates safe and appropriate positioning techniques for			
Bed	____	____	____
Chair	____	____	____
5. Client/caregiver demonstrates safe, effective, appropriate techniques for			
Bathing	____	____	____
Dressing	____	____	____
Feeding	____	____	____
Personal Care	____	____	____
Writing	____	____	____
6. Client/caregiver demonstrates effective and safe emergency skills			
Telephone use	____	____	____
Ability to get outside	____	____	____

______________________ ______________________

Client/Caregiver Occupational Therapist

Client # ____________ Date ____________

Comments: ______________________________________

CVA = cerebral vascular accident; DME = durable medical equipment.

Source: From Rex Home Services/Rex Home Care. Quality Management Committee. Raleigh, NC, 1991, with permission.

of client and caregiver outcome criteria to assess quality care. Additionally, many professional associations have published QA manuals and many agencies have developed their own forms.

Risk management involves monitoring an agency's potential risk factors, such as documentation, employee injuries and claims, employee performance, quality of care issues, client satisfaction surveys, incidents, and malpractice allegations. Each agency has a risk management committee and policies on risk management; one person is usually designated as the risk manager. Once problems are identified, it is possible to implement corrective action such as (1) in-service education, (2) probation or termination of employees and volunteers, (3) renegotiation of contracts with independent practitioners, (4) reallocation of resources, (5) review of credentials and privileges, (6) increased staffing, and (7) enhanced communication systems through beepers and electronic monitoring.[12] Initially the JCAHO manual

TABLE 2–6

Quality Management

Scope of Care ______________________

Survey Tool

Indicators

P+ Number	**1**	**2**	**3**	**4**	**5**	**6**	**7**	**8**	**9**

Source: From Rex Home Services/Rex Home Care. Quality Management Commmittee. Raleigh, NC, 1991, with permission.

TABLE 2-7
Tally Sheet

Important Aspect of Care: OT management of patients with diagnosis of CVA.

Name of Reviewer/Interviewer: __________ Date(s) of Review/Interview __________

Frequency of Data Collection/Time Frame Being Monitored: Collected on discharge

Relevant Data From Methodology: All clients with diagnosis of CVA who receive occupational therapy services will complete a discharge checklist with the occupational therapist to determine whether goals were reached. A copy of the D/C outcome criteria checklist is given to the QM coordinator. The QM coordinator or a designee will tally results and submit cumulative data monthly to the QM committee for evaluation, recommendations, and/or actions.

	Met		Not Met		
Indicator	**No.**	**%**	**No.**	**%**	**Comments**
1. Verbalize effects of immobility.					
2. Demonstrate therapeutic exercises as ordered and taught.					
3. Demonstrate ability to safely and effectively use properly DME, splints, and adaptive equipment.					
4. Demonstrate safe and appropriate positioning techniques for bed and/or chair.					
5. Demonstrate safe, effective and appropriate techniques for bathing, dressing, feeding, writing, and personal care.					
6. Demonstrate effective, safe emergency skills for telephone use and ability to get outside.					

Standard/Threshold for Evaluation: Reached __________ Not Reached __________

OT = occupational therapy; CVA = cerebral vascular accident; D/C = discharge; QM = quality management; DME = durable medical equipment.

Source: From Rex Home Services/Rex Home Care. Quality Management Committee. Raleigh, NC, 1991, with permission.

limited risk management to clinical and administrative activities designed to identify, evaluate, and reduce the risk of patient care. In 1988, the manual added new standards for risk management to include more active medical staff involvement in locating general risk areas in the clinical aspects of patient care and safety, in developing criteria for identifying specific cases at risk, and in helping to design programs to address these problems.[13]

Utilization Review

Utilization review (UR) is the retrospective and concurrent monitoring of client records to determine whether the services provided are appropriate and comprehensive in relation to the client's needs. UR helps to determine the necessity of care before, during, and at discharge, and thus saves

TABLE 2-8

Monitoring and Evaluation Worksheet

DATE: ____________________

Scope of Care and Services Offered: Occupational Therapy

Aspect of Care: Occupational Therapy management of patients with the diagnosis of CVA in the home setting.

Indicator: Client/Caregiver will correctly verbalize and/or demonstrate at the time of discharge: A. Immobility; B. Exercises; C. Proper use of DME, splints, and adaptive equipment; D. Positioning techniques; E. Techniques for bathing, feeding, writing, and personal care; F. Emergency skills.

Standard/Threshold for Evaluation: 95%/5%

Sample Size: 100%

Methodology: All clients with diagnosis of CVA who receive occupational therapy services will complete a discharge checklist with the occupational therapist to determine whether goals were reached. A copy of the D/C outcome criteria checklist is given to the QM coordinator. The QM coordinator or a designee will tally results and submit cumulative data monthly to the QM committee for evaluation, recommendations, and/or actions.

Review Results:

Problem Identified:

Opportunity for Improvement Identified:

Action Planned:

Date of Next Review:

Date Problem Resolved:

Comments:

Signature: ____________ Title: ____________ Date: ____________

CVA = cerebral vascular accident; DME = durable medical equipment; D/C = discharge; QM = quality management.

Source: From Rex Home Services/Rex Home Care. Quality Management Committee. Raleigh, NC, 1991, with permission.

TABLE 2–9

Quality Management 1991

Scope of Care/Services:

Aspect of Care:

Reporting Time Frame

☐ Weekly

☐ Monthly

☐ Quarterly

☐ Annually

INDICATORS	THRESHOLDS	JAN	FEB	MAR	APR	MAY	JUN	JUL	AUG	SEP	OCT	NOV	DEC

Source: From Rex Home Services/Rex Home Care. Quality Management Committee. Raleigh, NC, 1991, with permission.

TABLE 2-10

Discharge Outcome Criteria—Specific Diagnosis: Cerebral Vascular Accident (CVA)—Severe, Moderate, Mild (See Classification Sheet)

	Date	Signature
Visit Frequency Recommended		
No less than 2 twice weekly initially for skilled nursing, physical therapy, occupational therapy, speech therapy. All other services as needed.		
A. Knowledge, Understanding, Awareness		
1. Client, family, or caregiver is able to express correct understanding of disease and treatment regimen.		
B. Medications/Treatments		
1. Client, family, caregiver can correctly express:		
a. Types of medicines and their use		
b. Time medicines are to be taken		
c. Dosage and route of administration		
d. Interactions/side effects of all medicines/treatments (including "over-the-counter" drugs and home remedies).		
2. Client, family, or caregiver demonstrates that client is physically and cognitively able to take medications as prescribed.		
3. If client is taking an anticoagulant, he or she plus family or caregiver can correctly express:		
a. The need for blood studies		
b. Adverse reactions/interactions		
c. Emergency response as related to bleeding and/or embolus.		
C. Nutritional Status		
1. Client, family, or caregiver can correctly describe diet as prescribed by physician.		
2. Client, family, or caregiver can correctly express the importance of solid/liquid intake, so nutritional status is adequate.		
3. Client, family, or caregiver can express and demonstrate feeding techniques that are safe and effective.		
4. Client, family, or caregiver can express and demonstrate ability to prepare food for adequate nutrition.		
D. Home Programs		
1. Client, family, caregiver can effectively express the effects of immobility (total or partial).		
2. Client, family, caregiver can express as well as demonstrate:		
a. Therapeutic exercises as ordered and taught		
b. Safe and effective transfers and/or ambulation techniques		
c. Ability to safely and effectively use proper DME, splints, and restraints		
d. Safe, effective, appropriate positioning techniques (includes bed and/or chair)		
e. Safe, effective, appropriate techniques for bathing, dressing, feeding, and personal care		
f. Knowledge of bowel/bladder programs		
g. Skin checks for signs and symptoms of circulatory impairment		
h. Appropriate, effective communication		
i. Methods to control edema.		
3. Client, family, or caregiver can correctly express at time of discharge:		
a. Signs and symptoms of adverse reactions/complications as related to disease/disability		
b. Awareness of appropriate notification of physician		
c. Knowledge of regular physician contacts/appointments		
E. Psychosocial		
1. Client, family, or caregiver can express:		
a. Awareness of community resources and appropriate use of program resources (e.g., respite, council on aging, support groups, vocational rehabilitation, adult day care/day health, department of social services)		
b. Counseling as appropriate (e.g., mental health, financial)		
c. The need for continuous socialization.		
F. Safety		
1. Client, family, or caregiver can express and demonstrate:		
a. Communication (emergency measures/needs)		
b. Structural (ramps, rails, grab bars)		
c. Internal (lights, cords, scatter rugs).		

DME = durable medical equipment.

Source: Adapted from North Carolina Association for Home Care: Home health outcome criteria: A guide for quality care of the common home health diagnosis. Raleigh, NC, 1990, pp. 5, 6, with permission.

TABLE 2 – 11

Administration/Discharge Record

Patient's Name: ______________________

Start of Care Date:

Admission and Discharge Dates Per Discipline	Admission Date/Signature	Discharge Date/Signature
Nursing		
Physical therapy		
Occupational therapy		
Medical social worker		
Speech therapy		
Homemaker/home health aide		
Nutritionist		
Respiratory therapy		
Other		
Date discharged from agency		

COMMENTS:

Source: From North Carolina Association for Home Care: Home health outcome criteria: A guide for quality care of the common home health diagnosis. Raleigh, NC, 1990, p. 7, with permission.

TABLE 2-12

Cerebral Vascular Accident

(Classification by Severity)

Suggested frequency of visits per discipline based on diagnostic category—severe, moderate, mild

All disciplines are to evaluate CVA patients

Evaluation criteria: Profound/no problems

Areas addressed: Understanding, knowledge, medications, treatments, nutrition, home programs, self-care, psychosocial factors, safety

Teaching intent: Client/caregiver/family

Skilled care area:

1. Maximum—Assistance of two people needed
2. Moderate—Assistance of one person plus assistive device
3. Mild—Minimal assistance, assistive device, or one person as standby

	SEVERE	MODERATE	MILD
SN	Multiple system involvement Not teachable May have no communication skills Skilled care may include G/T, S/P, Lab, Foley, trach, Total care, unable to do self-care or comprehend disease/diagnosis Requires maximum assistance	Level of understanding Teachable Able to do limited self-care Assistance of one to two people needed Altered comprehension	Requires little assistance Communication good Not dependent Teachable Standby assistance may be needed
PT	Bedridden/wheelchair confined, unable to roll or come to sitting balance without maximum assistance Totally dependent Maximum assistance needed Maximum alteration in gait	Ambulates with moderate/minimal assistance May need assistance of person with transfers Altered sitting balance Altered gait disturbance	Ambulates with standby assistance Able to manage bed/wheelchair transfer for activity with standby Assistance needed for safety reasons Altered gait pattern
OT	Unable to do self-care without assistance of two people Altered physical and/or cognitive abilities Environmental hazards Visual/perceptual deficits Spatial defects	Able to do self-care with one person assisting or with an assistive device and/or verbal cueing	Able to do self-care with standby assistance and one person cueing

MSS	Assessment of social and emotional factors—counseling, financial, and placement assistance Meal program Assessment of home situation Response to crisis intervention	Assessment of social and emotional factors Assessment of home situation Counseling—financial, meal program	Assessment of social and emotional factors Assessment of home situation Counseling assistance
ST	Not understanding or communicating; severely impaired in carrying out all communication tasks Moderate success at visual matching Auditory input not functional Communicative skills may be good, but speech not functional	Beginning to understand and carry out instructions to the point he/she can function independently in a familiar environment Does well on tasks that offer most cues, such as copying, matching, and imitating Instructions and retention show significant problems Naming ability improves, but expression of names reveals problems	Minimal involvement Avoidance of difficult tasks, hesitancy in self-care, or distorted observations Output is usable. Lacks completeness in terms of syntax and grammar Attempts to respond quickly to perceptual error
Dietitian	Multiple systems management Tube feeding instructions Caloric intake according to need Teaching family	Diet instructions Diet management (Techniques for feeding)	Instructions only in a specific diet
RT	May involve wide-range activity May involve routine trach care May require CPT, assisted mechanical ventilation–IPPB or continuous mechanical ventilation	N/A unless extended confinement to bed—if so, lung consolidation must be considered, and CPT may be indicated	N/A
HM/HHA	Personal care ADL assistance	Personal care ADL assistance	Probably none needed

CVA = cerebral vascular accident; SN = skilled nurse; PT = physical therapist; OT = occupational therapist; MSS = master of social service; ST = speech therapist; RT = respiratory therapist; HM/HHA = homemaker/home health aide; CPT = carotid pulse tracing; IPPB = intermittent positive pressure breathing; ADL = activity of daily living; trach = tracheotomy; G/T = gastrostomy table; S/P = supra pubic catheter.

Source: From North Carolina Association for Home Care: Home health outcome criteria: A guide for quality care of the common home health diagnosis. Raleigh, NC, 1990, pp. 8, 9, with permission.

money for the agency. Donabedian states, "The net benefit to health must exceed the monetary cost incurred in obtaining the benefit" (ref. 14, p. 5). Internal staff or external consultants may conduct a UR. Team members can be, and often are, members of a UR committee.

SUMMARY

The health care provider has many functions in a home health care setting. Besides providing clinical services, the professional must be concerned with issues of communications, cost effectiveness, and quality assurance. The increased need for personnel to meet expanding service needs presents a challenge to health educators and society as a whole. Home health care is a demanding and stimulating professional arena with many challenges for the future.

REFERENCES

1. Employment Security Commission of North Carolina: Working towards tomorrow: Projections to 1995. Medical Life 1:49, 1990.
2. North Carolina State Occupational Information Coordinating Committee: Getting Started: North Carolina Jobs and Careers, ed 2. Medical Life 2:34, 1991.
3. American Physical Therapy Association: October, 1991, Professional Data Statistics. Rockville, 1991.
4. American Occupational Therapy Association: November, 1991, Professional Data Statistics. Rockville, 1991.
5. American Speech, Language, and Hearing Association: October, 1991, Professional Data Statistics. Rockville, 1991.
6. North Carolina Department of Human Resources, Division of Facility Services: The Rehabilitation System in North Carolina. Facing the Future. Raleigh, 1990, p 38.
7. North Carolina Association for Home Care: Quality Assurance Primer: An Introductory Guide to Quality Assurance for Home Care Agencies. Raleigh, 1988, pp 5, 6.
8. Meisenheimer, CG: Quality Assurance for Home Health Care. Aspen, Rockville, 1989, p 3.15.14, p 8.
9. Bassett, SS: Quality Assurance in Home Health: J.C.A.H.O.'s 10 Step Model. Cont Care 7:36, 1990.
10. Rex Home Services: Rex Home Care. Quality Management Committee, Raleigh, 1991.
11. North Carolina Association for Home Care: Home Health Outcome Criteria: A Guide for Quality Care of the Most Common Home Health Diagnoses. Raleigh, 1990, p 5.
12. Tehan, J and Colgrove, J: Risk management and home health care: The time is now. QRB Qual Rev Bull 5:179, 1986.
13. Innovative Health Group: Quality Assurance/Risk Management: The J.C.A.H.O.'s Ten Step Model. Innovative Health Group, Cary, NC, 1989, p 5.
14. Donabedian, A: The Criteria and Standards of Quality. Vol 2. Health Administration Press, Ann Arbor, 1982, p 5.

BIBLIOGRAPHY

Andreopoulos, S and Hoquess, JR: Health Care for an Aging Society. Churchill Livingstone, New York, 1989.

Bernstein, LH, et al: Primary Care in the Home. JB Lippincott, New York, 1987.

Brickner, PW: Home Health Care for the Aged. Appleton-Century-Crofts, New York, 1978.

Bulau, JM: Quality Assurance Policies and Procedures. Aspen, Rockville, 1989.

Crystal, S, et al: The Management of Home Care Services. Springer-Verlag, New York, 1987.

Friedman, J: Home Health Care. WW Norton, New York, 1986.

Innovative Health Group: Quality Assurance/Risk Management: The J.C.A.H.O. Ten-Step Model. Raleigh, 1989.

Lohr, KN (ed): Medicare: A Strategy for Quality Assurance, Vol 2. National Academy Press, Washington, DC, 1990.

Miller, SC: Documentation for Home Health Care: A Record Management Handbook. Foundation of Record Education of the American Medical Record Association, Chicago, 1986.

Monk, A (ed): Handbook of Gerontological Services, ed 2. Columbia University Press, New York, 1990.

National Academy of Sciences: Allied Health Services: Avoiding Crises. National Academy Press, Washington, DC, 1988.

National Association for Home Care: Quality Assurance in Home Care: Caring 10:3, 1988.

National Association for Home Care: Quality Assurance: Caring, 7:10, 1989.

Nassif, JA: The Home Health Care Solution. Harper & Row, New York, 1985.

Peters, DA: Consumer-Oriented Quality Assurance in Home Care. Pride Institute Journal 2:8, 1991.

Rabin, DL and Stockton, P: Long-Term Care for the Elderly: A Factbook. Oxford University Press, New York, 1987.

Spiegel, AD: Home Healthcare. National Health Publishing, Owings Mills, 1983.

Stewart, JE: Home Health Care. CV Mosby, St Louis, 1979.

Stuart-Sidall, S: Home Health Care Nursing. Aspen, Rockville, 1986.

Wagner, DM: Managing for Quality in Home Health Care: Effective Business Strategies. Aspen, Rockville, 1988.

Zucker, E: Being a Homemaker, Home Health Aide. Robert J. Brady, Bowie, 1982.

Chapter 3

Clinical Decision Making

Bella J. May & Jancis K. Dennis*

*The authors are both physical therapists; therefore, the sections reflecting the therapist's thinking processes reflect the physical therapist's point of view. However, the concepts relating to clinical decision making are equally applicable to all health professions.

As a home health therapist, I find that one of the more stimulating and challenging parts of my job is the varied decisions I must make. Walking in to the home health office on morning, I pick up two new referrals:

REFERRAL #1

Home Health Referral: To XYZ HH Agency	Referred: Yesterday
Name: Ms. Carrie Williams	SS#: 222-33-4455
Address: 2114 12th St., Site 16B, My City	Phone: 888-9900
Marital Status: W	Sex: F Race: B
DOB: 72 years old	
Caregiver: Anna N. Willow (daughter)	Address: 747 110th St., My City
Phone: 459-8120	
Physician: R. K. Farr, MD	Address: 354 Ames St., My City Phone: 656-0023
Hospital: ABC Hospital	Adm. date: 9 days ago D.C. Date: today

Significant HX/Diagnosis: Osteoarthritis, THR left
Supplies/equipment: Walker, commode
Services: Nursing, PT, HH Aide
Other: Going to daughter's house

REFERRAL #2

Home Health Referral: To XYC HH Agency	Referred: Yesterday
Name: Ms. Emily Lou Blaze	SS#: 999-99-7777
Address: 5678 Pine Tree Blvd., My City	Phone: 868-1111
Marital Status: M	Sex: F Race: W
DOB: 72 years old	
Caregiver: Walter Blaze (husband)	Address: same
Physician: R. K. Farr, MD	Address: 354 Ames St., My City Phone: 656-0023
Hospital: ABC Hospital	Adm. Date: 12 days ago D.C. Date: today

Significant HX/Diagnosis: Severe rheumatoid arthritis, THR left, HTN, COPD
Supplies/equipment: Walker, commode
Services: Nursing, PT, OT, HH Aide

THE NATURE OF CLINICAL DECISION MAKING

Home health therapists attend to different items when looking at a new referral. Some of us look first at the diagnosis and will note, in this instance, that each client has had a total hip replacement. Immediately a picture comes to mind on the basis of our past experiences with clients with total hip replacements. As experienced home health therapists we are familiar with total hip replacements and have an established set of decision rules to guide our actions. We note that Ms. Blaze is listed as having "severe" rheumatoid arthritis and that both occupational and physical therapy have been requested. Different pictures of each client will come to mind. We may also question the accuracy of the information.

We could look at other items first. Some therapists might look at the address. Experienced home health therapists have a map of their community in their heads and classify different neighborhoods. I know, for example, that Ms. Blaze lives in an older neighborhood where there are some substandard houses. Immediately I think about possible environmental hazards. Judgments and anticipated outcomes related to home area, although not necessarily biasing, are part of our knowledge and experience base and influence our preliminary decision making. Some therapists note the caregiver information and make hypotheses on the basis of expectations of support. Whatever we attend to, starting from our initial information, we begin to formulate hypotheses about the client's problems and possible interventions.

Decisions made by home health therapists can be categorized as falling along two continuums: from *familiar* to *unfamiliar* and from *standardized* to *open.* As Figure 3–1 indicates, decisions can fall in different areas of each continuum.

Familiar decisions are those in which a clinical pattern is readily recognized and the client fits the anticipated pattern. The therapist has a clear picture of the best management approach; the decision is "familiar" because it has been made many times before.

Unfamiliar decisions are characterized by individual parameters that make the situation highly idiosyncratic. Perhaps the optimal treatment for the problem is contraindicated because of other pathology or multiple pathologies, or perhaps the client's economic situation precludes appropriate intervention. The issue is that, with no readily available method of management, the situation requires adaption of ideas and some creativity.

Standardized decisions come to the therapist already fairly well defined by diagnosis or standard protocol. There are few variations of symptoms and the appropriate treatment is well documented. The treatments advocated and the decision rules that accompany them are usually well documented and supported by research data.

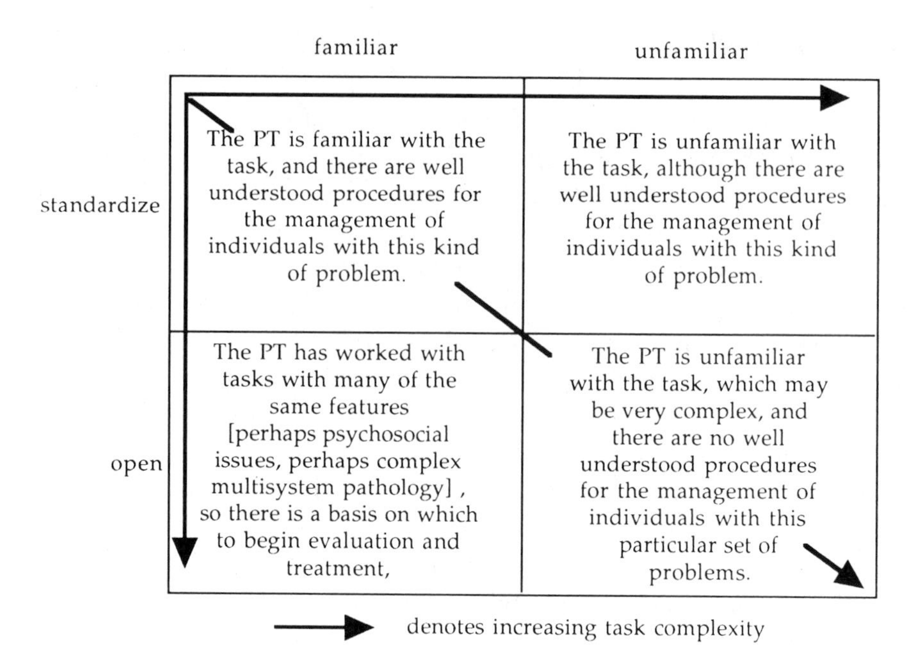

Figure 3–1. Complexity of problem type.

Open decisions come to the therapist with little structure. Either there is no established diagnosis or supporting medical information or the therapist does not know the diagnosis. Treatment is not well established in general practice or through research.

For me, Ms. Williams represents a familiar and standardized decision task; I have treated many patients with total hip replacements and am familiar with the literature regarding successful protocols for treatment. I have well-established decision rules about the management of clients following total hip replacements and have anticipated goals and a treatment plan already in mind. On the other hand, Ms. Blaze, with rheumatoid arthritis and chronic obstructive pulmonary disease (COPD), presents some possibly complicating factors that could make a standardized decision task more unfamiliar. I note the request for occupational therapy and wonder if her upper extremities are adequate for a walker.

Unfamiliar and open decisions are usually made slowly, often with careful consideration of all elements. Most decisions in home health care fall somewhere within each continuum. Categorizing decisions is a useful means of communicating about a generally internal and relatively subconscious process. Most therapists experience a variety of decisions in a day or week. Contrary to popular belief, clinical decision making is rarely the step-by-step, systematic process frequently advocated in the literature.

Forward and Backward Reasoning

Reasoning and decision-making processes interact. In familiar decisions, cues from the referral, client, home situation, or any other source cluster to form a recognized pattern from which we make inferences. We work from given observations and infer a still unknown diagnosis or problem. This is known as *forward reasoning* and is characteristic of expert behavior.[1] When we hear a clinician argue that, given features (a) and (b) together with feature (c), we should suspect (z), we recognize this inductive process in action.

In contrast, when decisions are unfamiliar—when we are unable to recognize patterns—we must work through more complex evaluations to build the picture gradually. We develop a hypothesis to test and work from the unknown (the hypotheses) to the known (the confirmed hypothesis). This is known as *backward reasoning* or, more commonly, as *problem solving*. It is what we do when no clear picture can be retrieved from encoded experience.[2]

In many cases, clinical decisions made in the domain of home health care are complex and require problem-solving capabilities. There are some familiar straightforward situations, but it is more common to encounter multiple pathologies and situations where we must factor in the socioeconomic context of the decision when projecting outcomes. Rarely, however, is a decision totally familiar or unfamiliar; our decision processes tend to fluctuate between inductive and deductive reasoning.

The model we describe accounts for just that kind of behavior. Hypotheses can be induced from a few meager facts or from many conflicting ones and subsequently tested. The decision maker must be opportunistic, responsive to new information, and able to handle a changing task environment as the nature of the clinical and socioeconomic issues unfolds.[3]

A Review of Research

There has been considerable research in the process of clinical decision making. In physical therapy, early study focused primarily on problem-solving models that described the behaviors of the clinician as a logical and linear progression from the presenting problem to its solution. A problem is stated, data are gathered in relation to hypotheses about that problem, an intervention is made, results are analyzed, and the outcome is evaluated for the appropriateness of the solution.[4] In 1980, May and Newman[5] synthesized the knowledge of problem solving in the psychological and educational literature to produce a model of the process in clinical physical therapy. The model, which recognized knowledge, skill, and attitudinal components, acknowledged the interactive elements of clinical problem solving. May and Newman emphasize that the process was not linear, but rather, that the components (problem definition, problem analysis, data management, solution development, solution implementation, and outcome evaluation) occurred again and again in a spiraling manner. The May/Newman model demonstrates the rich interrelationships between the affective and cognitive domains, describes the overt behaviors of the problem solver, and shows that pieces of clinical information can be combined and recombined before a final action is taken. The model, however, does not outline clearly the initial activities involved in defining the problem boundaries, nor does it address the structure of knowledge, which recently has claimed the attention of those seeking to model exemplary clinical decision making.

More recent activities have focused on the development of algorithms or expert systems to help physical therapists in their decision making.[6] Research is also focusing on the similarities and differences between novice and expert decision makers in attempts to gain a better understanding of how the expert organizes the knowledge base and structures the decision-making task.[7-9] While much is still to be learned about the activity, which takes place mostly in the mind of the decision maker, discussing the decision-making process in some detail may be useful in helping us improve our own function.

Differences between experts and novices have been found to be context dependent.[10] There are predictable differences between experts and novices functioning within the same domain. Experts in different areas of function exhibit similar behaviors. Experts in chess or physics, for example, demonstrate the same characteristics as experts in medicine, but the experts' behaviors become novicelike in other domains of knowledge. For example, a cardiologist does not display expert behaviors in the domain of orthopedics. Some general characteristics of experts include greater recall of relevant versus random information, greater use of forward reasoning, and easier integration of new knowledge.[10]

Only a few expert-novice studies exist in physical or occupational therapy.[7-9, 11-14] Data from studies of experts and novices in therapy suggest that, although some of the same behaviors may be exhibited, there are some specific differences that may reflect the complexity of the therapy task.[9, 11]

A MODEL OF DECISION MAKING

Over the years, on the basis of much research that has taken place, we have developed a model to schematize and explicate decision making. Basically, there is a task to be done, a decision maker, and eventually a decision that may be implemented and evaluated and that provides feedback for continuing the process. The model comprises three major sections: the *task universe*, the *decision maker*, and the *task environment* in which the decision process occurs (Fig. 3–2).

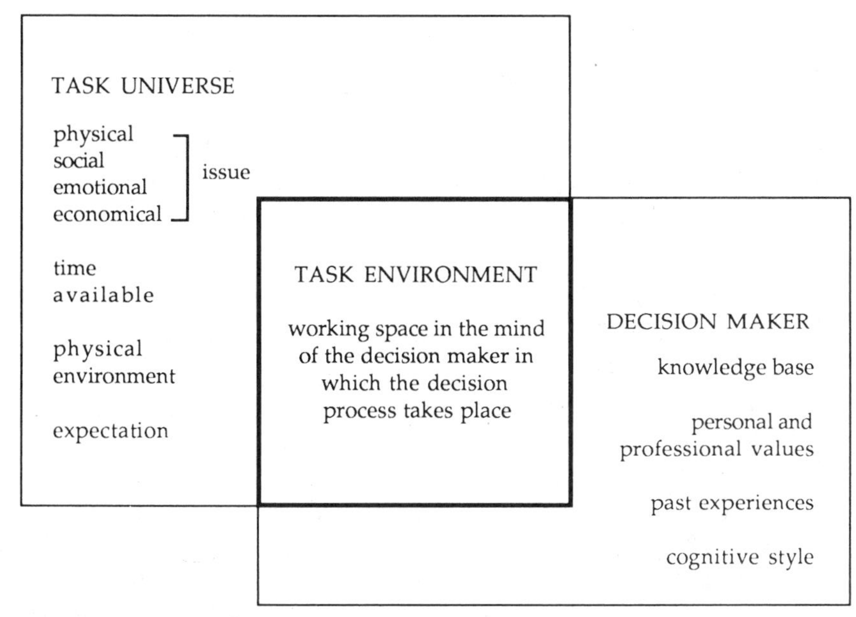

Figure 3–2. Interaction of the decision maker with the task universe.

My decision tasks are to assess the therapeutic needs of Ms. Williams and Ms. Blaze and to plan and implement a program of intervention.

In other situations, the decision task might be to determine whether intervention is appropriate, when to discontinue treatment, or what recommendations to make for referral to other services. Decision tasks are variable.

Definition of Terms

The *task universe* comprises all the potentially available information about the task and its context. It includes information about the client; the client's expectations, goals, and life-style; the environment in which the decision is to take place; the actual home setting; the time available for the client; and so forth. Within the task universe are the expectations of others (e.g., the home health administrator expects the therapist to be cognizant of Medicare guidelines; the physician expects the therapist to treat all clients referred.) Factors in the task universe exist independently of the decision maker. Some task universe factors for Ms. Williams and Ms. Blaze might include the home situation, Ms. Williams' relationship with her daughter and Ms. Blaze's relationship with her husband, their expectations of therapy, and feelings about their disabilities. All data regarding their pathologies, whether or not available to the home health therapist, are also part of the task universe.

The *decision maker* brings a knowledge base, feelings about being a decision maker, a well-established set of personal and professional values, a cultural background, a preferred style of thinking, and a variety of past experiences to the decision process. As experienced home health therapists we may feel confident about our ability to make decisions regarding the care of our two clients. On the other hand, we may be uncomfortable going into the home of clients from different cultures or may not feel knowledgeable about COPD. Those feelings may affect our decision process.

Scanning the referrals, I note that, although both clients have similar diagnoses, Ms. Blaze's referral suggests greater problems. The diagnosis states "severe" rheumatoid arthritis. How accurate is the information? Hypertension is fairly common among home health clients, but the COPD raises questions regarding Ms. Blaze's previous level of activity, endurance, and problems of secretion retention after surgery. Respiratory diseases are not my strengths, and I am somewhat concerned regarding my skills in handling her breathing problems if they are severe. She may not be able to tolerate a full initial evaluation and treatment. Mentally I prioritize the data I must obtain and the treatment I may want to initiate. I recall that she is married, her husband may be able to help with the home exercise program.

On the other hand, Ms. Williams has lived alone in a trailer park and will probably want to return to independent living. She may not be too comfortable in her daughter's home and may be able and willing to tolerate a more aggressive program. Already I have made tentative decisions regarding her management.

The *task environment* exists in the mind of the decision maker. In the few minutes it takes to read a referral, the home health therapist begins the process of decision making. Almost automatically we look at what we consider to be *critical cues* in the referral. The data evoke memories and patterns from our knowledge base and past experiences; we create a mental image of the decision task and make some hypotheses about the major problems and possible interventions. The focus of the decision process, then, is this interaction between the task universe and the decision maker which we call the task environment. The decision maker places boundaries on situations or frames the problem, and the decision process takes place within the frame. The task environment, then, is the working space in the mind of the decision maker in which the decision process takes place.

Critical cues can be defined as the keys in a set of data that access the clinician's memory for specific diagnoses or problems. The critical cues are linked with data in memory and are used to frame the task environment. The way we frame a particular problem, the cues we attend to in the task universe, and the particular relationships triggered in our memories all affect the decision process. Critical cues vary with different task universes. The client in the outpatient center presents somewhat differently than does the client in the home. There are a great variety of stimuli in the home environment that influence decision making. While reading the initial referrals, we have identified issues of caregiver support and home environment as well as the relevance of other diseases. These are issues we must attend to in our initial assessment.

The Decision Process

Decision making is presented as five major activities that may appear to be linear and logical but are actually ongoing and spiraling. Briefly, the therapists must identify and clarify the client's major problems, decide what to do and do it, and then determine if it worked. More formally, the activities include those illustrated in Figure 3–3.

Initial cues, usually critical cues, are key items that access the clinician's memory for specific diagnoses, problems, or actions. *Pattern recognition* is the phenomenon of making a judgment on the basis of a few critical cues. The patterns have been laid down in our memory through our past experiences and have been modified by our increasing knowledge and further experiences. *Hypotheses* are suppositions or assumptions about the client's diagnosis, major problems, and possible management. Critical cues in the task universe are interpreted in our memory on the basis of our knowledge and past experiences of similar situations; in many instances we recognize patterns and form hypotheses that help focus and guide further actions. We

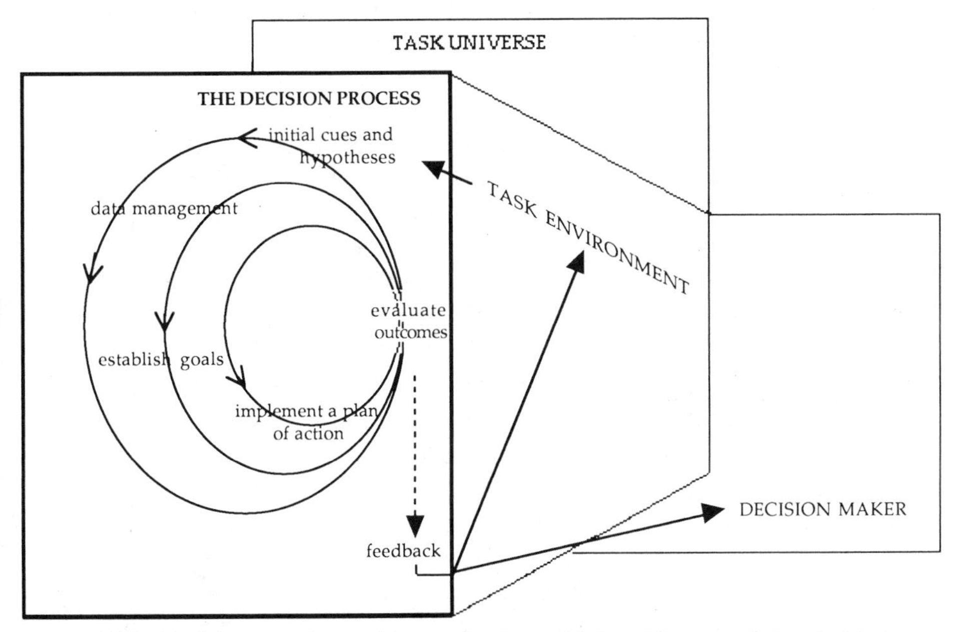

Figure 3–3. Model of decision making, indicating that the outcomes of the decision process are fed back to the current task environment and to the decision maker.

have already illustrated how the critical cues in the referral triggered hypotheses about Ms. Williams and Ms. Blaze. While driving to each home, we may create an actual mental image of each person.

When we arrive at the home, the *data management* process, which actually began when we read the referral, becomes the main emphasis of our activities. Data management is a complex cognitive process in which data are perceived, attended to, structured, and matched against other data stored in memory. Data management functions as a bridge between our hypotheses and our decisions regarding action. Some information is gathered to validate or rule out initial hypotheses and early decisions about treatment; other information is gathered to meet documentation requirements. We use a wide variety of information-gathering processes including routine history taking, formal assessment procedures, interviewing, and observation. Data management is an ongoing activity that permeates all aspects of decision making as new data are received and processed. The data management phase is actually never completed, although linear models suggest that data management ends when we set goals. Actually we are continually gathering data and revising actions accordingly.

I find that Ms. Williams' daughter lives in a large apartment complex on the second floor, but that there is an elevator. I note the one-curb step to the entrance door and automatically scan the external environment to see if critical cues come to my awareness. I am actually more interested in Ms. Williams' own home because I expect her to return to independent living.

Ms. Blaze, on the other hand, lives in a small house similar in structure to all the other houses in the block. Looking around, I see four steps with no handrails to a small front porch and file that information to use in setting treatment goals. I wonder if there is another entrance or if a family member could build a rail. I also question how she got in and out of the house before her surgery.

Mr. Blaze answers the door and takes me to a bedroom. Ms. Blaze is lying on her back with her knees bent, propped up by several pillows. She is quite thin and takes short shallow breaths using her accessory muscles of respiration. Her hands show typical rheumatoid arthritis deformities. I note Mr. Blaze hovering in the doorway and invite him to stay. I ask them how they are managing now and how things were before the surgery.

During this initial contact I am already beginning to readjust my initial thinking. The extent of her breathing problems and the hand and arm deformities suggest that ambulation might be difficult. The situation does not represent either a familiar or a standardized decision task; rather, it seems more open. I gather and analyze data more systematically, trying to find a pattern that will guide me toward relevant goals. The Blazes tell me that Ms. Blaze was able to transfer to the bedside commode with considerable assistance from her husband, who complains of back pain. Ms. Blaze indicates that she was not able to transfer on time on two occasions, which was very distressing (her personal care is important to her). The Blazes also tell me that she has not been out of bed since she came home from the hospital 2 days ago. Through questioning I learn that she was minimally ambulatory prior to her recent fall using a cane in her left hand because it is the stronger and less painful arm. She walked from the bedroom to the living room and back once a day and used a nearby bathroom. Mr. Blaze does the housework, but Ms. Blaze prepared an occasional meal. She enjoyed cooking but had not been able to do much in the kitchen recently. She also states that her hip has not hurt since the surgery.

By now I feel some ambivalence about my early ambulatory goals. Is it better to focus on wheelchair skills with minor ambulatory goals in the house? As we work together, could occupational therapy and physical therapy help her do some kitchen activities she would enjoy? I am beginning to organize the decision-making task around the rheumatoid arthritis rather than the total hip replacement.

At some point in our data management process we have enough information to conclude the investigations and *establish goals.* Again this is not a linear process, because we begin to establish tentative goals and make treatment decisions from our initial contact and refine them throughout the data management process. However, we finalize goals and treatment decisions after we have identified the client's major problems, made a diagnosis, or confirmed a given diagnosis. In practice, the treatment plan is designed to meet the long-term and short-term goals established in relationship to the client's defined problems.

We actually start *implementing the plan of action* early; we usually start some treatment on the first visit on the basis of our initial hypotheses and early data gathering. The formal plan of action can be defined as an externally observable behavior that evolves from a decision. The decision may be to perform a particular evaluation procedure, to initiate treatment, or to refer the client to another therapist. Implementing requires further judgments as we interpret client feedback and revise actions accordingly.

Finally, we *evaluate the outcomes.* Outcome evaluation provides feedback for further and more refined judgments and a continuation of the process. Clinical decision making is really a feedback loop system that requires ongoing determination of whether the outcomes are desired. Use of feedback has been shown to be problematic for some decision makers and will be explored later in this chapter. The evaluation of outcomes affects the decision maker's mindset or pattern for this type of problem; this in turn will influence subsequent decisions about similar clinical situations.

Effective outcome evaluation requires clear outcome measures, often lacking in home health care. Have we stated our goals in measurable terms? Have we identified clearly the level of independence, functional abilities, strength, and range of motion we expect the client to achieve? Outcome evaluation is an ongoing process because we are expected to document progress or its lack for third-party payers. Our need to succeed may lead us to focus more on positive outcomes. Looking at negative outcomes can be quite instructional. If we are teaching Ms. Blaze how to stand from her chair and she has difficulty with the method, we can either think that she just does not have the necessary strength or motivation, or we can think that the particular approach we are using may not be the best and try something else. It is sometimes difficult for therapists to consider negative outcomes.

There is much overlap and mental movement between the "steps" outlined above, depending on the clarity of the pattern. As was stated before, in familiar and many standardized situations, decisions are almost automatic and based on existing decision rules. In unfamiliar and open decisions we may have no pattern or conflicting patterns.

Ms. Blaze, for example, provides an excellent example of less familiar and more open decisions. She is not presenting with a "typical" pattern and our decisions must incorporate all her problems, not just the hip replacement. Our hypotheses about her capabilities will be continually revised by the way she responds to treatment and by the fluctuations in her condition.

Decision Rules

The extent to which the home health therapist actually goes through the decision-making process varies with the complexity of the situation. As the case of Ms. Williams exemplifies, many familiar and standardized decisions are actually made on the basis of decision rules, if-then relationships between cue and inference, or information and action developed through past experiences and education and modified by new knowledge and experiences. For example, *if* Ms. Williams shows at least a grade 3 quadriceps strength on evaluation, *then* we can begin straight-leg raise exercises and some weight bearing on ambulation. On the other hand, *if* the quadriceps strength is less than 3 or *if* there is pain, *then* we will concentrate on quadriceps strengthening and possibly limit weight bearing.

Decision rules can be given, discovered, or extrapolated. We are given decision rules in continuing education courses, articles, or books. Students are given decision rules throughout their educational activities. Discovered decision rules are the results of our own experiences; we successfully use a particular exercise or activity with several clients with left hemiparesis and develop a decision rule to use that exercise or activity with all such clients. Modified decision rules are adjustable in different clinical situations. For example, the decision rule to "always use a safety belt when walking a client the first time" is frequently modified when the client is apparently secure or is considered small enough for contact control. All therapists have decision rules that make decision making more efficient.

FACTORS THAT AFFECT DECISION MAKING

The decision-making process is affected by many elements. The process takes place within the decision maker's mind and is subject to interpretation by the decision maker's past experiences, values, and mindset.

Cue Perception

Each therapist frames similar problems differently. As discussed earlier, I attend to the environment from initial contact but do not automatically attend to the family situation unless something jumps out at me. Ms. Williams, who is using a walker, lets me in her daughter's apartment. As she walks back to her chair, I note that she is putting considerable weight on the left leg. The apartment appears large and airy; I can see the kitchen behind the dining area and a hallway going toward the bedroom area. Ms. Williams is dressed, has elastic stockings on both legs, and wears house slippers. I note the telephone cord crossing part of the room. Ms. Williams tells me that her daughter is at work but that she is managing "OK" alone. Her daughter has left something for lunch in the refrigerator. All of the data I have gathered so far support my initial hypothesis. On questioning, Ms. Williams indicates she was living alone in the trailer before she fell getting up in the night to go to the bathroom. She wants to go back to her trailer as soon as possible.

The way we frame a problem may influence which cues we attend to and which we overlook. We are likely to attend to cues that support our expected pattern rather than to discrepant cues in the task universe. Our past experiences and the extent to which cues are linked in our memory can influence our perception and the eventual outcome. Our attitudes, values, and beliefs can likewise influence our perception of the task universe. We can control the way we frame a situation. Sometimes, consciously changing our frame can help us visualize a difficult or complex situation in a way that clarifies it and guides us to see the relevant relationships.

Suppose that, instead of the scene above, when I enter Ms. Williams' home I find her slumped in a wheelchair wearing a hospital gown and her own dressing gown. She has on support stockings and slip-on slippers. She is somewhat obese and appears tired. There is no walker in sight. The daughter, who lets me into the home, quickly disappears into the back of the apartment.

I may be initially taken aback and start to search for familiar cues to guide my actions. The number of linkages between current cues and memory limits our ability to structure and restructure the problem. Students and inexperienced therapists may ignore what an experienced therapist would consider a significant piece of information. Such apparent neglect may mean that the cue or information has no meaning or linkage in memory. Failure to identify and attend to critical cues may lead the decision-making process astray. Our interpretation of cues and information is similarly linked to our past experience and values. We may believe that the daughter's quick retreat reflects her need to finish something in the back of the home and not give it much attention. Another therapist might interpret the behavior as an unwillingness to be involved in the care of Ms. Williams.

Representativeness

Representativeness refers to making a decision on the basis of case similarity.[15] This concept is especially useful for management decisions but may also apply to diagnostic or problem identification. Decisions are made on the basis of class membership; for example, a client may be designated "the typical arthritic." We enter Ms. Blaze's home and see her sitting in a wheelchair, her left leg propped on a pillow and her hands folded in her lap. We immediately remember several other clients with "severe" rheumatoid arthritis who had considerable difficulty doing bed-to-chair transfers because of hand and knee pain. We decide to start teaching Ms. Blaze how to transfer using a sliding board. Representativeness is a useful tool for processing situations with multiple inputs that do not fall into a known category. However, representativeness is based on personal experience rather than statistical concepts. To be effective we must remember that our experience may not be representative, and must be open to data that may lead us away from the case class.

Availability

Availability refers to the ease with which associations come to mind and are used by the decision maker to estimate frequency or probability.[15] Availability is highly influential in an individual's perception of the world and is acquired by exposure to a task.

As I discuss goals with Mr. and Ms. Blaze, my mind keeps turning to a recent client who had rheumatoid arthritis with similar disabilities. She wanted to walk but had not been able to achieve any ambulatory goals and had eventually gone to a nursing home. As I focus more on wheelchair goals for Ms. Blaze, I wonder if I am being biased by the availability of my recent experiences with the other client.

Availability helps us handle routine decisions with minimal mental effort, particularly with classes of problems that occur frequently; the strong associative bonds between cues and memory help us recall easily what to do. The problem arises when the strength of these cue-memory associations prevents us from seeing other nonfamiliar components of the familiar problem. Routine treatments and a lack of individual emphasis can result. We may even interpret a problem as familiar, attending to the available aspects and ignoring the unfamiliar, thus possibly misdiagnosing the causal elements or mismanaging the problem.

"Availability" also refers to the use of recently acquired information. Most of us have attended a continuing education course or read a journal article and implemented the new techniques immediately on our return.

The Law of Small Numbers

Isolated and unusual incidents have a stronger influence on our thinking than is statistically appropriate.[15] We remember the unusual situations and outcomes more than routine events. When we consider treatment options, outcomes experienced with two or three clients may lead us to expect all clients with similar problems to function in the same manner. The law of small numbers is affected by memory. Do we keep records to guide our memories? Do we know how many of our clients responded favorably to a particular treatment approach? We are more likely to remember positive than negative responses unless the latter are very negative. While good clinical research is necessary to validate our treatment approaches, informal individual records can help us avoid errors of small numbers. A check sheet can be used to note some treatment approaches, and a simple numerical code can identify client response on a plus-to-minus scale. A file of those sheets by major diagnosis refreshes our memories. A computer database can be developed for storing and retrieving such information.

Protocols

The term *protocol* is variously used in practice. Semantically, a protocol is a procedural document specifying the course of action to be followed under certain circumstances. In some centers, postoperative treatment protocols are developed by therapists and reviewed and signed by surgeons. Total hip replacement protocols suggest when to start which movements and when and for how long to avoid others. Our initial approaches to both Ms. Blaze and Ms. Williams may be based on such protocols.

Protocols are useful guides to efficiency in our evaluations and treatments. A protocol may guide us through a complex evaluation step-by-step or explain what to do if we find symptoms "a," "b," and "c" but not "d." Protocols provide a structure for a therapist who is inexperienced in a particular area, thus reducing the risk involved in complex decision making. They can be useful in the initial screening of a client who presents with a potentially critical situation (e.g., screening for thrombophlebitis).

However, protocols can be limiting. Used too rigidly, they can lead to a circumscribed database and inappropriate general decisions not designed for individual circumstances. Using a routine total hip protocol for Ms. Blaze would not address her major functional needs. Treatment protocols can discourage the consideration of alternative approaches if they are applied indiscriminately. Sometimes we accept the protocol of a recognized expert and apply it to our next client without a great deal of analysis, perhaps because it sounds like a good idea and we are anxious to "try it." If it does not work we may blame the protocol rather than make judgments about whether we applied it appropriately.

The Order of Impressions Received

A number of studies[16] have documented the influence on the decision outcome of whether information is received first or last. Initial information often makes a lasting impression, as does the source of the information.

Imagine that the morning I found the referrals for Ms. Blaze and Ms. Williams, I had been in the staff room, writing some notes and listening to two nurses discussing a new client. I hear one of them say: "That Ms. Williams I saw yesterday is a real complainer; nothing ever pleases her and she has her daughter wrapped around her little finger." A little later, I walk into the office and pick up Mrs. Williams' referral. What will my mindset be as I drive to the house? If I am let in by her daughter, who looks harried, my expectations of a complaining client may well be reinforced. All of Ms. Williams' responses and actions will be screened by the expectation of a "complainer" whether or not she turns out to be a cooperative and willing client.

It is not efficient to ignore information obtained in a referral, the client's medical records, or conversation with other health professionals; it is not even possible. It is important to be aware that the first information tends to have an anchoring effect on judgment. It is difficult to fully overcome the effects of the first impression; subsequent thinking takes place from a particular starting point and is affected accordingly. As we initiate our evaluation and begin treatment, we may interpret Ms. Williams' continued complaints of pain in the left leg and unwillingness to try to move the leg in relation to her being a "complainer."

The Client as an Information Source

Home health therapists rely on the client as a valuable source of information. May and Dennis[8] state that expert physical therapists in Australia and the United States found data from client interviews a very valuable source of information, although they were less enthusiastic about data from the client's family. When considering the client as a data source, we must consider reliability. How well does the client remember past events? How accurately is the person reporting his activities? Her pain? Client reliability varies with many factors including the disease itself, degree and perception of pain, and attention to what the therapist considers important information. The client presents her complaints from her own perceptual set, all influenced by culture, expectations, and fears. Fear is an important context for evaluation of symptoms. Is the client concerned that the lump in his leg may be a form of cancer? Does he ignore the symptom or belittle it, fearing to mention it directly, or does he magnify the size of the lump and mention it frequently during assessment and treatment? How many of us have experienced clients who were seen to magnify pain or a disability beyond what we thought reasonable? What is our usual response? On the other hand, how often does a client belittle an important symptom, fearing the loss of independence or even to be seen "as a baby"? Most of us have encountered the macho man or dependent woman, both presenting their symptoms from the context of their perceptual set. (See Chapter 12 for more information on the family.)

Positive or Negative Framing

Perceptions are influenced by the positive or negative framing of the information. Suppose the referral for Ms. Blaze had read:

> Client with severe COPD and rheumatoid arthritis who had a total hip replacement on the left. Probably will go to a nursing home but see what you can do.

I may look at that note with a feeling of hopelessness. If the client is going to a nursing home, why am I wasting my time? What will it take to keep her out of a nursing home and is it practical?

What if the referral had read:

> Client with rheumatoid arthritis who had a total hip replacement on the left and has a history of COPD. Needs to regain home independence.

The negative outlook of the first statement may influence me to propose fewer visits, set limited goals, or not even accept the client for treatment. The more positive outlook of the second statement may influence me in the opposite direction. A therapist's initial formulation of the task environment may well be influenced by whether the problem is framed positively or negatively.

Characteristics of the Decision Maker

Knowledge Base

The decision maker's knowledge and how it is encoded in memory is of major importance in attention to cues and development of initial hypotheses. Studies of experts and novices[16, 17] suggest that the rich networks of relationships in the memory of the expert allows information to be structured and restructured, with many permutations and combinations of the same data to suggest several different hypotheses. Errors that stem from knowledge base deficiencies include failure to generate the right hypothesis because the cues available did not trigger the appropriate schema, or because the actual disease schema was not encoded in the memory. In our practice we are often aware of difficulties with our knowledge base. We know there is something about a cue we should recognize but cannot quite remember what. We see something and realize that we do not have the ability to interpret or understand it.

Expanding our knowledge base is a continuous activity. Therapists attend continuing education programs, read books and journals, and generally seek information they have either forgotten or realize they do not know.

Affect and Values

A person's ego, self-concept, and emotional state all influence decision making. A therapist who is tense and frustrated may not structure the task environment as effectively as when feeling relaxed and integrated. Does the therapist value the decision-making role? Does she value the assessment and treatment planning roles or feel inadequately prepared to make diagnostic decisions? Does he feel threatened by the demanding elderly person or overwhelmed by a tiny infant? The therapist's self-concept permeates and affects cognitive and psychomotor functions, and thus decision making, in every situation.

Similarly, a person's value system and sociocultural background influence the structuring of the task environment. Does the therapist seek to understand the client's cultural background as a means of setting more relevant goals and teaching them in relevant ways?

> I may feel differently about Ms. Williams if she is motivated to return to independent living in her trailer than I will if she is content to stay in her daughter's home and be waited on.

Without necessarily changing our value system, we need to be aware of how it affects all of our decisions. To avoid potential errors we must also be aware of our mindset toward our clients. As Ramsden[18] reminds us: "When you look at a client whom you have never met before, and who reminds you of someone with whom you have had prior experience, you are prepared, probably at an unconscious level, to make inferences about the client's behavior based on your own experience" (ref. 18, p. 94). We place a value on the information gathered from a client on the basis of this unconscious recognition or association. (See Chapter 10 for an in-depth discussion of cultural influences.)

When we are faced with conflicting data from different sources we tend to credit the source most valued.

I may ask Ms. Williams (labeled as a "complainer") some questions about her leg pain and receive some nonspecific answers. She says the leg hurts "all over." I am now faced with some conflicting information. Ms. Williams has been labeled as a "complainer" by the home health nurse, but the pain she is describing could indicate problems with the prosthesis.

Studies indicate that client self-perception and reports vary greatly; some clients are excellent historians whereas others are not. What influences our perception of the client as a data source? Do we believe that all elderly people are a bit senile and so tend to discount some of their data? A study of medical students' perception of the reliability of a group of simulated clients revealed that the elderly person was consistently characterized as a poor historian regardless of other factors such as appearance, speech, and actual information provided.[19]

People are generally uncomfortable with uncertainty and seek ways of making the unfamiliar familiar. To some extent, effective decision making is related to the ability to function in a state of uncertainty and respond to the challenge created by the problem. The home health therapist is frequently faced with uncertainty. In such situations, the major risk for error is overconfidence. Overconfidence may lead us to overlook discordant information that might prompt us to reject likely hypotheses. We may also close on the problem early or select treatment options from a small sample of previously successful treatments. Experience allows us to be more cost effective and time effective in our approach to the problem; however, it is helpful to remember that such effectiveness and experience may prevent us from recognizing a situation that may require another approach.

SUMMARY

Home health therapists must consider many elements when making even routine decisions. Understanding the apparently intuitive and usually subconscious process increases therapists' awareness of their function, particularly when they are faced with unfamiliar or open situations. In this chapter we have described the clinical decision-making process, presented a model applicable to home health practice, and presented some elements that may affect the outcome. The reader can compare actual decision-making activities with the model and can identify areas in which function is satisfactory, as well as areas that might be altered to improve function.

REFERENCES

1. Groen, GJ and Patel, VL: Professional and novice expertise in medicine. Proceedings of the second International Symposium on problem based learning, Yogyarkarts, Indonesia, October 7–12, 1990.
2. Patel, VL and Groen, GJ: Knowledge based solution strategies in medical reasoning. Cognitive Science 10:91, 1986.
3. Turner, R: A schema-based model of adaptive problem solving. GIT-ICS-89/42. Artificial Intelligence Group, College of Computing, Georgia Institute of Technology, Atlanta, 1989.
4. Wolf, SL: Clinical Decision Making in Physical Therapy. FA Davis, Philadelphia, 1985.
5. May, BJ and Newman, J: Developing competence in problem solving: A behavioral model. Phys Ther 60:1140, 1980.
6. Rose, SJ (ed): Proceedings of the APTA Conference on Clinical Decision Making in Physical Therapy Practice, Education and Research, Alexandria, VA, 1988. Phys Ther 7, 1989.
7. Thomas-Edding, D: Clinical Problem Solving in Physical Therapy and Its Implication for Curriculum Development. Proceedings of the 10th International Congress of the World Confederation for Physical Therapy, Sydney, Australia, May 17–22, 1987, p 100.
8. May, BJ and Dennis, JK: Expert decision making in physical therapy: A survey of practitioners: Phys Ther 71:190, 1991.
9. Jensen, GM, Shepard, KF, and Hack, LM: The novice versus the experienced clinician: Insights into the work of the physical therapist. Phys Ther 70:314, 1990.
10. Patel, VM, Groen, GJ, and Arocha, JF: Medical expertise as a function of task difficulty. Memory & Cognition 18:394, 1990.
11. Dennis, JK: Decisions made by physiotherapists: A study of private practitioners in Victoria. Australian Journal of Physiology 33:181, 1987.
12. Rogers, JC and Masagatani, G: Clinical reasoning of occupational therapists during the initial assessment of physically disabled patients: Occupational Therapy Journal of Research 2:195, 1982.
13. Barris, R: Clinical reasoning in psychosocial occupational therapy: The evaluation process. Occupational Therapy Journal of Research 7:147, 1987.
14. Cohn, ES (ed): Special issue on clinical reasoning. Am J Occup Ther 45, 1991.
15. Kahneman, D, Slovic, P, and Tversky, A: Judgement under Uncertainty: Heuristic and Biases. Cambridge University Press, New Cambridge, 1982.
16. Hogarth, R: Judgement and Choice: The Psychology of Decisions. John Wiley & Sons, New York, 1980, p 167.
17. Gale, J and Marsden, P: Medical Diagnosis: From Student to Clinician. Oxford University Press, Toronto, 1983, pp 117–154.
18. Ramsden, E: Bases for clinical decision making: Perception of the patient, the clinician's role, and responsibility. In Wolf, S (ed): Clinical Decision Making in Physical Therapy. FA Davis, Philadelphia, 1985, p 94.
19. Johnson, SM, et al: Students' stereotypes of patients as barriers to clinical decision-making. Journal of Medical Education 61:727, 1986.

Chapter 4

Assessing Status and Function

MAREDITH SPECTOR

Every occupational and physical therapy practitioner who has worked in home health care for even a short time is familiar with the following scenario:

> The therapist enters the client's house and finds an elderly person who, until recently, had been living successfully at home. Now, disability has created an abrupt change in the client's ability to accomplish some or all of the basic living skills. The client may be unable to dress, bathe, or even move from bed to chair.

That client may need many services from diverse caregivers. One of the first requirements of the home health therapist is to establish the extent, amount, and types of services needed. In assessing overall client status, the professional considers the client's functional state in relation to physical impairments, mental and social well-being, and the particular living environment.

DETERMINING NEEDED SERVICES

The first skilled practitioner to enter the client's home often must assess the client's status on such basic a level as: "Is this person safe at home tonight?" Sometimes the answer is "No."

> Mr. Johnson, a medically stable, blind amputee, was discharged from the hospital after an illness and found that his wife, his only caregiver, had left him. When the therapist arrived the next day, Mr. Johnson was sitting in a chair in a cold, disorderly house. He lived in a small home on a lake, and it was winter. His only source of heat was a kerosene heater that was out of fuel. A brief assessment convinced the therapist that Mr. Johnson could not supply heat for his home or meals for himself, for both medical and emotional reasons, and that he was in danger of freezing without help.

While such problems are not therapy specific, status assessments are sometimes necessary and may require quick action. In the above example, the therapist contacted the home health agency and requested protective services. The agency responded with appropriate emergency care.

Sometimes the initial assessment reveals other health-related needs requiring the services of other practitioners. While doing an evaluation on a client following a cerebral vascular accident, an occupational therapist notices an open wound on the lateral malleolus. After the occupational therapist notifies the home health agency, the case manager can then mobilize the necessary services.

Narrowing the Need

The assessment is designed to define specific client needs. What will the home health therapist do for an individual client to enhance ability to function at home? The information obtained from a properly chosen and applied functional assessment instrument helps in determining a plan of care. Assessment instruments may be used to measure such activities as mobility, bathing, and transferring. The results will help determine what types of intervention, how much and how often, will best help the client. Assistance with bathing, for instance, may require only limited frequency of home health aide visits, whereas the client requiring assistance in personal care, transfers, dressing, and supervision of an established exercise program needs a different level of care.

Often the therapist bases the type and frequency of intervention on the ability and availability of informal caregivers. However, it should not be an automatic assumption that a spouse or family member either can, or will, provide the client with optimal care. It is best to determine ahead of time what the informal caregivers are able and willing to do (see Chapter 12).

Once a functional assessment is complete, the need for additional services not initially requested may become apparent. While each home health agency may have different procedures for requesting additional services, there is an area for such additional requests on Medicare's physician certification form, Form 485-487 (Appendix 4–1, Fig. A–1). Auxiliary help may be funded by Medicare A, Medicaid, some other local agency, or the family or various community services. As important as functional assessments are to the plan of care, they are equally important to both client and practitioner as a means of determining eligibility for funding for that care.

DETERMINING ELIGIBILITY

Eligibility for home health services is not automatically guaranteed in the presence of disease, disability, or even a referral for services. Federal, state, and area agencies define strict guidelines for determining service eligibility in the home. (See Chapters 13 and 14 for more specific details.) In general, the client must:

- Need services certified by a physician
- Be confined to the home
- Require part-time skilled care, for example, nursing or physical, occupational, or speech therapy
- Receive intervention services through a certified home health agency and demonstrate a potential for reasonable progress

Documented limitations in basic activities of daily living (ADL) or instrumental activities of daily living (IADL) support eligibility. Typically, ADLs include such activities as eating, transferring, toileting, dressing, and bathing. IADLs include common functions such as meal preparation, taking medication, telephoning, light housekeeping, going outside, grocery shopping, and money management. Clients who exhibit deficiencies in basic ADLs also need some help with IADLs, most often meal preparation and light housework. A man who cannot get to the bathroom from his bedroom is in no position to sweep his kitchen or carry groceries into the house; such functions should be assessed as independence is regained. There is a link between progression of sensory and musculoskeletal impairments and physical limitations in ADLs and IADLs.[1] Most clients will exhibit deficits in both ADLs and IADLs. However, if only IADLs are dysfunctional, the client is not likely to qualify for skilled therapy services under Medicare. Because home health care involves services other than therapy and may involve both physical and occupational therapists, the documentation must be easily understood by other medical professionals, health care agencies, and funding intermediaries. It is helpful to remember that funding intermediaries review therapy records to determine if the client's needs meet their funding criteria.

Ms. R., 77 years old, has diabetes and suffers occasional episodes of positional vertigo. While visiting her son in a different state, she fell leaving a restaurant and sustained a fracture of the proximal humerus on the right and a Colles fracture on the left. The hospital sent her home with her son. Since she could not feed, bathe, or dress herself, she decided to remain with her son's family until she was able to go home. She was referred for home health physical therapy. Following initial evaluation the physical therapist requested an occupational therapy evaluation as well. The Functional Status Index[2] was performed. The assessment determined that Ms. R. needed human assistance for all basic ADLs except eating, that she had pain in varying amounts, and that she had difficulty performing activities even with human assistance. In addition, she could not perform any IADLs. To return home and live alone again, which was her goal, Ms. R. had to be able to accomplish most of the ADLs, as well as some of the IADLs, without constant supervision.

The physical and occupational therapists worked together to help Ms. R. regain shoulder strength and range and, as the fractures healed, to regain basic ADL skills. Ms. R. was retested at 2-week intervals to document her progress. The periodic testing also provided a basis for a prognosis on returning the client to her home under a lower level of care.

Six weeks into therapy, the reassessment showed that Ms. R. could care for herself in most basic activities without assistance but would require help with bathing, light housekeeping, and meal preparation. If she went home, she could be considered homebound under Medicare A because of her positional vertigo and temporarily broken bones. She would not need constant care, and the interval assessments had demonstrated she could attain her functional goals within a reasonable time. The therapists advised the doctor that Ms. R. would need help with at least one ADL and two or more IADLs and continuing therapy for her temporary impairments. Ms. R. was referred to a home health care provider in her own town. The agency that had initiated the care sent the new agency a copy of her Functional Status Index records to ensure a carry-over of therapy and care. Because her case was properly documented, Ms. R. was able to return home and work toward her independence while receiving the services she needed.

Establishing the Basis for Skilled Intervention

Initially, the home health therapist determines if and why therapeutic intervention is required. The need for service is related to a specific problem as classified by the International Classification of Diseases (ICD-9) codes. The practitioner also establishes a plan of care to meet functional goals that have been identified by objective measurement data.

On this point a caveat may be helpful. It appears to be a common practice for the therapist to use subjective judgment on recertification forms supporting continued intervention. For example, the therapist treating a client with a broken hip may write "much improved" on line 16 of the Medical Update and Information form (Form 486; see Fig. A–2, Appendix 4–1). Such subjectivity is a mistake because it places ongoing assessment in the realm of intuition. "Feelings" about functional performance are difficult to document in concise fashion. How much is "much improved"? Instead the practitioner should retest the client with the assessment instrument used to document initial functional status. The updated assessment, measuring the level of improvement, can be attached to Form 486. Objective data available in the client's recent medical record may not be immediately available to the other practitioners or reviewers. Functional status assessment on admission and discharge, and regularly during therapeutic intervention, is necessary to support the need for continued service at home. It is helpful to remember that, regardless of client need, support for a continued services request ultimately may be in the hands of an intermediary reviewer who does not extract data from daily narratives. The reviewer makes decisions based on hard evidence from submitted documents designed for such progress (e.g., Medicare Form 486 or 487).

A client may be eligible for home care services without a hospital admission; the home health therapist must substantiate the need for such intervention. In this case, it is necessary to establish the level of function just prior to the episode as well as the changes in self-care that resulted from the episode. Careful interviewing of the client, family, or friends may be necessary if there are no medical records to consult. There are also instruments designed to broadly record retroactive functional status. These will be discussed later.

ASSESSMENT PROTOCOL

Although home care intake documentation forms are not standardized, most provider agencies require general categories of information. Usually some of the information is transcribed onto an appropriate physician certification form, such as Medicare Form 485-486 (Appendix 4–1). Assessment and care plans must be completed and submitted, with physician certification, to the home health agency within 7 days of the initial visit to comply with Medicare conditions for participation. If the home health therapist is evaluating a client who has not had a nursing assessment, baseline data must be determined, including:

Medications—Name, dosage, frequency, and mode of administration
Allergies—"No Known Allergies" may be used unless specific medicine, food, or environmental allergies are identified
Nutritional requirements—Type of diet; special needs such as low sodium intake or supplemental nutrition
Safety measures—available or needed
Durable medical equipment required—wheelchairs, commodes, and so forth

Baseline intake data also include the practitioner's clinical findings of the client's physical and functional limitations, rehabilitation potential, and prognosis. Prior physical or occupational services, and the client's progress during that therapy, are also documented at intake. Because these findings are the basis for supporting intervention measures, thoroughness is important. The addendum form, Medicare Form 487, (Appendix 4–1, Fig. A–3) may be used when space on the assessment plan is insufficient.

Documentation and Plan of Care

All of the above assessment information is used to develop the plan of care. The box on Medicare Form 485 for listing functional limitations (18A) can be used to record findings from the functional status instrument. Check the appropriate squares and name the instrument or instruments administered in box B (Other). Subfindings such as specific muscle strength scores or goniometric measurements may be marked on Form 486, box 17, or on Form 487. Specific measures are used to support clearly the therapeutic interventions, modalities, or home health agency services being requested on the plan of care. Essentially, the therapist is trying to identify certain functional test results as problems, which may be assigned ICD-9 codes and pinpoint the short-term goals for each problem. These results may be recorded in addition to medical diagnoses and surgical procedures.

For example, box 21 on Form 485 asks for the services requested, for example, physical therapy (PT), occupational therapy (OT), home health aide (HHA), and the modalities and therapeutic interventions for the listed problems. Assume you have administered the Katz Index of ADL[3] (which you have named in box 18A of Form 485) and have checked items "ambulation" and "other," specifying as ADL decrement, and score C on the Katz Index. You may infer that if the client cannot transfer, ambulation will require assistance. (Note: It is not the purpose of this chapter to teach how to score the assessment instruments mentioned. There is ample literature on the subject for anyone needing this information.) The problem or problems should be written in column format because it will be easier to transfer the information to a Plan of Care. The two problems identified above could be written as follows on Form 487:

PROBLEM	SERVICE AND MODALITY	SHORT-TERM GOAL
1. Gait instability (code 781.2)	PT: Gait training, therapeutic exercise HHA: Gait, exercise practice	Gait with contact guard Household distances
2. ADL deterioration (code 781.3)	OT: Self-care training	Independent bathing
a. Dependent bathing	HHA: Bathing assistance	Independent transfer
b. Dependent transfer	PT: Transfer training	Standby assistance in bathing

Long-term goals used for discharge planning are stated in box 22 of Form 486.

Functional Assessment

A definition of health based exclusively on observable physical manifestations and subjective symptoms is often too limiting and narrow for the home health therapist. Jette[4] notes that health is defined with respect to an individual's function. Measures of function and functional status represent the individual's interaction with his or her environment.

In fact, several realms of function can be tested for clinical purposes. These include physical, mental, emotional, and social function. While occupational and physical therapists generally concentrate on physical testing, other assessments are sometimes indicated. Testing the mental function of a person with observable dementia, for example, can aid the professional in determining the client's cognitive capabilities. Because thinking capacity affects functioning capabilities, occupational therapists, particularly in home care, frequently use instruments to assess cognitive and psychoemotional function (see also Chapter 11). Determinations from all realms of functional assessment can help support requests for additional professional help, if needed, or for a longer term of intervention by the home health therapist. Practitioners should become familiar with which of the many assessment instruments are most appropriate to their clients. The reader is referred to the publications of Jette[4] and Guccione and associates[5] for a more detailed review of physical function assessment instruments.

Choosing an Instrument

A measurement of basic ADL performance is often necessary for the client with generalized age-related decrements or "softer" manifestations of decline, regardless of whether there has been a PT-related or OT-related diagnosis. Many scales exist; several have been tested and adapted for use in the home. Many of the more commonly used forms are specific to each agency and have not been tested and published. These forms are designed by an individual agency or hospital. They are a response to the difficulty of finding and obtaining standardized forms such as those discussed later in this chapter.

While convenient, these "homegrown" assessment instruments may present certain disadvantages because they are not standard in the field. They have usually not been tested for validity and reliability and, since each agency uses a different one, they are difficult to cross-reference.

Suppose an elderly woman with a broken hip is treated by a home care agency using the Physical Therapy Initial Assessment form (Fig. 4–1) On the line labeled "Transfers: Toilet/Commode," the therapist writes, "Can accomplish." The client then goes to live with a relative and is seen by another agency, which uses the Physical Therapy Evaluation form (Fig. 4–2). The second form uses a 0 to 3 rating scale. The new therapist, seeking to compare client function, does not know if "can accomplish" is a 1, a 2, or a 3 on the current agency's form. The therapist will, of course, do a new functional assessment, but has no way of telling whether the move to another area has degraded the client's progress.

Lack of standardization or of a rating scale may also impede progress reporting on a client. The Occupational Therapy form (Fig. 4–3) has a line for "Pertinent Information."

Ms. Jones sustained a cerebral vascular accident 3 weeks ago and experiences considerable weakness on the left side. Discharged home and living with her husband, she is evaluated by an occupational therapist who notes "cannot bathe self" on the "pertinent information" line. A few weeks later another occupational therapist re-evaluates Ms. Jones and writes, "Does not bathe independently." Ms. Jones, while still not able to bathe independently, has progressed from total dependence to being able to participate in bathing and wash part of her body, a progress not reflected in the evaluation.

Some forms use descriptive phrases to describe the client's level of function. Statements such as "walks with assistive device; no guarding necessary" describes the client's ability to ambulate quite clearly. A statement under a dressing category might read: "needs verbal cueing only" and convey the level of help needed. However, "needs assistance with lower body dressing" does not indicate the scope of the assistance needed. Alternatively, an agency may require its therapists to define their judgments in more detail.

Another problem with nonstandard forms is their use in the client's medical record. Most hospitals and agencies have their own policies regarding what should be included in a client's record; few institutions have similar requirements. One suggestion for alleviating this problem is to write the name of the form used in the appropriate space on the agency's client record form. Sending a blank record form to a new agency when clients are transferred increases accuracy in documenting progress. This procedure also works on the Form 485 certification. In box 18A of the form, check "other," name the instrument, and attach a copy of the instrument.

Scoring and Validity

It is important to consider several characteristics when selecting an assessment form. Foremost is ease of administration within the home setting, both in testing time and in implementation. Avoid instruments requiring bulky equipment or lengthy written portions. Scoring should be simple. Be open to the self-administered questionnaires, which may have the advantage of targeting areas the client perceives as difficult and which can eliminate the time-consuming process of observing directly a group of ADLs or IADLs. A functional assessment form with a rating scale is more effective than a narrative form in measuring progress and supporting the need for skilled intervention.

The therapist must also consider the degree to which an instrument measures what it purports to measure. This concept is called "validity." Timing the performance of gait over a determined distance may be a valid measure of fall risk, for instance, but have little significance in determining a client's safety in the home.

Another important consideration is scoring reliability, or the degree to which a score measures performance differences rather than random error. One value of using published instruments is the prior performance of reliability and validity testing on sample populations and the availability of data.

Functional status instruments in home care are most often used for screening and assessment and for monitoring change of performance over time. Functional assessment instruments usually focus on ADL and IADL capabilities, but the home health therapist also assesses other areas. The Functional Assessment Questionnaire[6] encompasses multiconcept screening and targets physical function, mental capabilities, and other areas.

Physical Therapy
Initial Assessment

Patient Name ____________ Date of Birth ________ Date ________
Address ____________ Tel. No. ________
Physician ____________ Primary Diagnosis ________
Medical History ____________
Psychosocial, Family Support ____________
Medications ____________
Equipment ____________
Architectural Limitations ____________

Mentation ____________
Pain ____________
ROM ____________

Strength ____________

Posture ____________
Neuromuscular: Tone ____________
Balance ____________
Coordination ____________

Sensation ____________
Vascular/Skin ____________
Pulmonary Status ____________
Communication/Speech ____________
Vision ____________ Hearing ____________
Bed Activities: Rolling ____________
Supine to Sit ____________
Sit to Supine ____________
Transfers: Sit to Stand ____________
Bed ____________ Car ____________
Toilet/Commode ____________
Chair/Wheelchair ____________
Tub/Shower ____________
Weight Bearing Status ____________
Ambulation/Gait Quality ____________

Stair Negotiation ____________
Endurance ____________
ADL: Feeding ____________
Dressing ____________
Household Activities ____________
Other ____________
Home Health Aide? ____________

Figure 4–1. Physical Therapy Initial Assessment form.

Assessment

Rehab Potential

GOALS	PLAN
Short Term:	
Long Term:	

Signature ________________
Tel. No. ________________
Date Sent to M.D. ________________

Figure 4–1. *Continued.*

Agency ______________________ **PHYSICAL THERAPY EVALUATION** Date ________

PATIENT | NUMBER | DATE OF BIRTH

PHYSICIAN

DIAGNOSIS:

Physical Therapy Plan of Treatment has been reviewed with
_____ patient
_____ family
_____ other agency personnel involved with patient's care

PROBLEMS/FUNCTIONAL LIMITATIONS
1.
2.
3.
4.

FUNCTIONAL GOALS/TIME FRAME
1.
2.
3.
4.

REHAB POTENTIAL:

PHYSICAL THERAPY PLAN OF TREATMENT
1.
2.
3.
4.

FREQUENCY ______________ DURATION ______

The PT Plan of Treatment is recommended pending physician's approval

______________________ P.T.

The PT Plan of Treatment is amended and/or approved by:

______________________ Date ______
Physician

RETAIN THIS COPY FOR YOUR RECORDS

COGNITION/SUBJECTIVE

STRENGTH AND RANGE OF MOTION (Comments: pain, edema, tone, synergy, functional use):

PART/ACTION	STRENGTH		R.O.M.	
HIP	L	R	L	R
Abduction				
Adduction				
Rotation				
Flexion				
Extension				
KNEE				
Flexion				
Extension				
ANKLE				
Dorsiflexion				
Plantar flex.				

PART/ACTION	STRENGTH		R.O.M.	
Shoulder	L	R	L	R
Elbow				
Wrist				

SENSORY/SKIN CONDITION

HOME ENVIRONMENT and FAMILY SUPPORT

EQUIPMENT and SAFETY

POSTURE AND GAIT ANALYSIS (Assistive devices, assist, balance, etc.)

1. In and out of chair		6. Rolls		11. Transfers into car or cab	
2. In and out of bed		7. Assumes sitting over edge of bed		12. Walks all directions	
3. In and out of bath or shower		8. Can bridge		13. Walks on all textures	
4. Toilet independence		9. Assumes standing		14. Walks outdoors	
5. Down and up from floor		10. Wheelchair independence indoors		15. Climbs stairs	

Key

1	Normal /Independent	6	Moderate assist (50% of another person)
2	Independent but slow and/or difficult	7	Maximum assist (75% of another person)
3	Needs supervision	8	Dependent
4	Needs verbal cues and supervision	N/A	Not applicable
5	Minimum assist (25% of another person)	N/T	Not tested

PREVIOUS FUNCTIONAL LEVEL:

WHITE - CHART COPY YELLOW - M.D. COPY PINK - THERAPIST COPY

Figure 4–2. Physical Therapy Evaluation form.

Leonard Polar, 67 years old, lived alone in a one-story home following the death of his wife. He sustained a mild cerebral vascular accident and went to live with his son temporarily. He received home health services with the goal of returning to independent living in his own home. He was able to return to his own home 3 weeks after hospital discharge and continued to receive home health services for IADL training and nursing support. After several weeks of living alone he began to look disheveled, appeared not to be eating or fixing meals, and eventually stopped even getting out of bed. He was diagnosed as being depressed and returned to his son's home. Prior to his decline, no mental assessment was ever made although there had been subtle signs of stress. He would speak casually of "being better off dead," but this was not taken seriously. After his second return to his son's home and the diagnosis of "depression," he was placed on medication and showed improved function. The son, however, was concerned and convinced his father not to return to independent living. The staff conjectured later that if a mental assessment had been made earlier, Mr. Polar might have made a successful transition to independent living.

Review of Instruments

Some physical-function instruments have been in use over a long period and are particularly useful in home care settings. The original Katz ADL Index (Table 4–1) rates six basic ADLs: bathing, dressing, going to the toilet, transfers, continence, and feeding. A community-based version eliminates continence measures but includes walking and grooming. It can be used as a self-administered report. The Katz ADL Index has been broadly evaluated in the literature.[3,5,7]

An instrument that has appeared more recently in the literature measures the hierarchical difficulty of ADL and IADL tasks. The Groningen Activity Restriction Scale[8] (Table 4–2) elicits either separate ADL/IADL scores or a total numerical score. It may also be used as a self-reporting tool. Clients report task "independence," "dependence," and a middle category, "perform with difficulty," although no degrees of difficulty are measured.

Another self-assessment instrument useful in the community setting includes a pain rating scale along with the amount of assistance required or difficulty perceived in several specific ADL/IADL chores. The Functional Status Questionnaire[2] (Table 4–3), derived from the original Katz Index[3], assesses dependence on a five-point scale, where 5 indicates complete dependency. Pain and difficulty are assessed on seven-point scales, where 7 is the most severe intensity. Eighteen activities encompassing mobility, personal care, home chores, hand activities, and vocational and avocational areas are rated in three dimensions.

OCCUPATIONAL THERAPY: _______Initial _______Summary _______Discharge

Patient: ____________________

Address: ____________________

Telephone #: ____________________

Date of Assessment: ____________________

DOB: ____________________

Diagnosis: ____________________

Referred by: ____________________

Referred from: ____________________

Pertinent Information: (Medical, social, behavioral, psychological)

____

____

____

Home Environment: (Type of structure, barriers, family availability)

____

Mobility Statement: ____________________

Upper Extremeties: hand dominance ____________________

Non-dominant: ____________________

PROM ____________________

AROM ____________________

Muscle Tone ____________________

Muscle Strength ____________________

Coordination ____________________

Sensation ____________________

Note Abnormalities: ____________________

Dominant: ____________________

PROM ____________________

AROM ____________________

Muscle Tone ____________________

Coordination ____________________

Sensation ____________________

Note Abnormalities: ____________________

Visual Perception: ____________________

Figure 4–3. Occupational Therapy form.

Activities of Daily Living: ______

Eating ______

Dressing ______

Hygiene ______

Toileting ______

Avocational ______

Present Equipment: ______

Summary: ______

Short Term Goals: ______

Long Term Goals: ______

Plan of Care: ______

______
Signature

Sent to M.D. ______

20:PMR1317f

Figure 4–3. *Continued.*

TABLE 4–1

Katz ADL Index

Index of Independence in Activities of Daily Living

The Index of Independence in Activities of Daily Living (ADL) is based on an evaluation of the functional independence or dependence of patients in bathing, dressing, going to the toilet, transferring, continence, and feeding. Specific definitions of functional independence and dependence appear below the index.

A	Independent in feeding, continence, transferring, going to toilet, dressing, and bathing.
B	Independent in all but one of these functions.
C	Indepdendent in all but bathing and one additional function.
D	Independent in all but bathing, dressing, and one additional function.
E	Independent in all but bathing, dressing, going to toilet, and one additional function.
F	Independent in all but bathing, dressing, going to toilet, transferring, and one additional function.
G	Dependent in all six functions.
Other	Dependent in at least two functions, but not classifiable as C, D, E, or F.

Independence means no need for supervision, direction, or active personal assistance except as specifically noted below. This is based on actual status and not on ability. A patient who refuses to perform a function is considered as not performing the function, even when deemed able.

Bathing (Sponge, shower or tub)

Independent: Assistance only in bathing a single part (as back or disabled extremity) or bathes self completely

Dependent: Assistance in bathing more than one part of body; assistance in getting in or out of tub or does not bathe self

Dressing

Independent: Gets clothes from closets and drawers; puts on clothes, outer garments, braces; manages fasteners; tying shoes is excluded

Dependent: Does not dress self or remains partly undressed

Going to Toilet

Independent: Gets to toilet; gets on and off toilet; arranges clothes, cleans organs of excretion (may manage own bedpan used at night only and may or may not be using mechanical supports)

Dependent: Uses bedpan or commode or receives assistance in getting to and using toilet

Transfer

Independent: Moves in and out of bed independently and moves in and out of chair independently (may or may not be using mechanical supports)

Dependent: Assistance in moving in or out of bed or chair; does not perform one or more transfers

Continence

Independent: Urination and defecation entirely self-controlled

Dependent: Partial or total incontinence in urination or defecation; partial or total control by enemas or catheters, or regulated use of urinals and bedpans

Feeding

Independent: Gets food from plate or its equivalent into mouth (precutting of meat and preparation of food, as buttering bread, are excluded from evaluation)

Dependent: Assistance in act of feeding (see above); does not eat at all or needs parenteral feeding.

Adapted from Katz, S et al: Studies of illness in the aged. JAMA 185:914, 1963. Copyright 1963, American Medical Association, with permission.

TABLE 4–2
Groningen Activity Restriction Scale

Items, response categories and scores of the Groningen Activity Restriction Scale (GARS).

Scores and Response Categories for Each Item:

1. Yes, I can do it independently without any difficulty.
2. Yes, I can do it independently but with difficulty.
3. No, I cannot do it independently: I can only do it with someone's help.

ADL Items:

1. Can you, fully independently, dress yourself?
2. Can you, fully independently, get in and out of bed?
3. Can you, fully independently, rise from a chair?
4. Can you, fully independently, wash your face and hands?
5. Can you, fully independently, wash and dry your whole body?
6. Can you, fully independently, get on and off the toilet?
7. Can you, fully independently, feed yourself?
8. Can you, fully independently, get around in the house (if necessary with a cane)?
9. Can you, fully independently, go up and down the stairs?
10. Can you, fully independently, walk outdoors (if necessary with a cane)?
11. Can you, fully independently, take care of your feet and toenails?

IADL Items:

12. Can you, fully independently, prepare dinner?
13. Can you, fully independently, prepare breakfast or lunch?
14. Can you, fully independently, do "light" household activities (for example, dusting and tidying, up?)
15. Can you, fully independently, do "heavy" household activities (for example, mopping, cleaning the windows and vacuuming)?
16. Can you, fully independently, wash and iron your clothes?
17. Can you, fully independently, make the beds?
18. Can you, fully independently, do the shopping?

ADL = activities of daily living; IADL = instrumental activities of daily living.

Source: Adapted from Kempen,[8] with permission.

Specialized assessment of some functions is often required in home care. Mobility skills such as walking, balance, and fall risk can be germane to the independence of the client or to the need for more supervised living arrangements (see Chapter 5). A fast, easy rating system has been developed that uses videotaping to evaluate gait. The Gait Abnormality Rating Scale (GARS)[9] obtains a rating by totaling the points received on each of 16 variables, where 0 = normal, 1 = mildly impaired, 2 = moderately impaired, and 3 = severely impaired. The higher the total score, the more impaired the gait. Components in the rating system include the following categories: general (staggering, guardedness, etc.); lower extremity; and trunk, head, and upper extremity. Although the GARS[9] has shown to be a valid correlate of falls in nursing-home residents, significant differences in the variables between fallers and nonfallers have not been discerned in the community. Aside from the obvious need for a video camera and viewing monitor, the

TABLE 4–3

Functional Status Questionnaire

CATEGORY	ITEM
Physical Function	
During the past month have you had difficulty:	
Basic activities of daily living (ADL)	Taking care of yourself, that is, eating, dressing or bathing?
	Moving in and out of a bed or chair?
	Walking indoors, such as around your home?
Intermediate ADL	Walking several blocks?
	Walking one block or climbing one flight of stairs?
	Doing work around the house such as cleaning, light yard work, or home maintenance?
	Doing errands, such as grocery shopping?
	Driving a car or using public transportation?
	Doing vigorous activities such as running, lifting heavy objects, or participating in strenuous sports?
Responses: Usually did with no difficulty (4), some difficulty (3), much difficulty (2), usually did not do because of health (1), usually did not do for other reasons (0).	
Psychological Function	
During the past month:	
Mental health	Have you been a very nervous person?
	Have you felt calm and peaceful?*
	Have you felt downhearted and blue?
	Were you a happy person?*
	Did you feel so down in the dumps that nothing could cheer you up?
Responses: All of the time (1), most of the time (2), a good bit of the time (3), some of the time (4), a little of the time (5), none of the time (6).	
Social/role Function	
During the past month have you:	
Work performance (for those employed, during the preceding month)	Done as much work as others in similar jobs?*
	Worked for short periods of time or taken frequent rests because of your health?
	Worked your regular number of hours?*
	Done your job as carefully and accurately as others with similar jobs?*
	Worked at your usual job, but with some changes because of your health?
	Feared losing your job because of your health?
Responses: All of the time (1), most of the time (2), some of the time (3), none of the time (4).	
Social activity	Had difficulty vising with relatives or friends?
	Had difficulty participating in community activities, such as religious services, social activities, or volunteer work?
	Had difficulty taking care of other people, such as family members?
Responses: Usually did with no difficulty (4), some difficulty (3), much difficulty (2), usually did not do because of health (1), usually did not do for other reasons (0).	
Quality of interaction	Isolated yourself from people around you?
	Acted affectionate toward others?*
	Acted irritable toward those around you?
	Made unreasonable demands on your family and friends?
	Gotten along well with other people?*
Responses: All of the time (1), most of the time (2), a good bit of the time (3), some of the time (4), a little of the time (5), none of the time (6).	

TABLE 4–3
Functional Status Questionnaire—*Continued*

Single-Item Questions

Which of the following statements best describes your work situation during the past month? ***Responses:*** Working full-time; working part-time; unemployed, looking for work; unemployed because of my health; retired because of my health; retired for some other reason.

During the past month, how many days did illness or injury keep you in bed all or most of the day? ***Response:*** 0–31 days.

During the past month, how many days did you cut down on the things you usually do for one-half day or more because of your own illness or injury? ***Response:*** 0–31 days.

During the past month, how satisfied were you with your sexual relationships? ***Responses:*** Very satisfied, satisfied, not sure, dissatisfied, very dissatisfied, did not have any sexual relationships.

How do you feel about your own health? ***Responses:*** Very satisfied, satisfied, not sure, dissatisfied, very dissatisfied.

During the past month, about how often did you get together with friends or relatives, such as going out together, visiting in each other's homes, or talking on the telephone? ***Responses:*** Every day, several times a week, about once a week, two or three times a month, about once a month, not at all.

*Scores are reversed.

Source: Adapted from Jette et al,[6] with permission.

home environment needs a space approximately 1 m by 10 m for walking trials; this may be a drawback in the average home. However, consider using hallways in senior residences or nursing homes. Research subjects were tested on industrial-weight carpeting, but for individuals in the community, home floor surfaces will provide a more realistic performance. Videotaping can be educational and a morale booster. Consider renting a camera periodically and monitoring clients before, during, and after intervention for a visual proof of change. Some clients may enjoy showing their "tape" to friends and family.

Another simple and reliable instrument for observing balance and gait in the community-dwelling elderly was developed during investigations of risk factors for falls and serious injury. The Performance-Oriented Assessment of Mobility (POAM-I)[10] and the subsequently modified POAM-II[11] (Table 4–4) include gait maneuvers used during daily activity and reflect situations likely to be encountered during such activity. The POAM-I is used to assess balance. The POAM-II is meant to measure "usual function" rather than "standard function" and is designed to be used in homes, not laboratories. For instance, stair climbing is not rated in individuals who do not have to climb stairs in their living quarters. The POAM-II was developed to measure outcome following physical therapy intervention for fall risk. Therefore, each item is likely to improve with intervention, and the scoring directly reflects the safest means of performing the daily activities. A faster sit-to-stand task or faster walking pace is not encouraged even though slower paces may be associated with fall risk. The POAM-II has rating categories for balance in sitting and standing, transfers, gait, and timed walks. Instructions to the examiner and client are specific. For home use of the instrument, a tape measure and sticky tape are needed for marking distances. The POAM-II requires

TABLE 4–4

Performance-Oriented Assessment of Mobility II

Gait

Instructions: Subject stands with examiner. Subject walks down 10-foot walkway (measured). Examiner asks subject to walk down walkway, turn, and walk back. Subject should use customary walking aid.

Bare Floor (flat, even surface)

1. Type of surface
   1 = Linoleum/tile
   2 = Wood
   3 = Cement/concrete
   4 = Other ____________
   [not included in scoring]
2. Initiation of gait (immediately after command to "go")
   0 = Any hesitancy or multiple attempts to start
   1 = No hesitancy
3. Path (estimated in relation to **tape measure**). Observe excursion of foot closest to tape measure over middle 8 feet of course.
   0 = Marked deviation
   1 = Mild/moderate deviation **or** uses walking aid
   2 = Straight without walking aid
4. Missed step (tripping or loss of balance)
   0 = Yes and would have fallen **or** more than two missed steps
   1 = Yes, but appropriate attempt to recover **and** no more than two
   2 = None
5. Turning (while walking)
   0 = Almost falls
   1 = Mild staggering but catches self, uses walker or cane
   2 = Steady, without walking aid
6. Step over obstacles (to be assessed in a separate walk with two shoes placed on course four feet apart)
   0 = Begins to fall at any obstacle **or** unable to step over obstacles **or** walks around any ostacle **or** > two missed steps
   1 = Able to step over all obstacles but some staggering but catches self **or** one to two missed steps
   2 = Able and steady at stepping over all four obstacles with no missed steps

Source: Adapted from Tinetti,[11] with permission.

three shoes placed in the walking path as obstacles to step over. Gait performance may also be challenged by different surfaces—tile, hardwood, cement, carpet, and grass, for example.

Instruments for other specialized needs are also available, including, but not limited to, the Burke Stroke Time-Oriented Profile (BUSTOP),[12] the Rappaport Disability Rating Scale for Severe Head Trauma,[13] and the Jebsen Test of Hand Function[14] (Table 4–5).

Assessments of mental function may be the second-most-useful instruments for the therapist who is documenting required services. Cognitive decline is implicated first with IADL dysfunctions, but may also co-exist with mobility and ADL decrements and may affect the prognosis for intervention. The Mini–Mental State test[15] is often used by clinicians working with the elderly and is addressed in Chapter 11.

TABLE 4–5

Jebsen Test of Hand Function

Writing

Procedure—The subject is given a black ballpoint pen and four 8-by-11-inch sheets of unruled white paper fastened, one on top of the other, to a clipboard. The sentence to be copied has 24 letters and is of third-grade reading difficulty.* The sentence is typed in all capital letters and centered on a 5-by-8-inch index card. The card is presented with the typed side face down on a bookstand. After the articles are arranged to the comfort of the subject (see Instructions), the card is turned over by the examiner with an immediate command to begin. The item is timed from the word "go" until the pen is lifted from the page at the end of the sentence. The item is repeated with the dominant hand using a new sentence.

Instructions (if subject is right-handed)—"Do you require glasses for reading? If so, put them on. Take this pen in your left hand and arrange everything so that it is comfortable for you to write with your left hand. On the other side of this card (indicate) is a sentence. When I turn the card over and say 'Go,' write the sentence as quickly and as clearly as you can using your left hand. Write, do not print. Do you understand? Ready? Go."

Simulated Feeding

Procedure—Five kidney beans approximately ⅝-inch long are placed on a board† clamped to a desk in front of the subject 5 inches from the front edge of the desk. The beans are oriented left of center, parallel to and touching the upright of the board 2 inches apart. An empty 1-pound coffee can is placed centrally in front of the board. A regular teaspoon is provided. Timing is from the word "go" until the last bean is heard hitting the bottom of the can. The item is repeated with the dominant hand, the beans being placed right of center.

Instructions—"Take the teaspoon in your left hand, please. When I say 'Go,' use your left hand to pick up these beans one at a time with the teaspoon and place them in the can as fast as you can beginning with this one (indicate bean on the extreme left). Do you understand? Ready? Go."

*Different sentences were used when subsequent tests were given to a single individual. Available sentences were: (1) The old man seemed to be tired. (2) John saw the red truck coming. (3) Whales live in the blue ocean. (4) Fish take air out of the water.

†A wooden board 41½ inches long, 11¼ inches wide, and ¾-inch thick was secured to the desk with a C clamp. The front edge of the board (¾-in thick) was marked at 4-inch intervals for easy reference when placing objects. A center piece of plywood, 20 inches long, 2 inches high, and ½-inch thick, was glued to the board 4⅝ inches from the right end and 6 inches from the front (for a secretary-type desk with a right-sided kneehole). The front of the center upright should be marked at 2-inch intervals beginning 1 inch from each end for convenience in placing objects.

Source: Adapted from Jebsen, et al,[14] with permission.

Obtaining Author and Publisher Permissions

Having determined their value in formulating a plan of care, where does the skilled practitioner find the desired instruments? Journals and trade publications frequently discuss and often reproduce assessment instruments. The difficult part is obtaining permission to use the instruments because, once published, they are subject to copyright law and may not be legally used without proper consent from the author or publisher. There is no clearinghouse, book list, or catalogue where you can buy the instruments you need; this presents an often frustrating barrier to the professional seeking to use a published assessment form. Once permission is granted, however, the instrument can be used repeatedly. If the instrument has been published, permission to reproduce it must be sought from the book, journal, or magazine publisher. Unpublished materials require author permission for duplication. Several problems are inherent in the process of obtaining permission:

- Publisher addresses are different for each publication and listed addresses change from time to time.
- Locating author or publisher addresses is time-consuming. However, publishers provide author addresses, or you can check the inside pages in journals and compendiums of publishers, such as Gayle's, at libraries.
- Permission is sometimes granted with qualifications — the material may be reproduced only in English, for example.
- A sizable fee may be required.
- The publisher or author may fail to respond to the request.
- Publisher reprints of the original article, including the assessment instrument, may be available only from the primary author, necessitating another mailing.

Some steps can make the task easier:

- Have a request form printed on business letterhead, with blanks in the portion where the publisher name or article title can be inserted. This allows quick mailing of multiple requests.
- State clearly that the purpose of reprinting the material is only for assessing clients.
- Ask that permission be granted for all current and future versions of the instrument, and for current and future use by you or associates of your agency.
- Copy and date the original request and re-send the letter each month a reply has not come in. File and keep completed and returned forms.

Contact for permission to use referenced forms described in this chapter are listed in Appendix 4–2; permission to reproduce the nonreferenced forms may be obtained from the publisher of this book.

BROADER IMPLICATIONS OF ASSESSMENT

Recent changes in Medicare's reimbursement system have shifted the responsibility for elder rehabilitation away from acute-care hospitals and toward alternative settings, including home care. One repercussion from this shift is that regulations governing nonhospital settings continue to evolve. An example is the federal regulation (effective in October 1990) requiring that all nursing-home residents be evaluated for functional status on admission and periodically thereafter. To substantiate a claim for reimbursement, intervention aimed toward a functional outcome must be based on objective measurement data. Home care, rising in popularity among clients and congressional representatives alike, may be the next venue for reimbursement and its concomitant regulations. Congress has steadily expanded public coverage of home care, and private insurers are moving into the field. These funding sources will soon demand cost-effective strategies. Therefore, identifying chronic disablement and possible therapeutic intervention in the noninstitutionalized elderly may serve several purposes. It may reduce the need for institutionalization by allowing more clients who are at risk for nursing home placement to be served at home. Reassessment may also help reduce home-care costs by limiting use and preventing overuse of services. Accurate functional assessment may also affect the eligibility pool for home-care benefits. Altering eligibility criteria to include some or all ADLs and IADLs may increase the size of the eligibility pool. The beneficiary pool size may also forecast the need for specific types of providers.

Perhaps the greatest benefit from properly administered functional assessments comes in the satisfaction of seeing measurable progress in a client.

Ms. Fay, diagnosed with and treated for lymphatic cancer and hospitalized for a long time, was discharged from the hospital in a state of remission. She was extremely weak, lay most frequently in a semifetal position, and was totally dependent on family and home health aides for her care. Initial assessment by the physical therapist indicated total dependence in all areas of physical function and self-care. The occupational therapist indicated that Ms. Fay was not ready for OT intervention. She received PT for almost a year with periodic reassessment indicating areas of progress. Assessment data were used to justify continued care and the need for state medical support. After a year of treatment, Ms. Fay had regained considerable strength and could perform all her ADLs. Her energy level was too low to let her accomplish IADLS; she could not cook, clean house or drive a car. At this point, the physical therapist requested re-evaluation by the occupational therapist. The final PT assessment documented objectively that Ms. Fay needed continued home care. The OT assessment documented areas of IADL deficits and continued care was authorized. The occupational therapist designed a plan of care that included energy conservation measures and gradual withdrawal of HHA support. Throughout the year and a half that Ms. Fay received home health therapy, the skilled practitioners' accurate measurements of deficits and progress allowed for continued eligibility of services. Throughout that time, the objective data were also used with Ms. Fay herself and the family to help boost morale by depicting progress.

In the end, of course, for Ms. Fay and the professionals who came to know her well after so many months, the successful conclusion of her case is only hinted at by the written lines on various assessments. Ms. Fay now leads an independent life. She drives, she cooks, she readily accepts new challenges. That is worth all the paperwork that documentation demands.

REFERENCES

1. Jette, AM, Branch, LG, and Berlin, J: Musculoskeletal impairments and physical disablement among the aged. J Gerontol: Med Sci 45(6):203, 1990.
2. Jette, A: The functional status index: Reliability of a chronic disease evaluation instrument. Arch Phys Med Rehab 61:395, 1980.
3. Katz, S, Ford, AB, Moskowitz, RW, et al: Studies of illness in the aged; the index of ADL: A standardized measure of biological and psychological function. J Am Med Assoc 185:94, 1963.
4. Jette, A: State of the art in functional assessment. In Rothstein, J (ed): Measurement in Physical Therapy, Churchill Livingstone, New York, 1985.
5. Guccione, AA, Cullen, KE, O'Sullivan, SB: Functional assessment. In O'Sullivan, SB and Schmitz, TJ: Physical Rehabilitation: Assessment and Treatment. FA Davis, Philadelphia, 1988.
6. Jette, A, Davier, A, Cleary, P, et al: The functional status questionnaire, reliability and validity when used in primary care. J Gen Int Med 1:143, 1986.
7. Kane, RA and Kane, RL: Assessing the Elderly: A Practical Guide to Measurement. Lexington Books, DC Heath, Lexington, MA, 1981.
8. Kempen, GI: The development of a hierarchical polychotomous ADL-IADL scale for noninstitutionalized elders. The Gerontologist 30(4):497, 1990.
9. Wolfson, L, Whipple, R, Amerman, P, et al: Gait assessment in the elderly: A gait abnormality rating scale and its relation to falls. J Gerontol: Med Sci 45(1):12, 1990.
10. Tinetti, M: Performance-oriented assessment of mobility problems in elderly clients. J Am Geriatr Soc 34:119, 1986.
11. Tinetti, M: Personal communication, May–June, 1991.
12. Feigensen, J, Polkow, L, Meikle, F, et al: Burke stroke time-oriented profile (BUSTOP): An overview of client function. Arch Phys Med Rehabil 60:508, 1979.
13. Rappaport, M, Hall, K, Hopkins, K, et al: Disability rating scale for severe head trauma: Coma to community. Arch Phys Med Rehabil 63:118, 1982.
14. Jebsen, R, Taylor, N, Treischmann, R, et al: An objective and standardized test of hand function. Arch Phys Med Rehabil 50:311, 1969.
15. Folstein, MF, Folstein, S, and McHugh, PR: Mini mental state: A practical method for grading the cognitive state of patients for the clinician, J Psychiatr Res 12:189, 1975.

Appendix 4–1

Home Health Care Documentation Forms

Department of Health and Human Services
Health Care Financing Administration

Form Approved
OMB No. 0938-0357

HOME HEALTH CERTIFICATION AND PLAN OF TREATMENT

1. Patient's HI Claim No.	2. SOC Date	3. Certification Period From: To:	4. Medical Record No.	5. Provider No.

6. Patient's Name and Address

7. Provider's Name and Address.

8. Date of Birth:

9. Sex ☐ M ☐ F

10. Medications: Dose/Frequency/Route (N)ew (C)hanged

11. ICD-9-CM	Principal Diagnosis	Date
12. ICD-9-CM	Surgical Procedure	Date
13. ICD-9-CM	Other Pertinent Diagnoses	Date

14. DME and Supplies

15. Safety Measures:

16. Nutritional Req.

17. Allergies:

18.A. Functional Limitations

1 ☐ Amputation
2 ☐ Bowel/Bladder (Incontinence)
3 ☐ Contracture
4 ☐ Hearing
5 ☐ Paralysis
6 ☐ Endurance
7 ☐ Ambulation
8 ☐ Speech
9 ☐ Legally Blind
A ☐ Dyspnea With Minimal Exertion
B ☐ Other (Specify)

18.B. Activities Permitted

1 ☐ Complete Bedrest
2 ☐ Bedrest BRP
3 ☐ Up As Tolerated
4 ☐ Transfer Bed/Chair
5 ☐ Exercises Prescribed
6 ☐ Partial Weight Bearing
7 ☐ Independent At Home
8 ☐ Crutches
9 ☐ Cane
A ☐ Wheelchair
B ☐ Walker
C ☐ No Restrictions
D ☐ Other (Specify)

19. Mental Status:

1 ☐ Oriented
2 ☐ Comatose
3 ☐ Forgetful
4 ☐ Depressed
5 ☐ Disoriented
6 ☐ Lethargic
7 ☐ Agitated
8 ☐ Other

20. Prognosis: 1 ☐ Poor 2 ☐ Guarded 3 ☐ Fair 4 ☐ Good 5 ☐ Excellent

21. Orders for Discipline and Treatments (Specify Amount/Frequency/Duration)

22. Goals/Rehabilitation Potential/Discharge Plans

23. Verbal Start of Care and Nurse's Signature and Date Where Applicable:

24. Physician's Name and Address

25. Date HHA Received Signed POT

26. I ☐ certify ☐ recertify that the above home health services are required and are authorized by me with a written plan for treatment which will be periodically reviewed by me. This patient is under my care, is confined to his home, and is in need of intermittent skilled nursing care and/or physical or speech therapy or has been furnished home health services based on such a need and no longer has a need for such care or therapy, but continues to need occupational therapy.

27. Attending Physician's Signature (Required on 485 Kept on File in Medical Records of HHA)

Date Signed

Form HCFA-485 (U4) (4-87)

Department of Health and Human Services
Health Care Financing Administration

Form Approved
OMB No. 0938-0357

MEDICAL UPDATE AND PATIENT INFORMATION

1. Patient's HI Claim No.	2. SOC Date	3. Certification Period From: To:	4. Medical Record No.	5. Provider No.

6. Patient's Name	7. Provider's Name

8. Medicare Covered: ☐ Y ☐ N | 9. Date Physician Last Saw Patient: | 10. Date Last Contacted Physician:

11. Is the Patient Receiving Care in an 1861 (J)(1) Skilled Nursing Facility or Equivalent? ☐ Y ☐ N ☐ Do Not Know | 12. ☐ Certification ☐ Recertification ☐ Modified

13. Specific Services and Treatments

Discipline	Visits (This Bill) Rel. to Prior Cert.	Frequency and Duration	Treatment Codes	Total Visits Projected This Cert.

14. Dates of Last Inpatient Stay: Admission Discharge | 15. Type of Facility:

16. Updated Information: New Orders/Treatments/Clinical Facts/Summary from Each Discipline

17. Functional Limitations (Expand From 485 and Level of ADL) Reason Homebound/Prior Functional Status

18. Supplementary Plan of Treatment on File from Physician Other than Referring Physician: ☐ Y ☐ N
(If Yes, Please Specify Giving Goals/Rehab. Potential/Discharge Plan)

19. Unusual Home/Social Environment

20. Indicate Any Time When the Home Health Agency Made a Visit and Patient was Not Home and Reason Why if Ascertainable	21. Specify Any Known Medical and/or Non-Medical Reasons the Patient Regularly Leaves Home and Frequency of Occurrence

22. Nurse or Therapist Completing or Reviewing Form	Date (Mo., Day, Yr.)

Form HCFA-486 (C3) (4-87)

Department of Health and Human Services
Health Care Financing Administration

Form Approved
OMB No. 0938-0357

ADDENDUM TO: ☐ PLAN OF TREATMENT ☐ MEDICAL UPDATE

1. Patient's HI Claim No.	2. SOC Date	3. Certification Period From: To:	4. Medical Record No.	5. Provider No.

6. Patient's Name	7. Provider Name

8. Item No.	

9. Signature of Physician	10. Date
11. Optional Name/Signature of Nurse/Therapist	12. Date

Form HCFA-487 (U4) (4-87)

Appendix 4–2

Publishers of Assessment Forms

- Functional Status Index, BUSTOP, Disability Rating Scale for Severe Head Trauma, and Standardized Test of Hand Function. Published by Archives of Physical Medicine and Rehabilitation, Editorial Board, Suite 1310, 78 E Adams St., Chicago, IL 60603-6103
- Gait Assessment in the Elderly—gait abnormality rating scale. Published by Journal of Gerontology, The Gerontological Society of America, 127 K St., NW, Suite 350, Washington, DC 20005-4006
- Hierarchical Polychotomous–IADL scale for Noninstitutionalized Elders. Published by GIJ Kempen, PhD (gerontologist), Department of Health Sciences, State University of Groningen A, Deusinglaan 1, 9713 Av Sroningen, The Netherlands
- Katz Index of ADL: A Standardized Measure of Biological and Psychological Function. Published by Journal of the American Medical Association, 535 N. Dearborn St., Chicago, IL 60610
- Functional Status Questionnaire. Published by Journal of General Internal Medicine, Hanley and Belfus, Inc., 210 S. 13th St., Philadelphia, PA 19107
- POAM I and II. Contact Mary E. Tinetti, MD, 333 Cedar St., P. O. Box 3333, New Haven, CT 06510-8056
- Mini Mental State. Published by Journal of Psychiatric Research, Pergamon Press, Headington Hill Hall, Oxford OX3 OBW, United Kingdom

Chapter 5

Therapeutic Exercise in the Home Setting

LYNN ALLEN COLBY & BETTE HORSTMAN

The essence of home health rehabilitation is to maximize capabilities so that the client is able to function as independently as possible in the home. Therapeutic exercise, implemented to develop strength or endurance, improve flexibility, and prevent contractures, deformity, or circulatory complications, is one important aspect of a comprehensive rehabilitation program for the client receiving therapy at home. Home exercises directed to the achievement of specific functional activities can have a positive impact on the client's improvement rate after discharge from an acute care facility. An effective home exercise program may enable a client to develop enough functional capabilities to maintain independence and avoid the necessity for extended care at a nursing facility.[1–3]

To develop an effective exercise program for a client in the home setting, the home health therapist must have a thorough knowledge of the theoretical foundations and principles of therapeutic exercise. It is equally important for the therapist to understand the unique problems that a client or family may encounter with a home exercise program. Many clients who receive home therapy are elderly or have chronic disabilities. The therapist must understand the elderly client's special needs when designing an exercise program. Above all, the therapist must be creative and innovative when adapting exercises for a client at home.

The purpose of this chapter is to discuss a number of factors a therapist must consider when designing, implementing, and teaching a home exercise program. An overview of several conditions commonly seen in clients who receive home therapy is presented with the emphasis on appropriate goals and special considerations for exercise. Finally, the chapter describes the effective use of equipment in the home and a variety of exercises that a client can carry out independently or with minimal assistance from a family member.

EXERCISE FOR THE CLIENT AT HOME

The experienced therapist is aware of the basic goals and principles of therapeutic exercise and is well versed in evaluating clients and prioritizing functional goals, as well as choosing appropriate exercises to meet those goals. Before moving into home health care, most therapists also have a great deal of experience teaching clients how to perform exercises safely and effectively. To develop an exercise plan that will work for the client at home, however, the therapist must consider some special aspects of care that are unique to the home environment. The guidelines in this chapter for developing and teaching a successful exercise program illustrate some ways in which the home health therapist must modify a previously designed exercise plan, and how the exercises are taught to clients and family in the home.

Guidelines for Developing a Home Exercise Program

- Evaluate the client's status and the availability of support from the family.
- Ascertain the client's and the family's needs and functional goals and determine if they are compatible. Help the client prioritize the goals.
- Determine the client's and family's interest and willingness to regularly participate in an exercise program.
- Assess the home environment. Determine the best location for exercise and what adaptations may be necessary for carrying out a successful exercise program.
- Recognize the influence of temperature and lighting. If the room is too hot or too cold, the client may not be comfortable while exercising.
- Review any exercises or home instructions that the client may have been given by a therapist in a clinical facility.
- Develop a plan of care and select exercises directly related to achieving specific functional goals. Build in an appropriate warm-up or cool-down.
- Determine which exercises can be done only with the assistance of a therapist and which can be carried out independently by the client or with minimal assistance from a caregiver.
- Try to keep the number of home exercises to a minimum. Few clients will comply with a lengthy exercise routine.
- Determine the present or future need for equipment to be used in the exercise program.
- Help the client determine the best time of day to do the exercises considering the family's daily routine.
- Explain to the client what type of clothing will be best for exercise.
- After a few sessions, re-evaluate the exercise plan. Ask what the client thinks about the program. Try to determine the level of compliance.
- Assist the client in developing a sense of self-responsibility for the exercise plan and overall rehabilitation.

Teaching a Home Exercise Program

- Find an area of the home where exercise can be performed safely and with a minimum of distractions for the client or caregiver. Stable and firm but comfortable surfaces are usually best.
- Explain the purpose or benefit of each exercise and how it will help the client reach a particular functional goal.
- Demonstrate the exercise to the client or caregiver. It is usually helpful to guide the client through the desired movement to provide vi-

sual and proprioceptive cues that will enhance learning. Point out how far or at what speed the movement should occur. If isometrics are being performed, indicate the correct intensity of the contraction. Point out substitute motions that should not occur during the exercise.

- Ask the client or caregiver to perform the exercise several times as you assist or watch. Provide visual and tactile cues and verbal feedback as necessary. Some elderly or disoriented clients may react slowly and will need more time to respond to the instructions. Have the client practice the exercise a reasonable number of times.
- Always remind the client to breathe while exercising.
- Have the client perform the number of repetitions you have recommended and see how the client responds.
- After going through an entire exercise session, evaluate the client's response to the exercises. Modify the number, intensity, or duration of exercises if necessary.
- Teach the client or caregiver to evaluate responses such as heart and respiratory rate, fatigue, or delayed-onset muscle soreness. It may be useful to teach the client or caregiver to monitor vital signs before, during, and after exercise.
- Try to make the exercise program a pleasant experience. Some clients may enjoy exercising to music.
- Provide written and illustrated instructions for each exercise. Indicate the number of repetitions and the frequency of each exercise during the day and the week. A chart helps the client keep track of the frequency and extent of exercise.
- Explain the value of rest between exercise sessions and the importance of warm-up and cool-down periods. Instruct the client about the appropriate use of heat or cold before or after exercise.
- Teach the client how to recognize improvements in strength, endurance, and flexibility as they apply to desired functional goals. Find simple ways to measure improvement quantitatively; for example, how far up the wall the client can reach or how many repetitions of an exercise can be done before fatigue sets in.
- On a return visit, have the client or caregiver demonstrate the exercises. You may have to review or re-explain the exercise. Different clients have different learning and memory capabilities, which will affect how the exercises are done.

Precautions in a Home Exercise Program

When carrying out a home exercise program, the client must be aware of the following precautions:

- Do not exercise immediately after a meal.

- Do not exercise in very high humidity or high temperatures.
- Do not hold breath with exercise exertion.
- Stop exercises if dizziness, severe pain, nausea, blurred vision, or profuse sweating occurs. Persistent joint or soft-tissue pain that lasts more than 30 minutes after exercise, or joint swelling that develops the next day, may mean the exercise program is too strenuous or aggressive.
- Perform isometric exercises cautiously. Vigorous isometric muscle contractions can cause dramatic increases in blood pressure. Generally, clients with a history of hypertension, cardiovascular accident (CVA), or heart disease should do isometric exercises at a very low intensity.
- Be sure that all commercial or home-made equipment is safe and in good working condition.

COMMON CLIENT PROBLEMS: GOALS AND HOME EXERCISE PLANS

The home health therapist observes many types of clients who require instruction or assistance with exercise in the home. One report suggests that, of the clients observed in home therapy, 50 percent have orthopedic problems, 25 percent have disabilities of neurologic origin, and the remainder have problems arising from multiple conditions.[4] Some conditions commonly seen in clients receiving home health care are amputation, arthritis, CVA, and fractures. In addition, many clients seen by home health therapists are also elderly. This section highlights the main problems of clients with these conditions and prioritizes rehabilitation goals as they relate to developing a home exercise plan. Most of the concepts described here can be applied to treating other conditions.

Amputation

Amputee care in the home must emphasize psychological as well as physical rehabilitation. The psychological adjustment to the loss of a limb is difficult. Loss of an upper extremity is much more difficult than loss of the lower extremity.[5] Unless the client develops a healthy attitude toward the disability and prosthesis, rehabilitation will be compromised.

Clients who have undergone amputation of a lower or upper extremity may be discharged from an acute care facility as early as 1 week after surgery and will require postoperative therapy, including exercise, in the home. Most clients with amputations treated by home health therapists have had one or both lower extremities amputated as the result of chronic peripheral vascular disease. These clients often have a history of other chronic problems such as diabetes and heart disease. Many have had a great deal of pain, due to intermittent claudication before the amputation. These clients are often elderly and may have been sedentary before the surgery.[6] Many have associated pulmonary problems, visual deficits, or renal disease. Occasionally a therapist may see a client who has had an upper extremity amputation as the result of trauma or disease who will also require therapy.[7] The goal of rehabilitation for both the lower-extremity and upper-extremity amputee is to return the client to the highest level of functional independence possible.[7-9] For the lower-extremity amputee this may mean independent ambulation with a prosthesis. For the upper extremity amputee the ultimate goal is restoration of bimanual capabilities with a prosthesis. Goals for the client with bilateral above-knee amputation will be very different than for the client with a unilateral amputation above or below the knee. The age of the client, the extent of associated medical conditions, and the chronicity of the problem prior to amputation will determine whether or not the client is a candidate for a prosthesis and will affect the outcome of a rehabilitation program in the home.

An effective postoperative exercise program can prevent contractures, maintain or improve strength in the residual limb and the uninvolved extremities, maintain balance and coordination, and prepare the client for effective use of a prosthesis. Proprioceptive neuromuscular facilitation (PNF) exercises for the trunk and extremities[10] are an excellent means of strengthening key muscle groups and can be used effectively by the skilled home therapist. Cardiopulmonary conditioning exercises to improve endurance may also be necessary, particularly in elderly or sedentary clients.

Lower Extremity Amputation

General Goals and Exercise Plan[6-9,11-14]

1. **Prevent hip and knee flexion contractures.** The hip is vulnerable to flexion, adduction, and external rotation contractures, and the knee is vulnerable to flexion deformities. Gentle active exercises of the residual limb may be initiated almost immediately after surgery. When wound healing is not yet complete, range of motion (ROM) may cause some discomfort at the site of the incision. If a preexisting hip or knee flexion contracture is present, the therapist or caregiver should not initiate passive stretching until the incision is well healed. The client should be encouraged to lie prone for at least some time each day. Lying prone while watching television or resting for 20 to 30 minutes each day will help maintain adequate hip or knee extension and prevent flexion contractures.
2. **Increase strength in the residual limb.** Key muscle groups to be strengthened are the hip extensors and abductors and the knee flexors and extensors if the knee is intact. The hip extensors must be at a Fair/Three (F or 3) strength level and the hip abductors at a Good/Four (G or 4) level for effective ambulation with a prosthesis.

Abductor muscles maintain the stability of the pelvis during ambulation. Various resistance exercises to strengthen the residual limb can be done in a supine or side-lying position with a rolled towel under the residual limb. Most clients can do these exercises independently; body weight is the source of the resistance as the client attempts to lift the hip and buttocks off the floor. Elastic resistance materials or belt exercises, described in the last section of this chapter, are also very useful for strengthening the residual limb.

3. **Maintain or increase strength in the uninvolved extremities and trunk.** Unilateral lower-extremity amputees require assistive devices such as a walker or crutches for ambulation without a prosthesis. Bilateral lower-extremity amputees need strong upper-body muscles for independent wheelchair transfers. The exercises should strengthen the elbow and shoulder extensors and scapular depressors. The client can do partial push-ups while sitting in an armchair or lying prone. Strengthening the hip and knee extensors and hip abductors of the intact lower extremity is also important for ambulation with or without a prosthesis.
4. **Maintain or improve balance and coordination.** After amputation of one or both lower extremities, the client must adjust to a change in balance and motor control in the upright position. Balance activities can be performed in a wheelchair or standing at a kitchen counter. Dynamic balance can be improved by sitting in a chair or standing with minimal support and reaching for objects on a low table or on the floor. PNF exercises that involve combined movements of the trunk and lower extremities and emphasize rhythmic stabilization also improve balance and upright control. Adequate balance and coordination are necessary for independent ambulation with or without a prosthesis or independent mobility in a wheelchair. More detailed information on planning a program for progressive mobility in the home can be found in Chapter 6.

Upper Extremity Amputation

General Goals and Exercise Plan[7,11,15]

1. **Maintain mobility of the joints above the site of the amputation.** To use an upper extremity prothesis effectively and perform bimanual activities in daily living, the amputee must have normal ROM of the shoulder. After an above-elbow amputation, contractures can develop that will decrease shoulder abduction, flexion, or extension. Scapular mobility is also necessary for use of an upper-extremity prosthesis. In the below-elbow amputee, an elbow flexion contracture can develop and impair normal reaching with the prosthesis. Exercises should include elbow flexion and extension and forearm

supination and pronation motions. The client can be taught self-assisted and, later, active exercises that require little to no supervision after instruction by the therapist.

2. **Increase strength and improve isolated muscle control in the residual limb.** Emphasis should be placed on strengthening the scapular depressors, shoulder flexors, extensors, and abductors, and the elbow flexors and extensors if the elbow is intact. Isometric exercises can be done to strengthen the shoulder by having the client stand next to a wall and push the residual limb against it. Scapular depressors can be strengthened by pushing the well-healed limb into the padded arm of a chair. A caregiver can also be taught to do gentle manual resistance exercise for the residual limb. By performing isometric muscle contractions, the below-elbow amputee can also practice isolated control of the key muscles, such as the wrist flexors and extensors, that will operate the terminal device of a myoelectric prosthesis. For a better understanding of which muscle is to contract isometrically, the client can practice bilateral contractions as the therapist palpates the belly of the contracting muscle.
3. **Maintain normal postural alignment and symmetry.** A client with an upper-extremity amputation can develop postural asymmetry. Postural awareness training and active exercises of the neck or trunk will help the client maintain normal mobility and postural alignment.

Arthritis

Although "arthritis" is a general term associated with a wide variety of inflammatory and joint diseases, the client with arthritis usually develops varying degrees of joint inflammation, stiffness and pain, limitation of motion, deformity, muscle weakness, and atrophy.[16,17] Joint deformities often develop in positions of comfort. The main goals of a home exercise program for the client with arthritis are relief of pain, restoration or maintenance of joint mobility and muscle strength, and prevention of joint deformity.[17,18]

When developing an exercise program for the client with arthritis, the therapist must consider the degree of inflammation or stage of the disease (acute, subacute, or chronic) at the time exercise is to be performed. During the acute and early subacute stages, the client has significant joint swelling and effusion, pain with motion, and limitation of motion, and he or she tires easily. As inflammation subsides in the late subacute and chronic stages, limitation of motion often persists due to joint and soft-tissue tightness, but pain is experienced at the ends of the ROM. The therapist may note evidence of chronic deformity, muscle atrophy, and weakness at this time. Clients with a long history of arthritis or prolonged use of steroids may also have developed osteoporosis and are more susceptible to pathologic fractures.

General Goals and Exercise Plan[16–19]

1. **Relieve pain and muscle guarding and promote relaxation.** When significant inflammation is present, the use of cold or heat may decrease pain. Contrast baths, a warm bath or shower, or the application of a warm moist towel covered by a heating pad can relax muscles and decrease pain prior to exercise. Icepacks are often preferable for relief of pain during the acute inflammatory stage if the client can tolerate the cold. One very effective form of exercise that the therapist can employ to decrease pain is gentle joint traction or oscillation techniques (Grade I) with the affected joint in a comfortable resting position. Gentle setting exercises of muscles that surround an inflamed joint can promote relaxation, decrease muscle guarding, and reduce pain and stiffness.
2. **Maintain joint ROM and prevent deformity.** Active assisted or passive ROM exercise of affected joints can help maintain joint and soft-tissue mobility and prevent or minimize joint deformity and contractures. Passive or assisted exercises need not be performed repetitively to maintain range. In fact, repetitive motions may irritate the already inflamed joint further and delay recovery. Care must be taken not to stretch a swollen joint; this can contribute to joint instability. Therefore, stretching techniques are not indicated during the acute inflammatory stage. The therapist may have to set priorities to decide which joint motions are most important to maintain. For example, it may be more desirable to maintain normal elbow flexion for eating and dressing than to try to maintain full elbow extension. Full knee extension is more important for walking than full knee flexion.
3. **Prevent muscle weakness and atrophy.** Antigravity muscle groups weaken rapidly if the client is confined to bed for even a brief period of time. When acute signs and symptoms of arthritis are present, the safest way to strengthen muscles that cross an inflamed joint is with isometric exercises. Multiple-angle isometrics held for 6 to 10 seconds maintain static strength throughout the available range. Isometric exercises will not irritate an already painful and swollen joint. They can be performed against resistance without any equipment, using only the client's unaffected extremity, or by pushing against an immovable object such as a door frame or heavy padded piece of furniture. As mentioned previously, clients performing isometric exercises should consciously breathe while exercising to minimize the effect of the Valsalva phenomenon and its impact on the cardiovascular system. Isotonic exercises against resistance can cause excessive joint compression, pain, and further irritation and are contraindicated during the acute or subacute stages of arthritis.

4. **Protect inflamed joints.** The therapist must teach the client ways to protect inflamed joints, particularly the weight-bearing joints. Use of assistive devices for ambulation is often indicated at this stage of the disease. The client can also be shown how to adapt furniture to minimize stresses to involved joints. For example, the client can raise the chair height a few inches with a stable platform to make it easier to get up from the chair (see Chapter 7). Appropriate use of splints may also help protect and rest a painful, inflamed joint.
5. **Avoid excessive fatigue.** Although exercise is important for the client with arthritis, the home health therapist must help the client understand that if exercises are performed too vigorously or too frequently, this can cause greater pain, joint irritation, and excessive fatigue.

As joint swelling, pain, and muscle guarding subside, the goals of treatment can be modified and the exercises progress. High-impact activities causing joint compression must be avoided.

General Goals and Exercise Plan[16–18]

1. **Increase joint ROM.** When inflammation has subsided, stretching techniques such as joint mobilization and muscle stretching can be initiated. Caution must still be used because tendon deterioration, ligamentous instability, and osteoporosis are often associated with long-standing arthritis. Low-intensity, long-duration stretching techniques are safer and usually more comfortable for the client and keep postexercise muscle soreness to a minimum. Various self-stretching techniques that the therapist or client can use safely and effectively are discussed later in this chapter.
2. **Increase muscle strength.** Both static and dynamic resistance exercises are appropriate when inflammation has subsided. If isotonic exercises are used, resistance should be light (low load) and a high number of repetitions should be emphasized. This minimizes compressive forces to joint surfaces and prevents further joint deterioration. Light weights and light grades of elastic resistance material are appropriate forms of resistance. If the client experiences pain during the exercise, the resistance or arc of motion should be decreased. If pain persists with motion the therapist must rely on isometrics to maintain strength. If the therapist or client notices any postexercise swelling or pain, the intensity or frequency of the strengthening exercises should be decreased.
3. **Improve general conditioning and endurance.** A client whose arthritis is not in an acute flare or severely involved can participate safely in a nonimpact, low-intensity aerobic conditioning program. Modified aerobic activities can promote a feeling of general well-

being and improve endurance for daily living activities. Cycling on a stationary bicycle and swimming are both excellent forms of exercise for general body conditioning. The Arthritis Foundation also publishes a variety of pamphlets dealing with exercise and videotapes developed specifically for the client with arthritis who wants to participate in a safe and effective fitness program

Fractures

The long-term goal for any client who has sustained a fracture and requires a postfracture exercise program is to return to a prefracture level of activity. Postfracture pain, the time and method of immobilization, the rate of radiologic healing, and the age of the client all affect the the scope and intensity of an exercise program. Clients who are up and about as quickly as possible after sustaining a fracture have the best prognosis and the fewest postfracture complications.[20,21] Some types of fractures, such as a Colle's fracture or a fracture of the tibia, may be managed with external immobilization, generally applied for a minimum of 6 weeks postreduction.

Other types of fractures, such as hip fractures, can be managed by surgical reduction with internal fixation and no external immobilization. The most common type of fracture occurring in elderly people who will require home therapy is hip fracture. It is estimated that one of five women 80 or above has sustained or will sustain a hip fracture.[20] After surgical reduction of a hip fracture, most patients are discharged from the hospital 1 week postoperatively and require extensive home rehabilitation to return to a reasonable level of function. Hip fracture rehabilitation can be a challenge for the home health therapist. A study by Barnes[22] demonstrated that only 40 percent of the clients with fractures of the hip reach prefracture ambulation status at the end of their rehabilitation program.

Common problems during the acute phase of rehabilitation of a postfracture client may include pain at the fracture site or incisional pain after an open reduction, decreased ROM of the involved extremity due to external immobilization or pain, decreased circulation in the involved limb, and possible restricted weight bearing and decreased functional mobility.[17,21,22] If long-term immobilization is required, common problems that can develop and affect later rehabilitation include soft tissue contractures, joint immobility, muscle weakness, atrophy, and cartilage degeneration in immobilized joints.[17,21]

General Goals and Exercise Plan Acute Phase Fracture Rehabilitation (Immediately After Fracture Reduction)[13,17,21]

1. **Maintain normal ROM of all joints of the fractured limb where movement is permissible.** Active or active assisted exercise for all

nonimmobilized joints. Initially the client may experience pain at the fracture site and must be assisted with exercise and assured that some discomfort is normal in the early phase of rehabilitation.

2. **Prevent muscle weakness or atrophy.** If one or more joints are immobilized, isometric exercises of muscles that cross immobilized joints are indicated. If the client experiences pain at the fracture site, start with low-intensity muscle setting. As fracture pain or incisional pain decreases, isometric setting exercises can be performed more vigorously and against resistance. The client may also perform isotonic exercises against light resistance at areas of the involved extremity that are not immobilized. *Precaution*: Until radiologic healing is complete, the therapist must avoid placing any vigorous stress (resistance or stretch forces) distal to the fracture site.
3. **Increase or maintain strength in uninvolved extremities.** This goal is important for the client who has sustained a lower-extremity fracture and must restrict weight bearing on the fractured lower extremity and use an assistive device for ambulation. Various strengthening exercises, described later in this chapter, are appropriate for the upper and lower extremities.
4. **Increase circulatory exchange in the involved extremity.** Active ankle-pumping exercises, performed regularly during the day, minimize the incidence of thrombophlebitis while the client's mobility is restricted. Elevation of the involved extremity also decreases venous stasis and peripheral edema.

General Goals and Exercise Plan[17]

1. **Restore normal ROM of immobilized joints.** Joint mobilization and soft tissue stretching techniques are usually necessary to restore normal ROM when immobilization is removed. When stretching a contracture, if possible, try to place the stretch force proximal to the fracture site so it will be more comfortable for the client. Long-term immobilization weakens muscle, connective tissue, and cartilage, so apply stretching techniques cautiously and gently.
2. **Increase strength and endurance in the involved extremity.** Significant weakness develops in a fractured extremity as the result of immobilization. Progressive resistance exercises are indicated as soon as the immobilization is removed. Strength and endurance are particularly important in the lower extremity for safe and efficient ambulation and in the upper extremity for lifting and carrying objects. Since joint cartilage is fragile after an extended period of joint immobilization, use low loads (light weights) initially to minimize compressive forces at the moving joint.
3. **Improve balance after immobilization of the lower extremity.**

When a joint is immobilized for a long time, proprioception and kinesthetic sense can be impaired. Static and dynamic lower-extremity balance activities under varying sensory conditions (stable and unstable surfaces, with or without visual cues, etc.) are often required to maximize functional mobility.

Cerebral Vascular Accident

Recovery of function after a CVA is often slow. Most clients require an extended period of rehabilitation, much of which will occur in the home. A client who has sustained a stroke encounters extensive problems that affect physical function profoundly. Some common problems directly related to the neurologic deficit include impairment of motor control, balance, and coordination; loss of selective movement coupled with abnormal tone, reflexes, and synergic movements; impairment of proprioception and exteroceptive sensation; cognitive deficits; receptive or expressive language disorders; perceptual dysfunction; and emotional lability.[8,14,22,23] Secondary problems can also develop; these include contractures, muscle weakness, atrophy, and pain. In addition the client may have associated cardiovascular problems such as hypertension, heart disease, chronic pulmonary disorders, or renal disease.

After a comprehensive evaluation by a therapist, a rehabilitation program is carefully designed for the client in the home. The ultimate goal of a rehabilitation program for the post-CVA client is to restore motor control and the highest level of function possible. To function effectively, the client needs an appropriate balance of postural stability and functional mobility.[8,22–24] Although therapists use many techniques and approaches to therapy that incorporate inhibition, facilitation, and practice of motor skills during different stages of recovery,[8,10,14,22,23,25] current research consistently suggests that a motor relearning approach may be the most practical and efficient means of helping a client regain functional mobility for activities of daily living.[22,25,26] An in-depth discussion of the restoration of mobility can be found in Chapter 6 and should be the basis of a rehabilitation program for the post-CVA client.

Isolated exercises as discussed in this chapter are one small aspect of a functional mobility program. Selective active exercises that involve assisted or resisted movements of the head, trunk, or extremities should be used to practice the components of a specific functional activity. Individual exercises or PNF patterns can also maintain length in spastic muscles that are likely to develop contractures or to increase strength in weak muscles. Inhibition techniques are preferable to passive stretching in maintaining normal length of spastic muscles. Isolated exercises alone will not help the client relearn functional tasks. Isometric exercises should be emphasized to promote stability and may be particularly important at proximal joints. Dynamic exercise with or without resistance can be used to promote controlled mobility and to practice components of functional, coordinated motor skills. Several exercises described in the last section of this chapter are appropriate as part of a total rehabilitation program designed to help the client regain functional mobility.

EQUIPMENT FOR HOME EXERCISE

Equipment is necessary in most home exercise programs. Unlike choosing from the great variety of equipment types available for patients in rehabilitation centers or therapy departments, the home health therapist uses equipment that is compact and portable and can fit into the back seat or trunk of a car. Before having a client purchase commercial exercise equipment, it is helpful to bring some sample equipment to the home to try it out. Because many clients cannot afford to purchase exercise equipment or because equipment will only be needed for a short period of time, the therapist must also be able to design exercise equipment from items commonly found around the home.

Commercially Available Equipment

- TheraBand[R] or elastic tubing
- Velcro cuff weights
- Vinyl-covered hand weights
- Overhead pulley system for a door frame
- Elastic bandages

Improvised Equipment

TREATMENT SURFACES—STABLE AND COMFORTABLE

- Small pad or foam rubber for the floor or stable table
- Firm couch or bed
- Firm chair with or without arms
- Padded stool or footstool

SUPPORTS FOR STANDING ACTIVITIES AND EXERCISE

- Kitchen counter, bathroom sink or vanity edge
- Back of a couch or heavy upholstered chair
- Wall or door frame
- Bottom of stair railing or newel post

WEIGHTS

- Cans of soup, packages of dried beans or peas placed in nylons or socks, and so forth. The following weights can be placed over or tied around a limb, or held.
- Woman's handbag or plastic shopping bag, filled with weight and hand held or placed on client's foot
- Fishing tackle box or small tool box with weights inside

WANDS—30-IN LENGTH

- Cane
- Broomstick handle
- 1-in plastic pipe
- Towel or curtain rod
- Umbrella

HAND EXERCISERS

- Rubber bands
- Spring loaded clothespins
- Small plastic bottle

MISCELLANEOUS EXERCISE EQUIPMENT

- Rolled bath or face towel secured with adhesive tape (diameter will vary with use). Useful for thigh support during knee strengthening exercises or under buttocks for bridging.
- Two- or three-liter soda bottle wrapped with a bath towel and secured with tape or a rubber band for short-arc quadriceps exercises
- Thick hardbound books for practicing push-ups while seated
- Pulley glove made from cotton work glove pinned at wrist. Fingers can then be curled around a handle and pinned down to the palm.
- Belts, useful in several ways for isometric exercise for upper or lower extremities or for assisted sit-ups
- Elastic car tie-downs

HEAT OR COLD APPLICATION

- Hot water bottle
- Heating pad placed over a towel
- Immersion of painful area in warm water
- Warm bath or shower
- Ice cubes or crushed ice in plastic bag, covered with dish towel
- Contrast baths for hand or foot. Two buckets, one containing warm water, the other ice water

SELECTED EXERCISES

The exercises in this section generally allow the client to perform independently or with minimal assistance from a caregiver.[3,13,15,17,27–29] Every effort has been made to incorporate appropriate stabilization to maximize safety and minimize substitute motions. Exercises have also been adapted so that the elderly client can perform them safely.[27,29]

All exercises should be carried out on a firm, comfortable surface. If exercises are performed on soft surfaces or in the sling seat of a wheelchair, the client is less stable and exercise will be more difficult. Examples of exercises include isometric and isotonic (concentric and eccentric) strengthening exercises and self-stretching and self-mobilization techniques.

Strengthening exercises are performed in both open- and closed-chain positions, using body weight, free weights, or elastic materials[30] for resistance. Initially during isotonic exercise, movements are done slowly with emphasis on controlling the motion. Although speed may be increased somewhat as the client learns the exercise, movements with free weights can never be performed safely at very fast speeds, as is possible with isokinetic equipment. Since the variety of weights and elastic resistance material is much more limited at home than in the clinical setting, the same weight can provide greater resistance during exercise if it is moved from a proximal area of the limb to a more distal position.

Isometric resistance exercises are easily carried out in the home by pushing against an immovable object such as a wall or doorframe. During isometric exercises, the client is taught to contract the muscle for 6 to 10 seconds for each repetition.[13,15,29] Whenever possible, isometrics are performed at multiple angles to increase strength throughout the ROM. However, isometric exercises may not be advisable for elderly clients with high blood pressure or cardiac disease.

Isotonic exercises use light weights to minimize compressive forces on joints. Since most activities of daily living require endurance rather than a great amount of strength, emphasis is placed on increasing repetitions, rather than significantly increasing resistance, during home exercises.

Exercises to increase functional ROM are a frequent part of the therapeutic intervention and home program. The safest form of stretching is a static, low-intensity, long-duration stretch. Low-intensity, long-duration stretch (as long as 20 to 30 minutes) also appears to be the most comfortable and may be the most effective method for treating chronic contractures.[27,31] However, long-duration stretching may not be practical. Clients often do not tolerate a stretching position for the necessary length of time and an appropriate place or desired positioning may not be possible. Active stretching is therefore a more frequently used alternative for increasing ROM. Self-stretching can be effective if the client learns proper techniques. Clients must be taught to avoid bouncing during a stretch maneuver. Soft-tissue trauma is more likely to occur with high-intensity ballistic stretch. Sometimes it is possible to incorporate muscle inhibition (contract-relax) into the stretching procedure. Most stretching techniques described in this section are self-stretching procedures using body weight as the stretch force. Simple weights can also be constructed and used to apply a sustained mechanical stretch force to tight structures. Loads should be kept very light (2 to 3 lb) so that the client will remain relaxed and tolerate the stretch for an extended period. Finally, as was mentioned earlier, prior heat (warm-up) or cold may make stretching exercises more comfortable. Heat also makes soft tissue more extensible; cold decreases muscle guarding. Cold after stretching lessens delayed muscle soreness.

The exercises presented in this chapter do not represent even a small portion of the many options available to the therapist. Numerous publica-

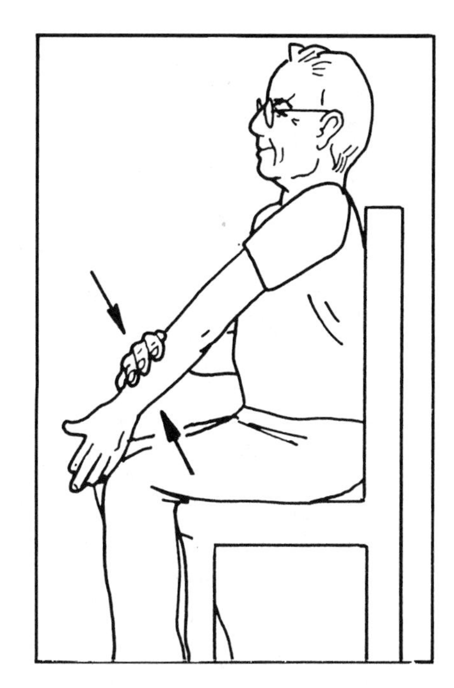

Figure 5–1. Self-resistance for shoulder flexion.

tions depict a wide array of exercises, programs, and adaptions many of which are listed in the references. The exercises and illustrations represent some suggestions for exercising in the home. The emphasis is on using available materials. Well-known exercise programs and exercises performed in a hospital bed are not included because they are described well in other publications.

Techniques illustrated for one part of an extremity can often be used for other parts. For example, Figure 5–1 shows a man applying self-resistance to strengthen the shoulder flexors. The same kind of self-resistance can be used for other shoulder, elbow, hand, or wrist movements. Exercises depicting equipment such as elastic resistance bands can be used for other movements as well. Various weights can be used for more than the joints presented. Variability is limited only by the client's condition and therapeutic needs and the imagination of the therapist.

Trunk and Upper Extremity

Active Movements

To increase shoulder and upper chest flexibility:

1. Stand in a corner with arms in a V or reverse T position; place hands on each wall and lean into corner (Fig. 5–2). This can be done unilaterally by holding onto a door frame and leaning into the open doorway.
2. While sitting erect on a stool, clasp hands behind back. Slide clasped hands up the back as far as possible (Fig. 5–3).

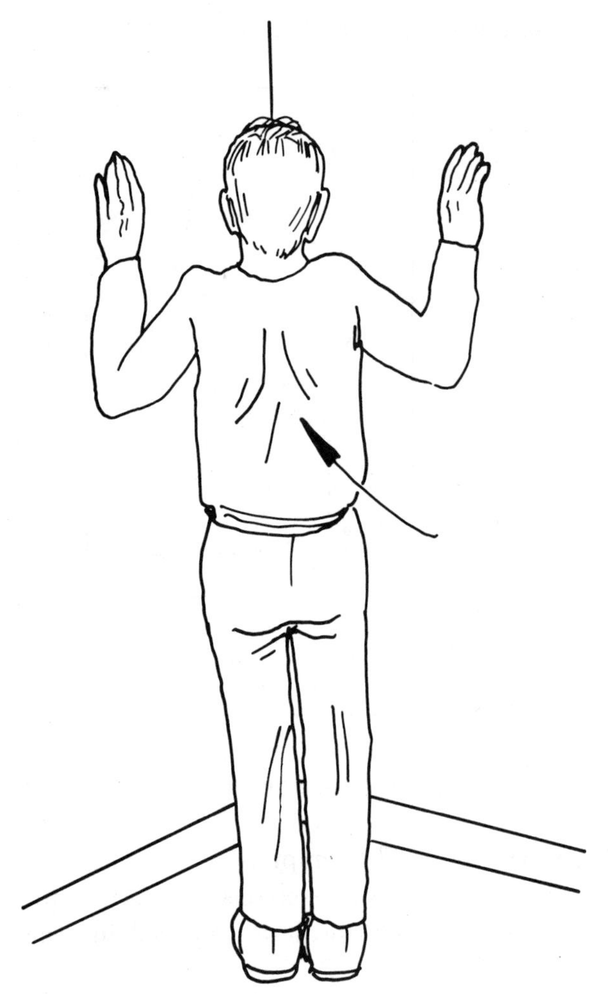

Figure 5–2. Standing bilateral shoulder stretch.

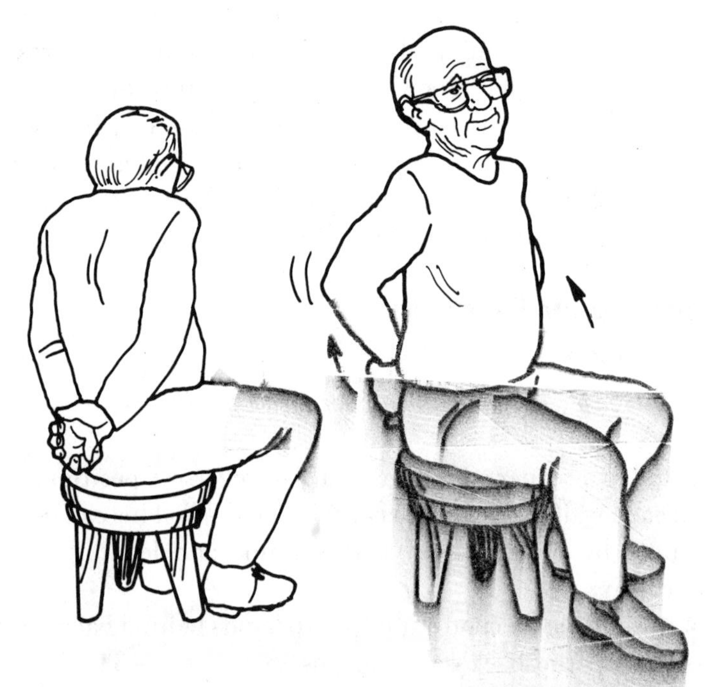

Figure 5–3. Sitting bilateral shoulder and upper trunk stretch.

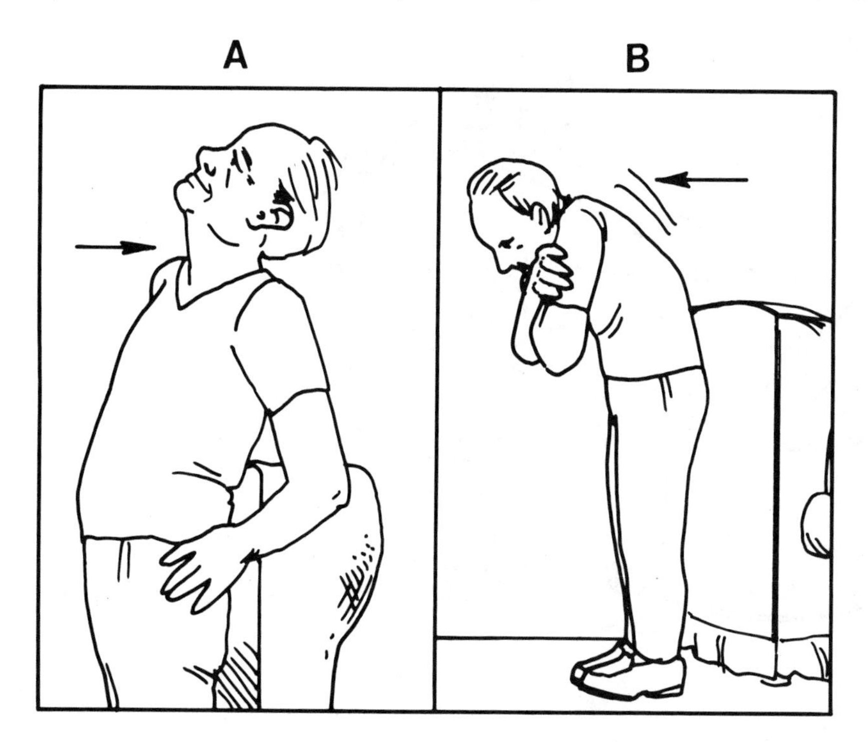

Figure 5–4. Increasing trunk flexibility in flexion and extension.

To increase trunk flexibility:

1. With hands on hips, bring head and upper trunk backward within a comfortable range (Fig. 5–4A). Take care to maintain proper balance.
2. Cross arms in front of chest and curl forward (Fig. 5–4B). This exercise can also be done in a sitting position for upper back flexibility.

To increase low back or hamstring flexibility:

1. Sit in a straight chair, one foot flat on the floor and the other leg on a stool either lower than or even with the seat of the chair. Reach forward toward the toe, keeping the knee as straight as possible (Fig. 5–5). If hamstring stretch is desired, the back should be straight and the head up looking straight ahead. Another method, which may not maintain pelvic stabilization, is long sitting, preferably on the floor with feet against a wall. Reach forward slowly toward the feet, keeping the back straight and the head up.

To strengthen the upper extremities and upper trunk:

1. While sitting in a wheelchair, feet flat on the floor, grasp the armrests and lift the buttocks (Fig. 5–6). To make the exercise more difficult, extend the knees.

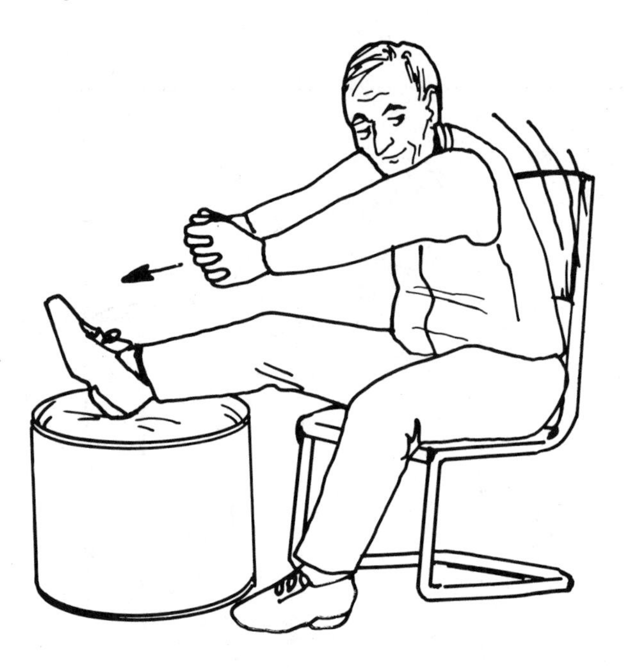

Figure 5–5. Increasing hamstring flexibility.

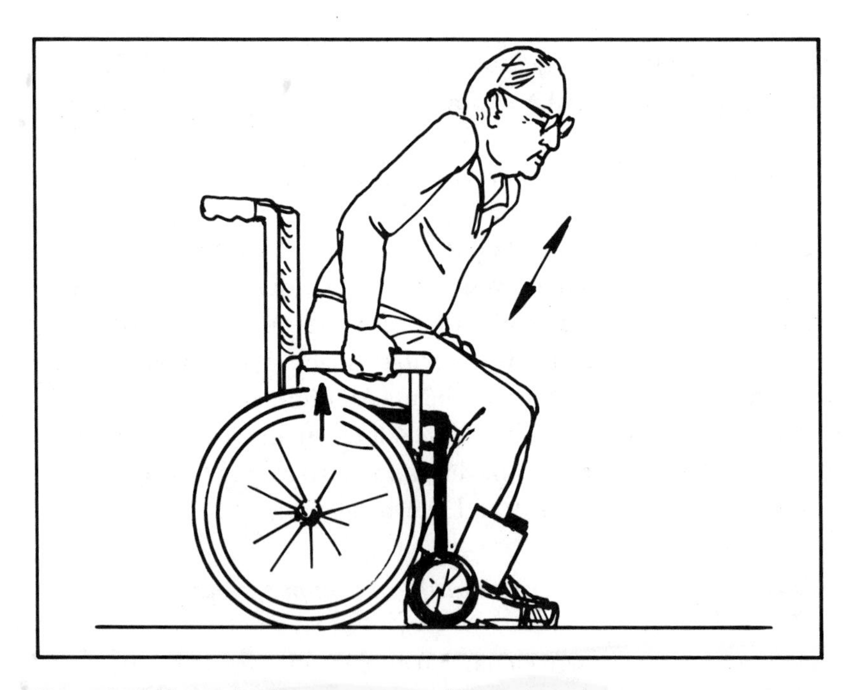

Figure 5–6. Strengthening upper extremities and trunk.

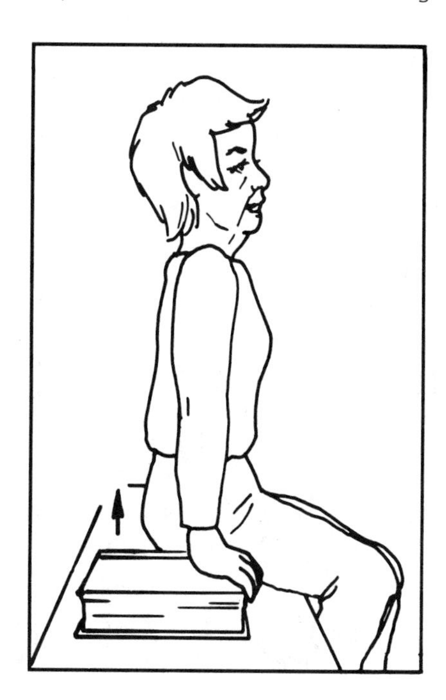

Figure 5–7. Strengthening upper extremities and trunk.

2. While sitting on a low bench, place thick books on either side of the hips. Push on the books and lift the buttocks making sure to fully depress the shoulders (Fig. 5–7).

To increase shoulder or elbow strength:

1. Sit, using the opposite hand for resistance. Apply resistance to distal humerus, proximal or distal forearm (see Fig. 5–1).

Pulleys

Pulleys can be used to strengthen or increase shoulder ROM.

1. A single pulley can be purchased commercially or can be made using an eye hook, clothesline, and wooden dowel and a plastic bag as a weight (Fig. 5–8). The specific motion is determined by the client's position under the pulley and the direction of the shoulder movement.
2. Using a double pulley, either perform self-stretching for a shoulder or use a strong upper extremity to provide resistance to a weaker extremity (Fig. 5–9).

Cane, Wand, or Broomstick

Canes or other straight sticks can be used for assistive, resistive, and ROM exercises.

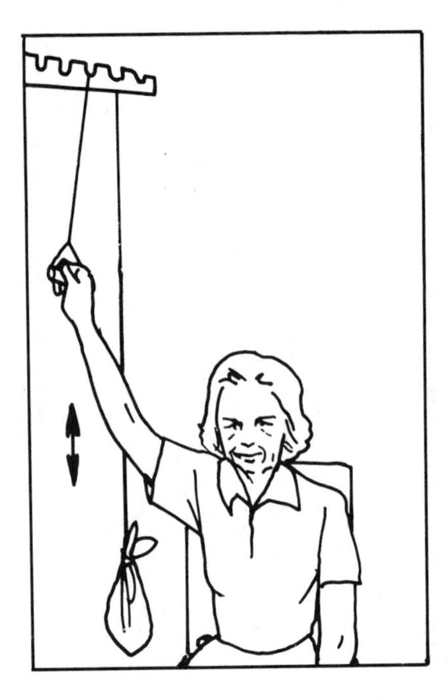

Figure 5–8. Single pulleys to increase shoulder strength or mobility.

1. Sit on a stool and grasp a cane with both hands behind the back. Raise extended arms behind the back (Fig. 5–10). A small weight around the cane can be used for added resistance.
2. While sitting in a chair, grasp a cane with both hands. Keeping

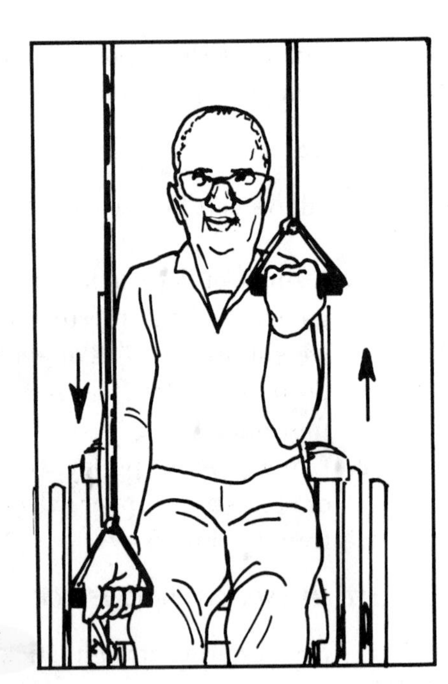

Figure 5–9. Double pulley for shoulder strenthening or mobility.

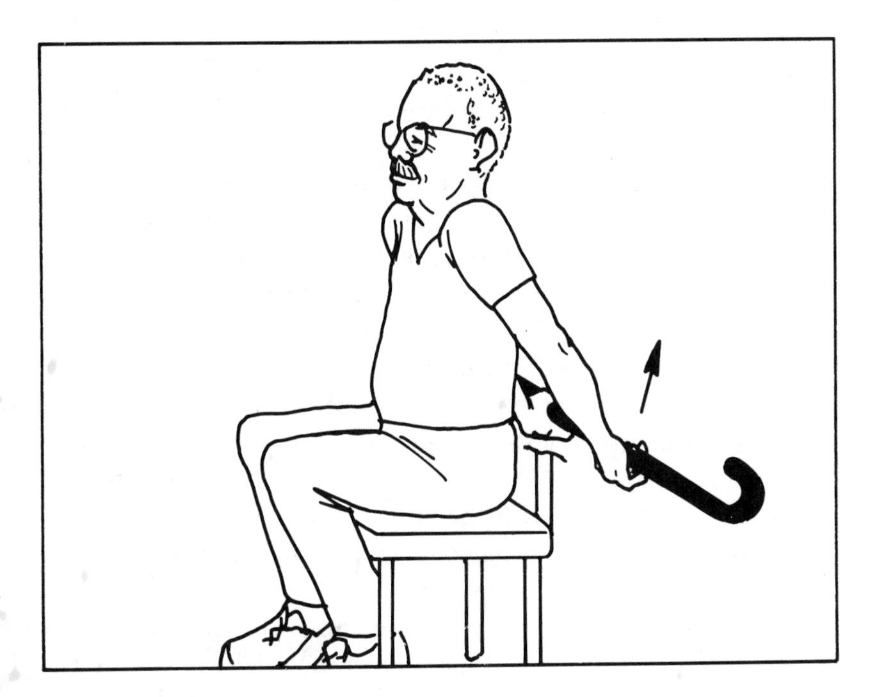

Figure 5–10. Using a cane for shoulder exercises.

elbows in contact with the body, lift and lower the cane over the head or bend and straighten the elbows depending on the desired exercises. This exercise may be done with or without a weight for resistance. It can also be used to increase shoulder ROM (Fig. 5–11).

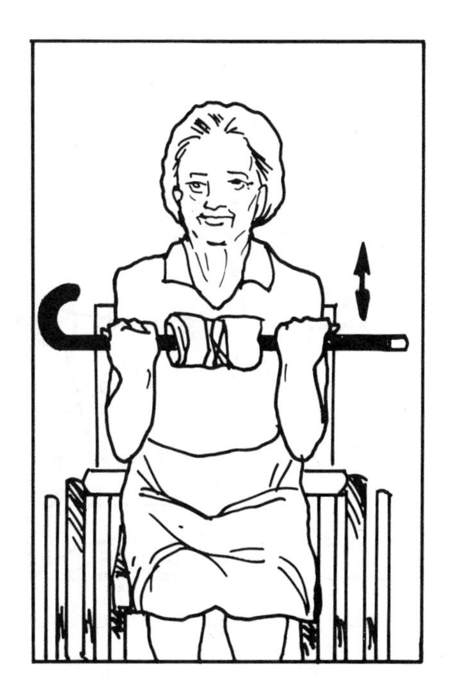

Figure 5–11. Using a weighted cane for elbow strengthening.

Bags, Cans, and Other Weights

Many household items can provide resistance for exercises.

1. To strengthen various upper extremity muscles, hold a soda bottle filled with water, a can, or a grocery bag containing such weights while performing the desired motion. Care must be taken that the client has the ability to hold the weight securely and that progression in weight can be documented (Fig. 5–12).
2. To resist or increase flexibility in supination and pronation, place the affected elbow at 90° and in contact with the body; hold a screwdriver or hammer with the heavy end out, then pronate and supinate slowly (Fig. 5–13). The same implements can be used for resistive wrist motions with the arm resting and stabilized on a table.
3. To resist wrist flexion and extension, wring out a washcloth until it is taut (Fig. 5–14) while flexing one wrist and extending the other.
4. To resist finger flexion or extension, place the hand in a container of warm water; squeeze and spread a washcloth by flexing and extending the fingers (Fig. 5–15). Resist flexion only by squeezing a sponge.
5. Strengthen finger flexion by pinching a spring-loaded clothespin together with the thumb and index finger (Fig. 5–16). Place

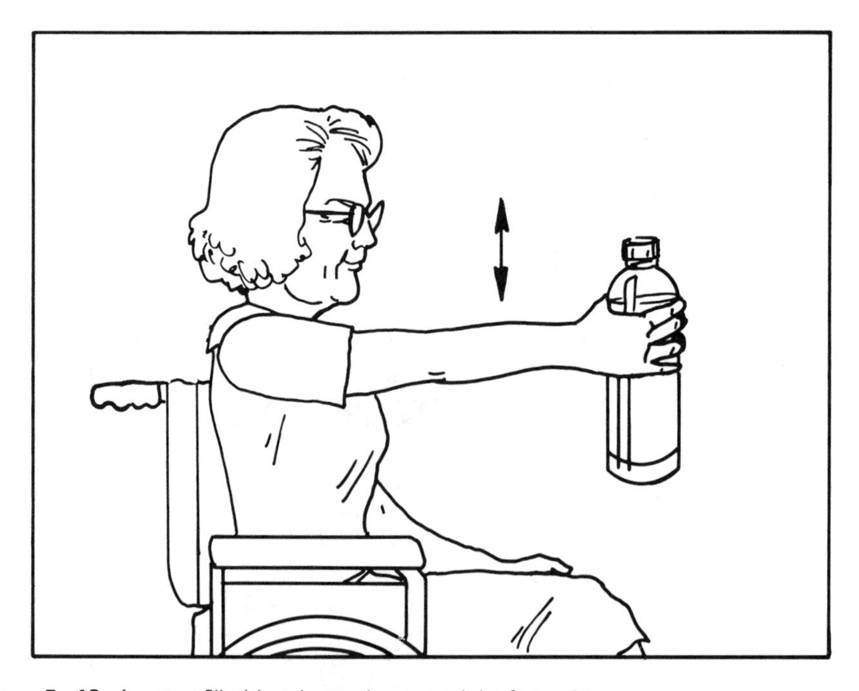

Figure 5–12. A water-filled bottle used as a weight for resistance.

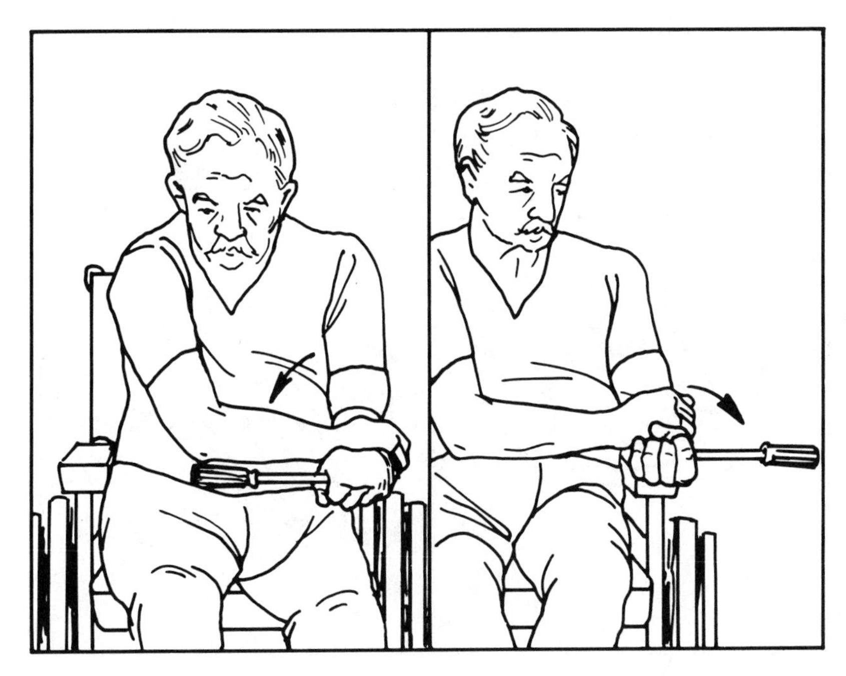

Figure 5–13. A screwdriver provides resistance to supination and pronation.

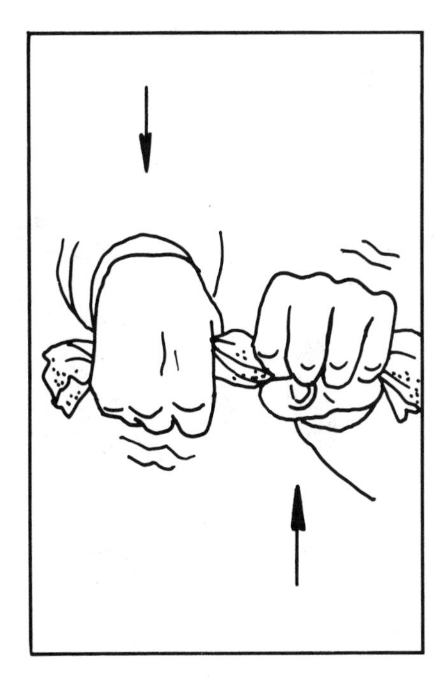

Figure 5–14. Wringing a washcloth for wrist strengthening.

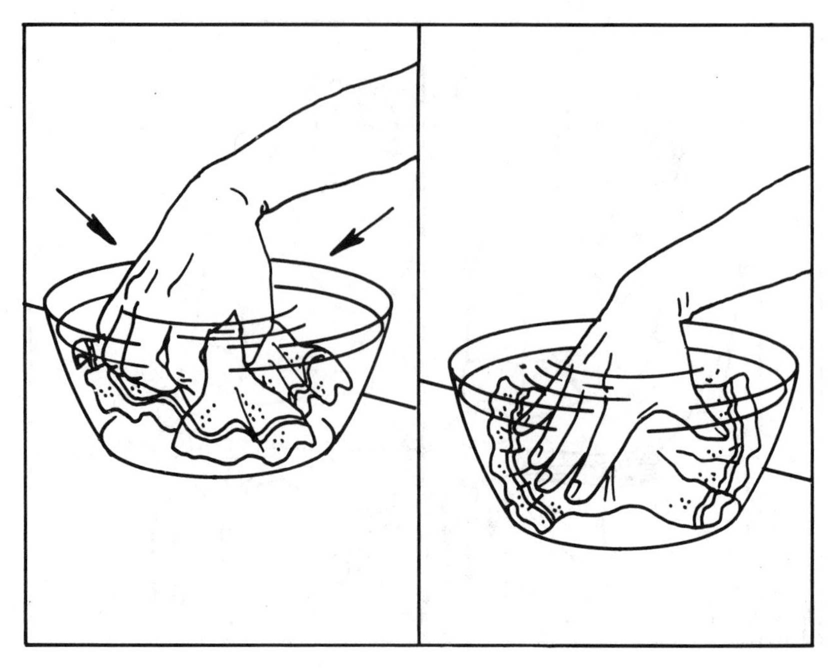

Figure 5–15. Squeezing and spreading a washcloth for finger exercises.

clothespins horizontally on a rope or ruler and vertically on a yardstick as high as possible for combination movements.

Elastic Bands

Elastic resistance bands can be commercially purchased in different resistance levels or made from plastic tubing or the inner tubes from bicycle tires. Many exercises can be developed using elastic bands, which are usually formed into a loop by tying in a knot. Loops of different resistances are commercially available.

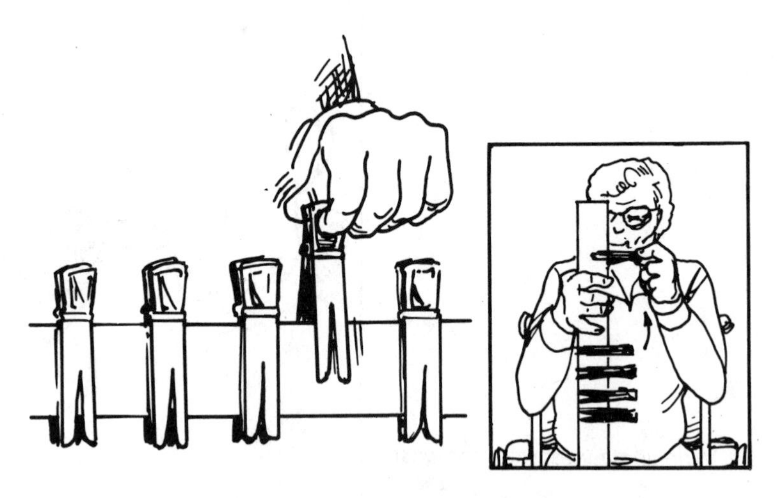

Figure 5–16. Resisted pinch using spring-loaded clothespins.

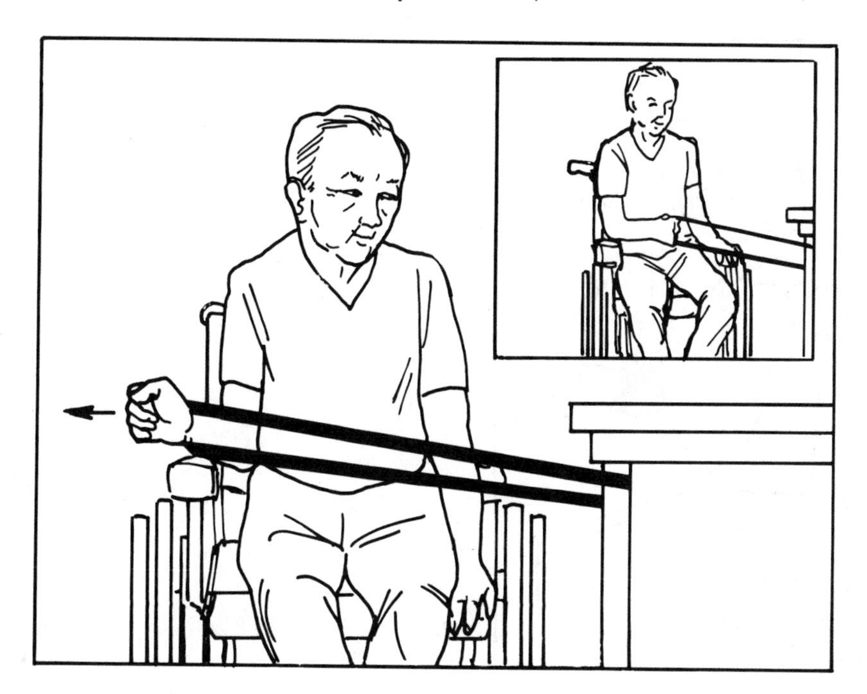

Figure 5–17. Using an elastic band for shoulder resistance.

1. To resist shoulder, elbow, wrist, and finger motions, either use both arms against each other or have one end of the loop tied to a stable object (Figs. 5–17 to 5–19).
2. Combination upper-extremity and lower-extremity exercise can be achieved by holding the elastic band with the foot for upper extremities and with the hand for lower extremities. Figure 5–20 depicts

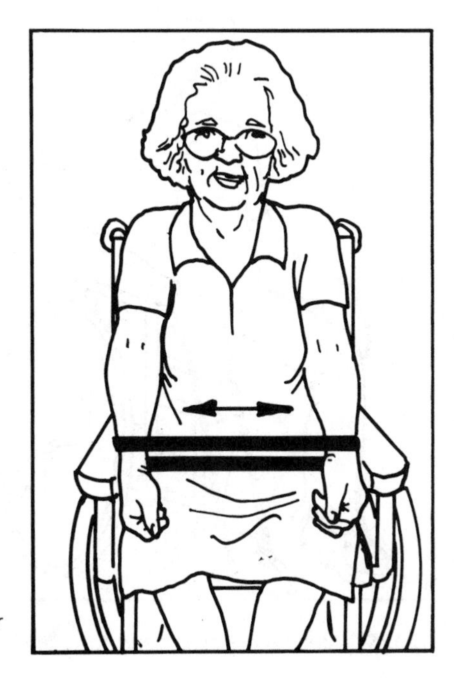

Figure 5–18. Using an elastic band for shoulder exercises.

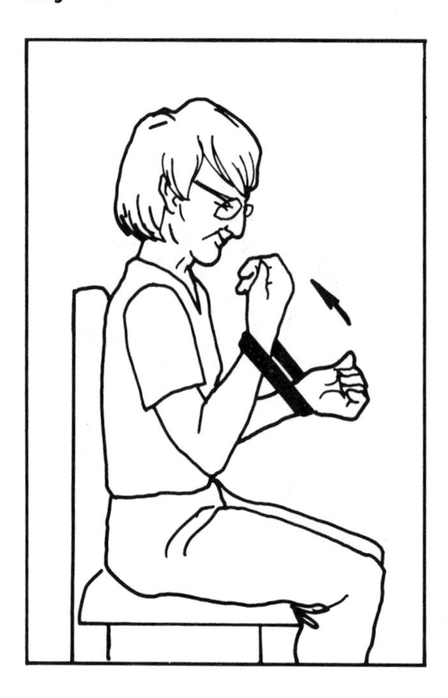

Figure 5–19. Bilateral arm exercises with elastic band.

the client holding the band with his foot while performing wrist extension. The action could be reversed using a heavier band if he held the loop with the hand on the armrest of the chair and performed hip and knee flexion and extension with the foot.

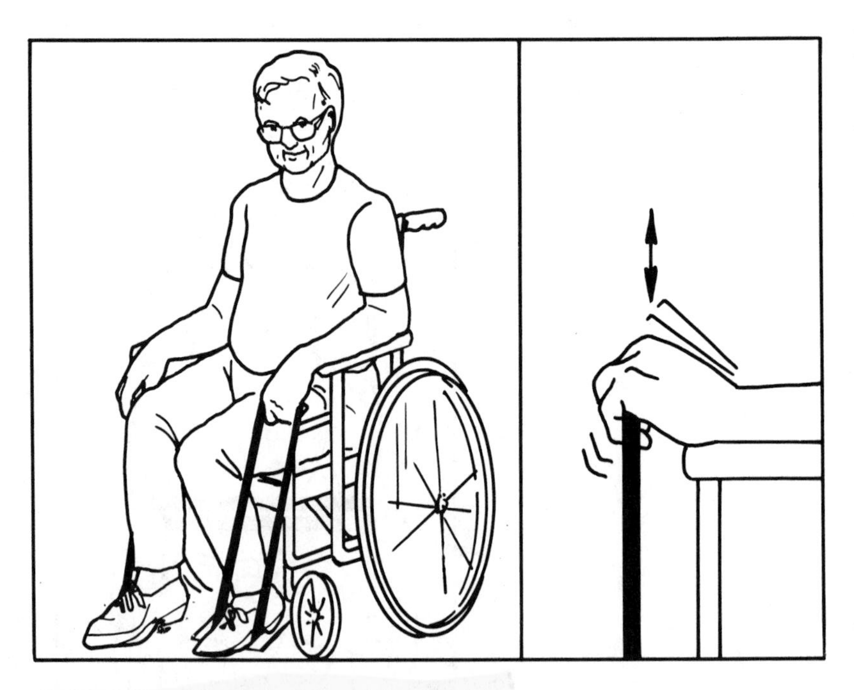

Figure 5–20. Self-stabilized elastic band for exercising.

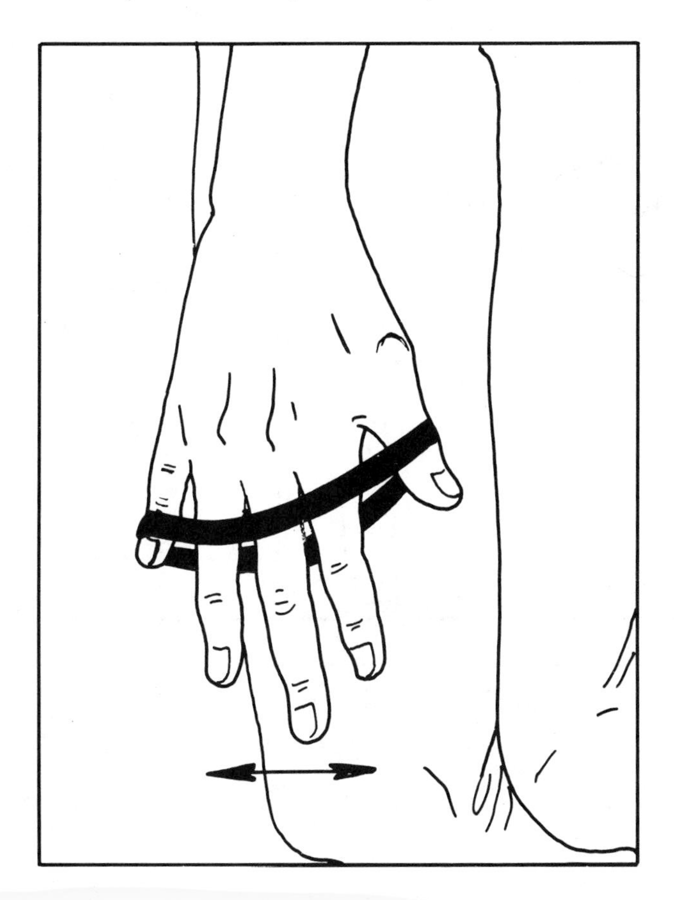

Figure 5–21. Using a rubber band for finger exercises.

3. Regular heavy rubber bands can provide resistance for finger motions (Fig. 5–21).

Lower Extremity

Many well-known lower-extremity exercises, such as quadriceps setting or bilateral buttock raises (sometimes called "bridging"), will not be illustrated or discussed here. Their exclusion reflects their familiarity rather than their value. As with upper-extremity and trunk exercises, highlighted exercises have been specifically adapted for the client in the home setting.

Active Movements

To strengthen hip extension:

1. Bend forward and lean the chest on a console television or countertop with a pillow for comfort. Raise the affected leg toward the ceiling (Fig. 5–22). To progress this exercise, place a weight around the ankle.

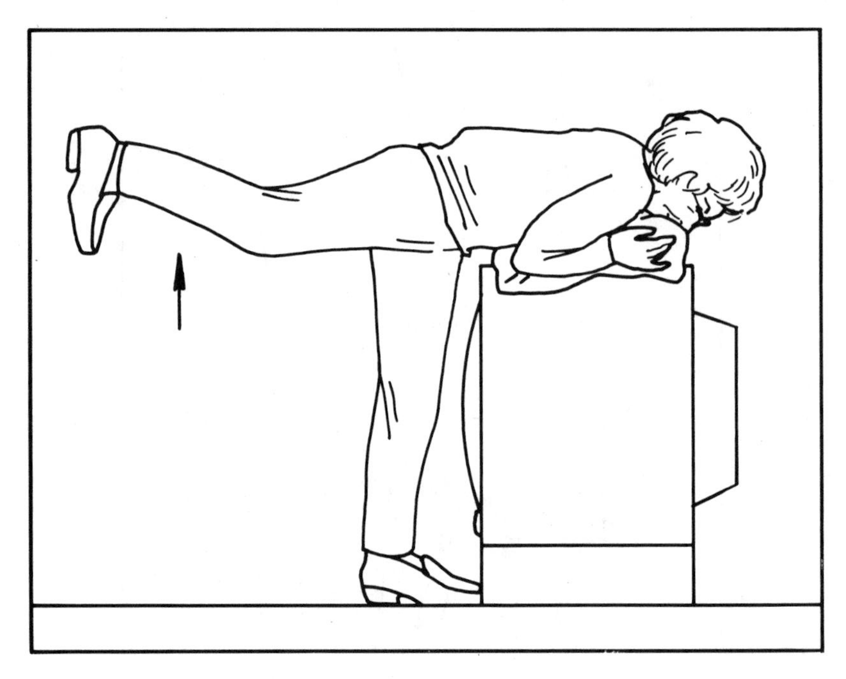

Figure 5–22. Gravity resisted hip extension.

To strengthen or increase the flexibility of hip, knee, and ankle musculature:

1. Stand next to a counter and hold on for support. Slowly squat down and then return to a standing position. Make sure to stay in an upright position and do not flex the knees more than about 30 to 35 degrees. This exercise is not recommended for anyone with arthritis or limited weight bearing (Fig. 5–23).
2. Place a footstool or large book on the floor next to a counter. Step up onto the stool with the affected leg and step back down. The counter is used for balance only (Fig. 5–24). This exercise can also be done on a stair step if there is a rail for balance.
3. Lie prone on a couch or bed (Fig. 5–25). Place a folded towel under the distal thigh to avoid compression of the patella during knee motion. Flex and extend the knee actively against gravity and with or without a weight around the ankle. To increase the range of knee flexion, a long belt or sheet can be tied around the ankle. Hold the end of the belt or sheet and provide a gentle continuous stretch at the end of the range of flexion. Take care to be properly aligned.
4. Lie supine with the affected leg off the bed on a stool. Press down on the stool with the whole foot and tighten the buttocks muscle (Fig. 5–26). Slight elevation of the buttocks is acceptable, but care must be taken not to put undue strain on the low back.

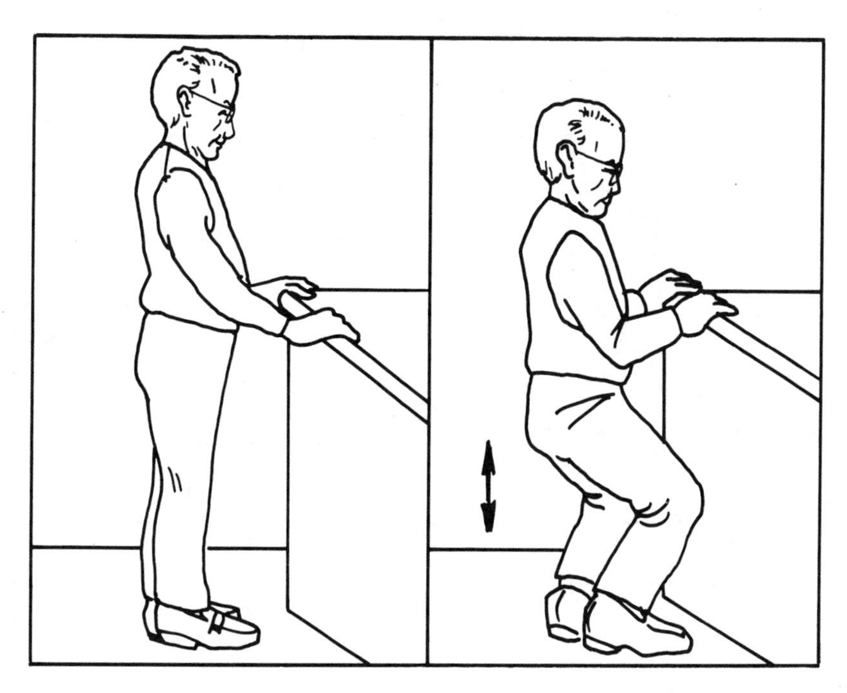

Figure 5–23. Squats for strengthening using a counter for balance.

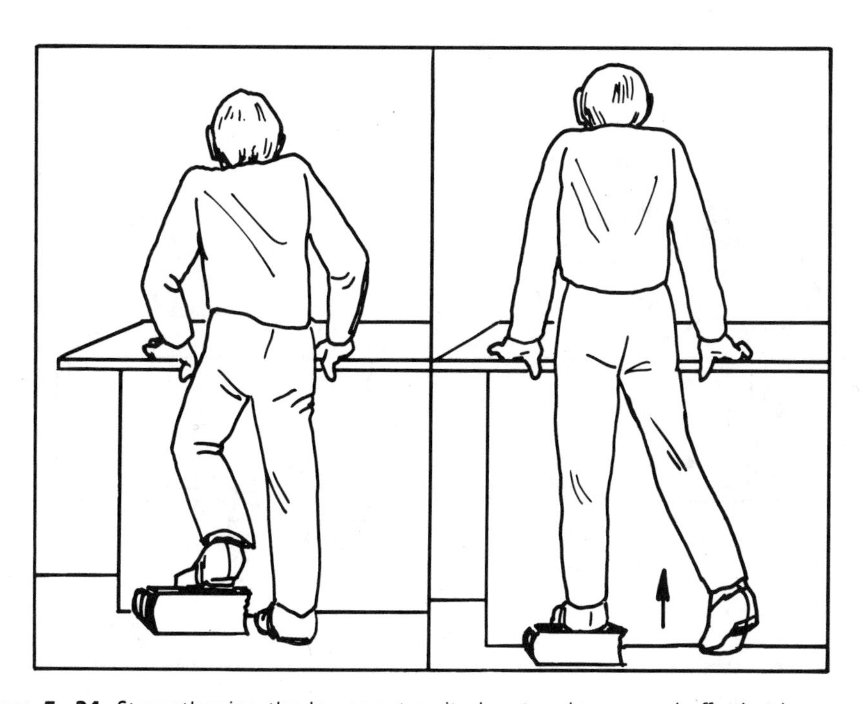

Figure 5–24. Strengthening the lower extremity by stepping on and off a book.

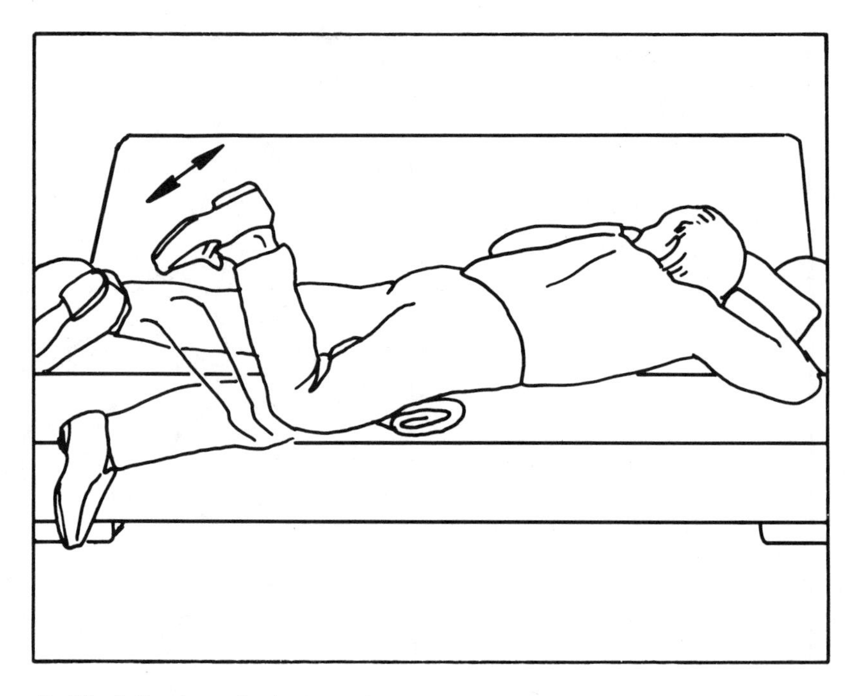

Figure 5–25. Active knee flexion exercises.

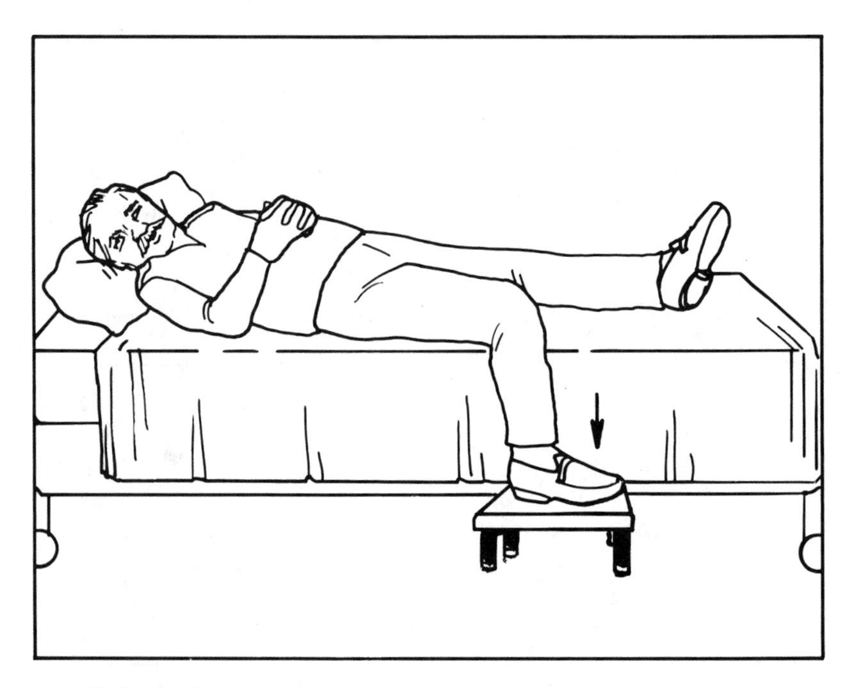

Figure 5–26. Resisted hip extension.

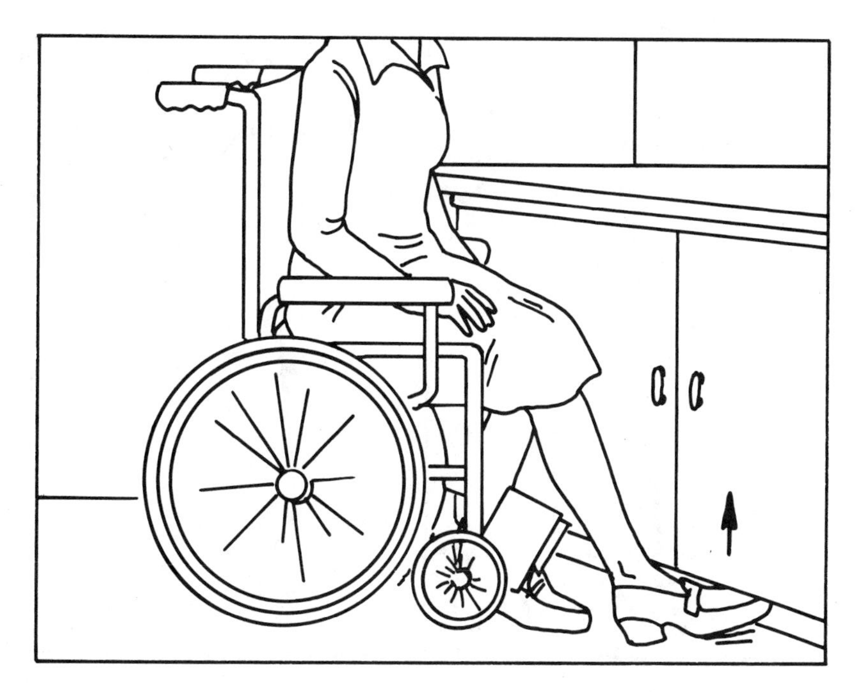

Figure 5–27. Using a counter for resisted knee extension and dorsiflexion.

To resist knee extension or ankle dorsiflexion (Fig. 5–27):

1. Sit in a chair and position the affected foot under the lip of a cabinet, then attempt to straighten the knee. Alter the angle of knee flexion. A cabinet lip can also be used to resist ankle dorsiflexion.

To increase knee flexibility in flexion:

1. Sit in a straight chair and actively flex the knee to the end of the available range. Place the unaffected foot on top of the affected foot and exert a gentle continuous stretch (Fig. 5–28).

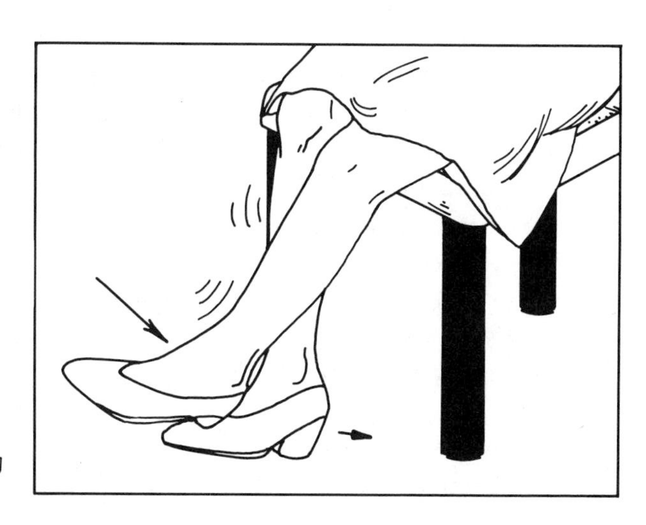

Figure 5–28. Self-stretching of knee in flexion.

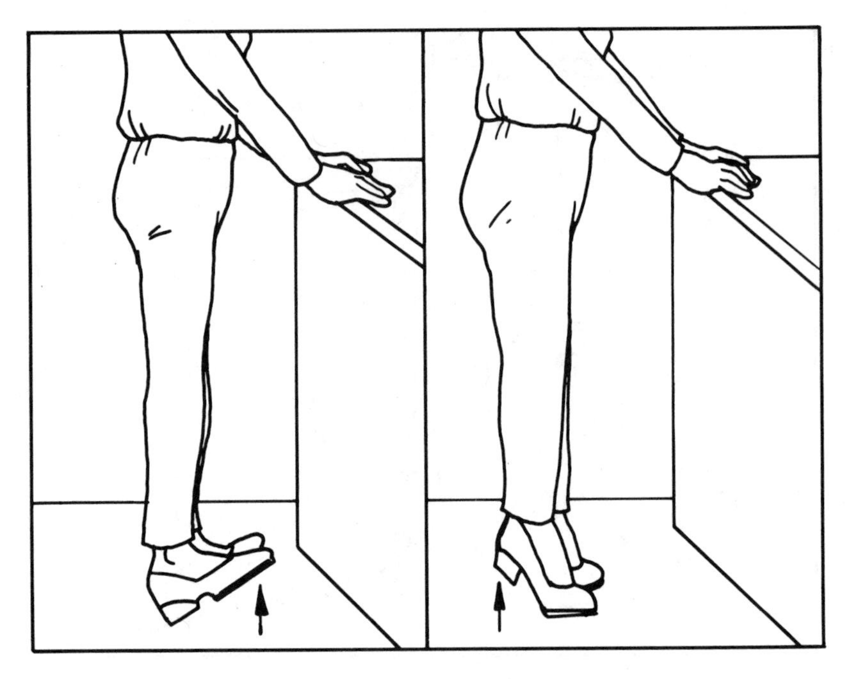

Figure 5–29. Active ankle exercises using a counter for balance.

To strengthen ankle muscles and increase flexibility:

1. Stand and hold onto a counter. Raise toes off the floor; raise heels off the floor; stand on the outside of the feet. Body weight provides resistance (Fig. 5–29).

Bags, Blocks, and Elastic Bands

To resist knee flexion:

1. Position a heavy object in front of a chair leg. While sitting, press the back of the heel against the object and attempt to bend the knee (Fig. 5–30).
2. Stand at a counter and place a weighted plastic bag around the affected ankle. Bend the knee; lift the weight and then lower it back down to the floor (Fig. 5–31). Care must be taken to keep the weighted part of the bag close enough to the ankle to actually lift off the ground through most of the range of knee flexion. This exercise is particularly useful for individuals who cannot lie prone but who are able to stand with minimal support for balance.

To resist knee extension:

1. There are numerous ways to provide resistance for knee extension. The client can lie on a bed or couch with a roll under the knee and

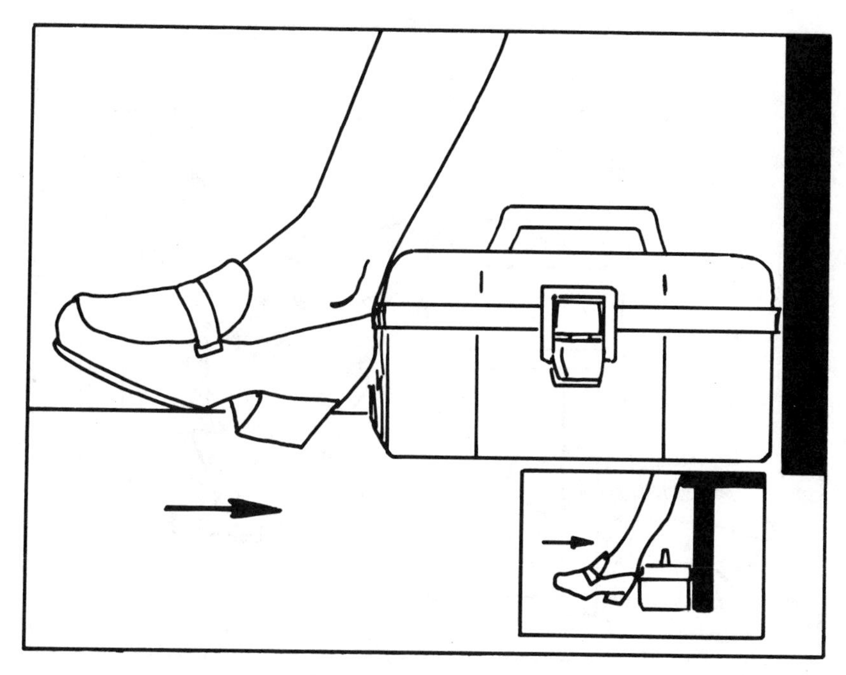

Figure 5–30. Resisted hamstring strengthening using a box.

the affected leg off the bed. Extension can be done actively through the range or a weight can be added to the ankle. An elastic band secured around a stable object can also provide resistance. Knee extension can also be done sitting with a weight or elastic band for resistance (Fig. 5–32).

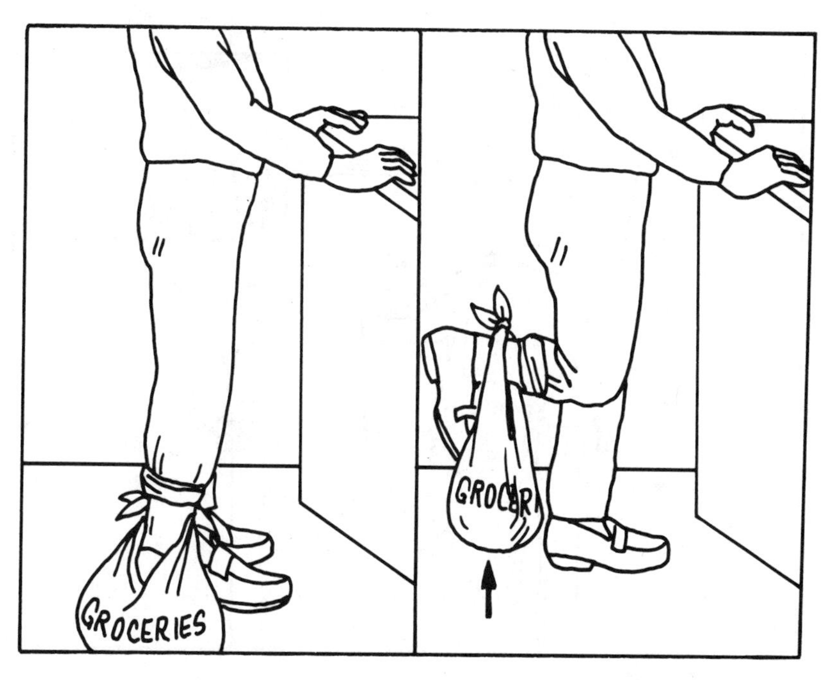

Figure 5–31. Resisted hamstring strengthening using a bag of groceries.

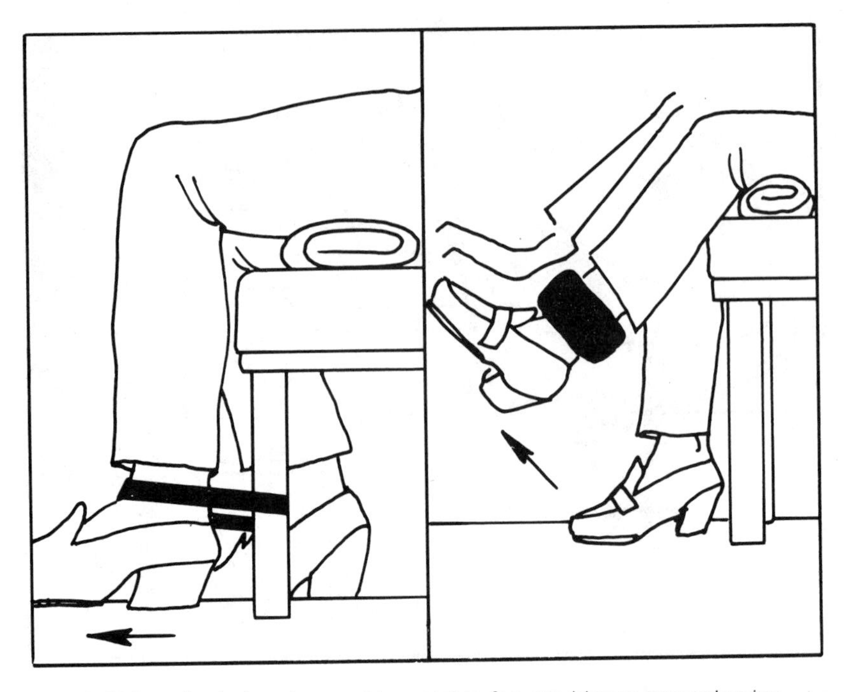

Figure 5–32. Using elastic bands or ankle weights for quadriceps strengthening.

To resist hip adduction:

1. Sit and squeeze a rolled towel or newspaper between both thighs (Fig. 5–33).

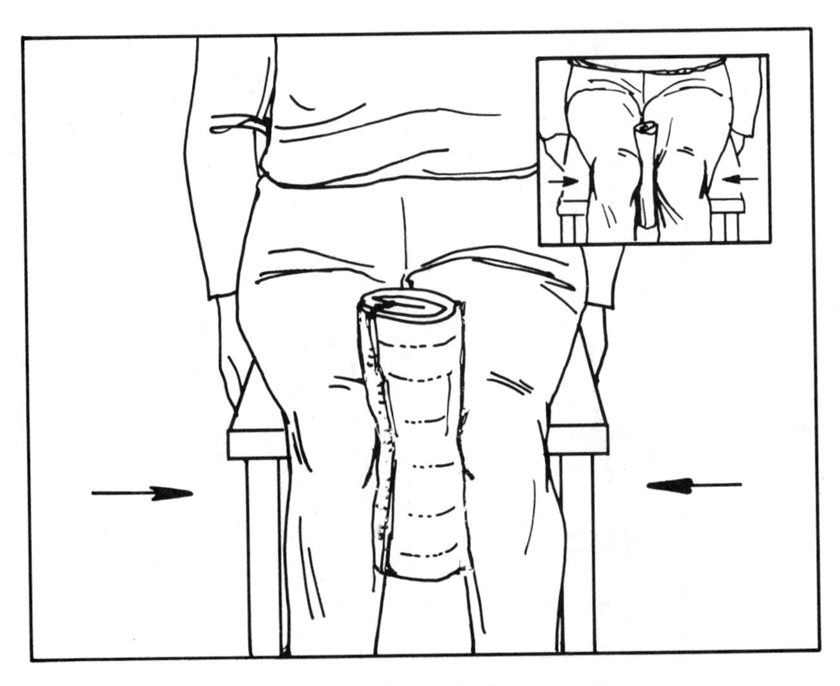

Figure 5–33. A towel or newspaper used to resist hip adduction.

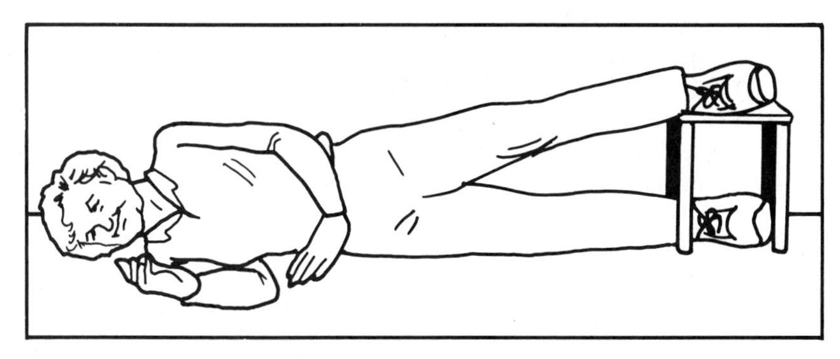

Figure 5–34. Using a stool for resisted hip adduction.

2. Lie on the affected side and place the unaffected leg on a footstool. Raise the affected leg off the floor and push it against the bottom of the footstool or, if resistance is desired, push down with the top leg (Fig. 5–34). Resisted hip abduction can be performed in the same position by placing a rolled pillow or pillow-covered book under the distal thigh of the underneath leg and raising the hip off the bed.

SUMMARY

Therapeutic exercise is one of the building blocks of an effective rehabilitation program for many clients who are assisted by therapists in the home setting. A home rehabilitation program with appropriate instruction and follow-up by a therapist may mean the difference between a client's being able to live independently at home or going to an extended-care facility. To apply a high level of professional care for the client at home, the therapist must be able to recognize and prioritize the functional needs of the client and family and structure an exercise plan that will meet those needs as efficiently as possible.

This chapter has reviewed the basic principles of developing, adapting, and implementing exercises for clients in the home, and has focused on how exercises must be modified to work for such clients. The problems discussed represent common orthopedic and neurologic conditions of clients who often require home therapy. The goals of exercise and the specific priorities of an exercise plan have been summarized for each clinical condition. Several creative ideas for designing and using equipment in home exercises have also been discussed. Finally, a variety of exercises appropriate in a home exercise program have been described and illustrated.

REFERENCES

1. Harrington, J: The case for home health specialization. Clinical Management in Physical Therapy 3:17, 1983.
2. Jackson, BN: Home health care and the elderly in the 1980's. Am J Occup Ther 38:717, 1984.

3. Jackson, DE and Wilhoire, MJ: Home health physical therapy: Considerations for the provision of care. Clinical Management in Physical Therapy 5:10, 1985.
4. Schaefer, K and Lewis, CB: Marketing geriatric programs — A home care example. Clinical Management in Physical Therapy 6:14–17, 1986.
5. Friedman, LW: The Psychological Rehabilitation of the Amputee. Charles C Thomas, Springfield, IL, 1978.
6. Cirullo, JA: Prosthetic training for the elderly amputee in the home: Two case studies. Clinical Management in Physical Therapy 5:30, 1985.
7. Keagy, RD: Amputations of the upper extremities. In Nickel, VL (ed): Orthopedic Rehabilitation. Churchill Livingstone, New York, 1982.
8. Davies, PM: Right in the Middle: Selective Trunk Activity in the Treatment of Adult Hemiplegia. Springer-Verlag, New York, 1990.
9. May, BJ: Preprosthetic management for lower extremity amputation. In O'Sullivan, SB and Schmidtz, TJ (eds): Physical Rehabilitation, ed 2, FA Davis, Philadelphia, 1988.
10. Voss, D, Ionta, MJ and Meyers, B: Proprioceptive Neuromuscular Facilitation, ed 3, Harper & Row, Philadelphia, 1985.
11. Mensch, G: Exercise for amputees. In Basmajian, VJ and Wolf, SL (eds): Therapeutic Exercise, ed 5, Williams & Wilkins, Baltimore, 1990.
12. Sanders, GT: Lower Limb Amputation: A Guide to Rehabilitation. FA Davis, Philadelphia, 1986.
13. Schneider, L and Cecil, J: Progressive Individualized Exercises. Therapy Skill Builders, Tucson, 1989.
14. Steinberg, FU, Sunsoo, I and Roettger, RF: Prosthetic rehabilitation of geriatric amputee patients. A follow-up study. Arch Phys Med Rehabil 66:742, 1985.
15. Mills, D and Fraser, C: Therapeutic Activities for the Upper Limb. Therapy Skill Builders, Tucson, 1988.
16. Guccione, AA: Rheumatoid Arthritis. In O'Sullivan, SB and Schmitz, TJ (eds): Physical Rehabilitation, FA Davis, Philadelphia, 1988.
17. Kisner, C and Colby, LA: Therapeutic Exercise: Foundations and Techniques, ed 2. FA Davis, Philadelphia, 1990.
18. Gerber, LH and Hicks, JE: Exercises in the rheumatic diseases. In Basmajian, JV and Wolf, SL (eds): Therapeutic Exercise, ed 5, Williams & Wilkins, Baltimore, 1990.
19. Michelsson, JF and Riska, EB: The effect of temporary exercising of joints during an immobilization period. Clin Orthop 144:321, 1979.
20. Crane, JG and Kemek, CB: Mortality associated with hip fractures in a single geriatric hospital and residential facility: A ten year review: J Am Geriatr Soc, 31:472, 1985.
21. Mooney, V: Major fractures. In Nickel, VL (ed): Orthopedic Rehabilitation, Churchill Livingstone, New York, 1982.
22. Duncan, PW and Badke, MB: Stroke Rehabilitation: The Recovery of Motor Control. Year Book Medical Publishers, Chicago, 1987.
23. O'Sullivan, SB: Strategies to improve motor control. In O'Sullivan, SB and Schmitz, TJ (eds): Physical Rehabilitation, ed 2. FA Davis, Philadelphia, 1988.
24. Sullivan, PE and Markos, PD: Clinical Procedures in Therapeutic Exercise. Appleton and Lange, Norwalk, 1987.
25. Carr, JH and Shepherd, RB: Motor Relearning Programme Following stroke, ed 2. Aspen, Rockville, 1987.
26. Carr, JH, et al: Movement Science. Aspen, Rockville, 1987.

27. May, BJ: Principles of exercise for the elderly. In Basmajian, JV and Wolf, SL, (eds): Therapeutic Exercise, ed 5. Williams & Wilkins, Baltimore, 1990.
28. Pfau, J: Adult Exercise Instruction Sheets: Home Exercise for Rehabilitation. Therapy Skill Builders, Tucson, 1989.
29. Sallade, J and Adam, L: Geriatric exercise booklet. Clin Manag in Phys Ther 6:32, 1986.
30. Thera-band[R] Resistive Exerciser Instruction Book, Hygienic, Akron, 1985.
31. Light, KE, et al: Low-load prolonged stretch vs. high-load brief stretch in treating knee contractures. Phys Ther 64:330, 1984.

Chapter 6

Mobility

JANCIS K. DENNIS & D. MICHAEL MCKEOUGH

It is common for therapists to think of transfers and ambulation as synonymous with mobility. In this chapter we present a more global view of mobility, expanding the concept to include the movements necessary for the activities of daily living. We begin by presenting a taxonomy of motor tasks.* A taxonomy is a classification system; in this case, a system is presented to classify motor tasks according to their difficulty. The taxonomy is used to explore the training conditions required to attain different levels of functional mobility. We then discuss the implications of motor learning theory for mobility training. The chapter concludes with case presentations that exemplify mobility training for four individuals with different predicted outcomes.

DEFINITION OF MOBILITY

Mobility is defined in terms of the skills required to solve movement problems confronted during the activities of daily living. It includes problem recognition, goal selection, development of a strategy to meet the goal, formulation of a motor plan, and implementation of the strategy, or response. Feedback is then available to the performer: Was the goal met? Was the strategy effective? Was the motor plan the most efficient and effective one? Figure 6–1 illustrates the flow of recognition of a movement problem and its solution.[1]

For example, a woman is watching television and perceives a feeling of thirst. She decides to act to quench her thirst. Because she remembers there is water in the kitchen sink, she is then faced with the movement problem of getting from the sofa to the kitchen. The specific component skills required include:

Problem Recognition and Goal Selection

The woman watching television must have the cognitive ability to recognize the problem (thirst). Having recognized the need, she must then decide whether or not to resolve it. If she chooses to ignore the need, she con-

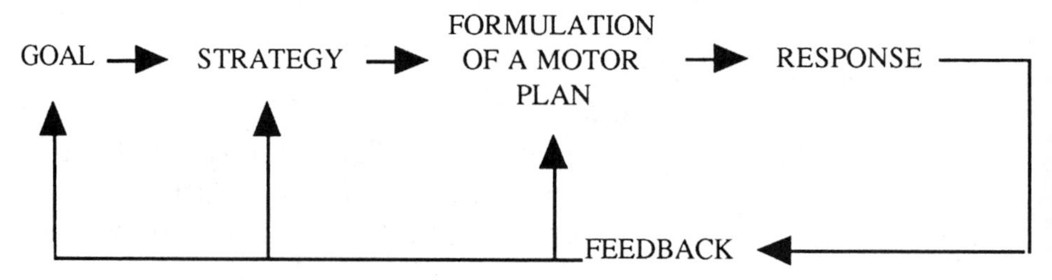

Figure 6–1. Components of a response to a motor problem. (Adapted from Gentile.[1])

*This chapter extends the work of Gentile, as cited in references 1 and 3, on the nature and classification of goal-directed movements.

tinues to watch television. If she chooses to resolve the problem, the goal of her future movement becomes "Quench the thirst!" Having chosen to quench her thirst, she must select a strategy to meet that goal.

Strategy Development

All strategies that would meet the goal involve some type of movement. Therefore, selection and execution of a movement strategy become the means for solving a motor problem. The woman may relieve her thirst using one of many different strategies. For instance, she may call out for someone to bring her a glass of water or she may decide to get it herself. Selection of the most appropriate alternative requires decision-making capabilities and insight.

Formulating a Motor Plan

Each strategy involves several motor components. The strategy of getting the drink for herself requires standing up from the sofa, moving to the kitchen, reaching into a cupboard, taking out a glass, moving to the sink, turning the faucet, filling the glass with water, and finally drinking the water. As you read the text you may have developed a different strategy, for example, drinking a soda, and your motor components would include going to the refrigerator and selecting a soda. For each of the motor components described, such as reaching into a cupboard, a motor plan must be developed. Persons with motor planning problems may have selected a goal and an appropriate strategy but are unable to plan its essential components.

Response

Once having decided to enact the strategy, the woman needs the ability to adapt to morphologic, environmental, and biomechanical constraints.[2] Morphologic constraints are imposed by an individual's functional ability and include both physical and psychological factors. Height, strength, range of motion, and motivation are examples of morphologic constraints. Strategy implementation first requires the motivation to carry it out. It is possible to develop strategies but decide not to carry them out; the television may be too interesting, or the person may decide there is no hurry to complete the strategy—that delay is all right. Environmental constraints are the features of the environment itself, including such critical factors as the height of the sofa, the distance to the kitchen, floor coverings, the width of the kitchen door, the height of the cupboards, the stiffness of the faucet, and any obstacles along the intended route.

Biomechanical constraints stem from the intended movement pattern. These interact with morphologic constraints to determine the types of transfers and gait patterns that would solve the movement problem successfully. To stand from the sofa, walk to the kitchen, and fill a glass with water, the woman must generate adequate forces given the stability and mobility requirements of the intended movement pattern. It is also necessary to initiate and terminate the forces at appropriate times if the movement is to be smooth, efficient, and safe. The environment must be perceived accurately and movement adapted to avoid bumping into furniture, tripping over cords, and stepping on the dog's tail. It is clear that impairment, whether motivational, musculoskeletal, neurologic, cardiovascular, pulmonary, cognitive, or perceptual, could reduce mobility by interfering with any of the stages of acquiring a particular goal.

When mobility is defined in terms of skills required to solve a movement problem, it becomes clear that the motor components involve not merely translation of the body's center of mass in space, as in a transfer, or walking, but the ability to control the body within its base of support. In the example above, the woman needs control of standing balance to reach for a glass and to hold it in one hand while turning on the faucet with the other. Gentile[3] developed a taxonomy of motor tasks that helps us analyze movement problems according to whether they are stability or body transport tasks. The taxonomy also addresses the varying degrees of perception and information processing required for performance in different environments.

THE TAXONOMY

Factors Determining Task Difficulty

Gentile's taxonomy identifies two dimensions along which motor tasks progress from simple to complex: the desired outcome of the action being taken, that is, body stability or body transport; and the environmental conditions, closed or open, under which the movement is performed.[3]

The Desired Outcome of the Action

Along the first dimension, the desired outcome of the action, tasks become more difficult as they progress from requiring body stability to requiring body transport. These tasks can be graded further by superimposing independent limb manipulation in addition to stability or transport. So, in only this dimension, a simple task would require body stability with no independent limb manipulation, for example, maintaining static, erect sitting posture. A complex task would require body transport with simultaneous independent limb manipulation, for example, walking from the kitchen to the sofa while carrying a full glass of water. For real task difficulty, consider juggling while riding a bicycle (see Fig. 6–2).

Conditions of the Performance Environment

The second dimension of the taxonomy, environmental conditions, progresses from simple to complex on the basis of whether the environment

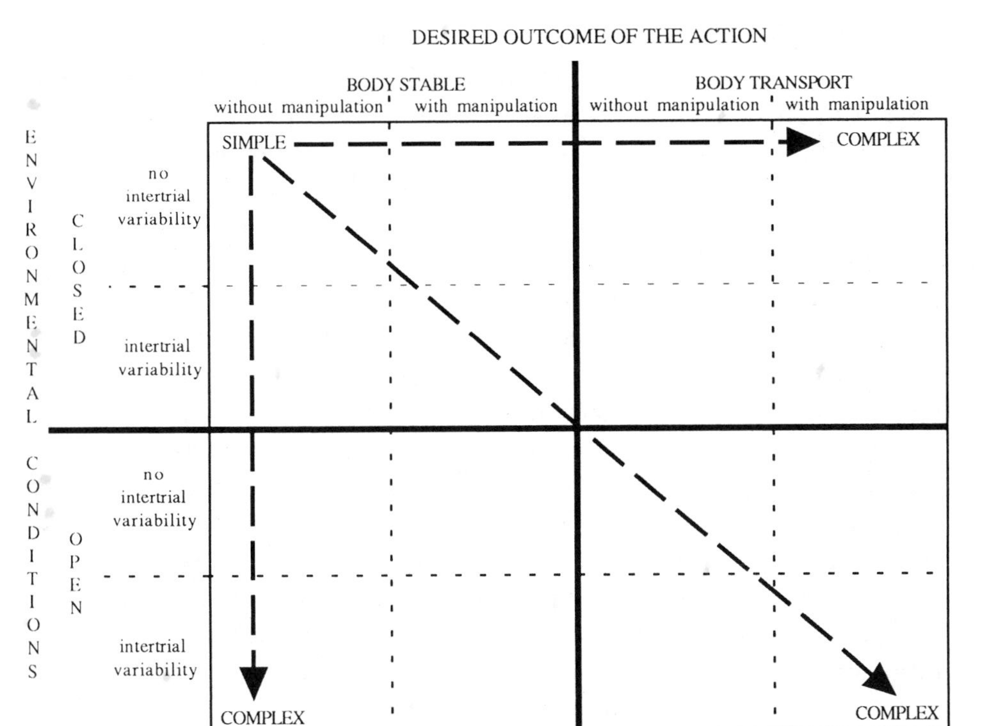

Figure 6–2. *Taxonomy of motor tasks: dimensions of task difficulty. (Modified from Gentile.[3])*

changes in time and space during performance. The nature of the performance environment places informational processing demands on the performer. As home health therapists we encounter widely varying movement environments in patients' homes.

If objects in the environment critical to a successful performance are stationary, it is referred to as a "closed environment."[4] Here a performer is free to focus attention on planning and executing the desired movement pattern without regard to objects moving in the environment. A furnished room is a closed environment regardless of how much furniture is present. Crowded spaces with narrow passageways present the same type of fixed environmental constraints on the organization of an effective movement pattern as a spacious environment does. Because the crowded environment provides less working space, the movement performance must be more precise, which increases performance difficulty. One service that therapists can perform is to arrange the movement environment in a way that best suits the client's abilities. First, however, the interaction between the space and the client's movement strategies must be carefully evaluated. A more spacious movement environment is not automatically more advantageous; furniture may have been placed strategically to assist in movement performance, and the pattern may incorporate the furniture as an essential part of the movement. For example, a strategically placed piece of furniture may provide an essential support surface for making a turn. It is also important to consider that the person may have an emotional attachment to the furnishings and their arrangement. Under these circumstances it is important to evaluate the desirability of changing the environment versus teaching the client to operate in a less than optimally safe environment. If the client cannot be persuaded that a scatter rug is a hazard, it can be taped down and the client taught to lift the walker and feet high enough to accommodate it. Although the performance may be slightly less safe, it is still closed.

The second type of performance environment is one in which objects are moving. Poulton[4] calls this an "open environment." Performance in an open environment is more difficult because interaction with moving objects requires predictive ability. Because of built-in time delays in our motor control system (reaction and response time), if a performer waits until an event occurs in an open environment, the response will necessarily occur at some time after that event. For example, if we cannot predict the speed of a car that is moving toward us, we cannot plan how fast we need to move out of its way. The performer must predict what the conditions will be in the immediate future, then plan and initiate a response based on that prediction. If the prediction and response execution are both correct, the response will coincide with the event in a changing environment and the goal will have been achieved. A good example of this is the way a child learns to catch a ball. If the child waits for the ball's arrival before initiating a catching response, the response will necessarily be too late and the child will surely get a sore nose! Until the child learns to watch the flight of the ball, predict when it will arrive, and plan and initiate the catching movement with proper timing, she will not be able to catch the ball as it moves in space.

The presence of children or animals in the home may create an open environment because a performer must predict the environmental change to respond adaptively. Consider, for example, the woman carrying the glass of water across the living room. If her dog jumps up to greet her while she is moving to the sofa, she must be able to predict the timing of the impact and meet it with appropriate force to avoid being knocked over. If the movement response is poorly timed or scaled, she may lose her balance or spill the water.

The environmental conditions can be modified further by changing the specifics of the task from performance to performance. This is known as "intertrial variability." Every motor task has a specific plan—the plan for standing from a chair varies, for example, with the chair height and the softness of the seat. In an effort to make the practice of the sit-to-stand skill more transferable between different seating surfaces, it is important to practice from many different chairs and on different floor surfaces. It may be easier to start with one simple condition and move to incorporating many different heights and surfaces after one condition has been mastered. An individual may not find it easy to transfer in and out of chairs of different types unless confronted with a large variety of environmental conditions.

Combining the two dimensions of task difficulty, the desired outcome of the action and the environmental demands, creates a taxonomy that can be useful in classifying mobility skills. The complexity of the task being performed (body stability or body transport with or without independent limb manipulation) combines with the information processing demands due to the performance environment (open or closed environment with or without intertrial variability) to determine task difficulty. If tasks fall into the same cell in the taxonomy, their demands on the performer are known to be similar. Examples of several types of activities may be seen in Figure 6–3.

The taxonomy can be used to structure within-session activities as well as long-term rehabilitation goals. A therapist may choose to structure the treatment session using activities that require similar classes and levels of difficulty. Because each dimension of the taxonomy specifies a progression of difficulty, a therapist can progress the treatment program and continually challenge a client's functional ability by moving to more difficult tasks from the next cell in the taxonomy.

		BODY STABLE		BODY TRANSPORT	
		without manipulation	with manipulation	without manipulation	with manipulation
CLOSED	without intertrial variability	Maintaining balance in sitting on bed while caregiver combs hair Maintaining balance in standing in hallway as caregiver buttons coat	Sitting at the table and eating a meal Sitting doing household accounts Sitting at desk to write a letter	Rolling over in bed Sit <=> stand from bed Tub transfers Bed <=> bathroom, using same route daily	Carrying a tray of food or drinks from the kitchen to the living room, using same tray and same route each time
	with intertrial variability	Maintaining sitting balance on different chairs in the room e.g., rocker, straight-backed chair, sofa. Maintaining standing balance on different surfaces: carpet, wood	Standing in the kitchen unloading a dish-washer Sitting on a low stool in the yard, bending over to weed the vegetable garden	Rolling over in a twin bed and a queen bed Sit <=> stand from different heights and surfaces Up and down curbs of different heights	Carrying a tray of food or drinks from the kitchen to the living room, using different trays and routes each time
OPEN	without intertrial variability	Maintaining balance in a moving elevator	Rearranging packages while standing in a moving elevator	Walking up or down a moving escalator or a moving sidewalk.	Rearranging packages while walking up or down the moving escalator
	with intertrial variability	Maintaining sitting or standing balance in a moving bus.	Drinking a cocktail on the deck of a cruise ship	Community ambulation Walking through a living room where children are playing	Shopping in the supermarket Walking a precocious pet on a leash

Figure 6–3. Activities of daily living represented in the taxonomy of motor tasks.

Consider next the systematic progression of task difficulty throughout a rehabilitation program. For example, once the client has achieved independent control of sitting balance (body stability in a closed environment), the therapist may increase task difficulty by asking the client to move and stack objects while seated (superimposing independent limb manipulation on a stability task). This change in treatment activities progresses the treatment program to the next cell in the taxonomy, thereby increasing task difficulty. The task becomes more difficult because a successful performance requires independent limb manipulation on top of weight shift and maintenance of dynamic stability. If appropriate, the same activity could be performed in standing. During standing, the type of task remains the same (body stability with independent limb manipulation is a closed environment), but the task specificity changes to include control of balance. This entails different biomechanical constraints, which in turn increase task difficulty. Finally, task difficulty can again be increased by opening the performance environment progressively. First, intertrial variability is introduced in a closed environment. Ask the client to stack different types of objects from different sitting surfaces; then to grasp objects that are moving at a constant rate along a constant path (reach to catch an object that is swinging from a fixed point in a pendular manner). Next, introduce intertrial variability into the open environment by asking the client to grasp different types of objects moving at varying speeds along varying paths (play Nintendo™; catch a ball). Finally, superimpose body transport on top of independent limb manipulation in an open environment with intertrial variability (e.g., balancing a tray of food while walking to find a seat in a crowded kitchen).

MOTOR LEARNING

Motor learning theory offers several principles that can be applied to mobility training. Many of these principles are familiar to therapists but other principles are less widely incorporated into treatment.[5]

Task Specificity and Transfer of Training

When considering the transfer of learning between a treatment session and daily life, therapists should be aware of the results of recent research in motor control that clearly support the view that learning and performance are task specific. That is, the best training for a task is the task itself.[4] Training of a mobility goal is, therefore, best attained by practice or training of the activity itself. Consider a client with grade 3+ strength of the quadriceps and gluteals who is having difficulty with a sit-to-stand transfer. Task specificity predicts that the client will learn the transfer more efficiently by using sit-to-stand activities to learn the movement pattern (and increase muscle strength) than if the therapist focuses on strengthening the weakened muscle groups using traditional exercises. Motor plans are as important to the transfer as the appropriate strength. Strengthening alone will not automatically carry over to the transfer activity.

In planning rehabilitation programs it is often impossible or unsafe to apply this principle without modification. Because of concern for safety, rehabilitation programs, even those with long-term goals in an open environment, begin treatment activities in a closed environment. Because open environments have higher information processing demands than closed environments and may require rapid response times from the performer, they constitute a more difficult performance environment. In many cases it would be unsafe for a therapist to place a patient with reduced functional capacity in an open environment initially.

The Principle of Whole-Part-Whole

Wherever possible, therapists should use the mobility task as the treatment activity, but in some situations the activity is too difficult or complex. In such cases the activity can be segmented into components and the principle of whole-part-whole applied. This principle involves practice of the whole task, of its components, and finally of the whole task again. Components should be large chunks of the task and as few in number as possible. The sit-to-stand transfer itself is performed once or twice, with as much assistance or guidance as is required. It is then segmented into the following components: the most effective starting position for the transfer (buttocks near the edge, feet back, etc.); forward weight transfer, and finally elevation. Once each component has been addressed within the session, the client performs a complete sit-to-stand transfer, thus putting the components back together.

Feedback

Feedback is a critical element in the learning process. Initially, feedback may need to be augmented by visual, auditory, or other means. Mirrors and key words are the means most commonly available to therapists working in the home, but sometimes families with video cameras can tape performances that can be used to illustrate the needed changes and keep a record of progress. As performers progress, augmented feedback can be withdrawn gradually until performers are able to accurately and independently assess and correct their own performance.

The Progression of Learning

Three phases of learning outcomes are sometimes described: cognitive, associative, and autonomous[6].

Cognitive Learning

The client learns best initially if the goals, outcomes, and processes are made explicit. Begin by teaching on the cognitive level. Explain the components of the movement, demonstrate, have the client explore the "feel" of an efficient performance, give accurate feedback on the performance outcome, and begin to teach self-evaluation of performance. If the therapist persists in providing constant feedback and performance correction, the client will come to depend on external feedback. To promote self-evaluation the therapist may choose to stop correcting the client and ask, for example, "How did that go?" or "How did that feel?" The client begins to develop a feel for the movement if the therapist highlights the sensation, for example, the feeling of weight through the feet. The feeling of the movement is a very important component of self-evaluation. Golf or tennis players will relate to feeling a good swing, or ball players to feeling an accurate throw. In the same way, the person relearning mobility skills after injury or neuromuscular pathology will learn the feeling of correct gait pattern with a walker.

Associative Learning

During the associative phase of learning, the therapist withdraws external feedback further and allows time for the client to process performance outcomes. For example, the client transfers from a wheelchair to a bed. The transfer was poorly executed. The therapist makes no comment. The client in the associative phase of learning may offer: "I don't think I did that too well." The therapist then asks how the performance could have been better, thus encouraging the client to identify movement components that need improvement. This also encourages the client to take more responsibility for the rehabilitation program. A client in the associative phase of learning will self-correct as errors are detected.

Autonomous Learning

The therapist can progress to making the task more automatic by imposing distractors, such as independent manipulative tasks, on the basic skill. At first the client's attention may need to be drawn to performance error if the distractor indeed distracts, but, once the movement has been truly learned, the client will be able to maintain accurate performance in spite of distractors.

Verbal Cues

One form of verbal cueing that the therapist can provide is to identify which elements of the intended movement pattern are essential to a successful performance. For example, a successful sit-to-stand movement must include sufficient weight shift and extensor force generation to displace the center of mass anteriorly and superiorly from the sitting to the standing base of support. To meet these biomechanical constraints, the therapist might instruct the client to "lean forward until your nose is over your knees and push hard with both legs."

Visual Imagery and Mental Practice

The therapist can also encourage clients to rehearse the movements visually, kinesthetically, or both. The trajectory of the distal segment of the movement can be cued visually and rehearsed mentally. Similarly, the client can be asked to recall the feeling of the movement. Maring[7] demonstrated greater changes in timing variables, leading to more efficient movement, among an experimental group using mental practice in contrast to a control group who used only physical practice. This suggests that we should be open to the idea of incorporating mental practice into mobility training for those individuals with intact cognitive processing.

Structure of the Treatment Session*

Evidence from research in motor learning suggests that scattering the practice of a skill throughout the treatment session may result in better learning and carryover of the skill, but that blocking the practice of the skill may be better for a within-treatment performance.[5] Blocked practice may be preferable when the client is first learning the skill. It is more traditional for therapists to block the practice of different mobility skills throughout the treatment. For example, if the mobility goals are: [I] bed mobility, [I] supine to bedside sit, [I] sit to stand, [I] bed-to-wheelchair transfers, and ambulation with contact guard, the treatment may be performed as follows: practice bed mobility, then supine to sit, then sit to stand, then bed-to-wheelchair transfers, then walking. Randomized practice might be: roll [L] and practice supine to bedside sit, sit to stand, sit to supine, bridging across the bed, supine to sit, sit to stand, walking around the room, sit to stand from a bedroom chair, and so forth.

Because the research findings are not clear about whether these principles apply equally to normal persons, the disabled, and those with cognitive dysfunction, we can apply the principles and evaluate the effects in the home. If the client is cognitively impaired and always requires some cueing, we may not want to introduce too much intertrial variability, but the treatment order can still be randomized.

*[I] = independent; [L] = left.

INDIVIDUAL EVALUATION AND GOAL SETTING

Mobility goals set for each client depend on the synthesis of the evaluation data and the predictive factors related to the client's disease or dysfunction. Critical information that helps determine these goals includes both physical and psychosocial elements including:

1. Previous mobility status, in particular ambulatory status, and changes in the past 12 months
2. Cognitive status including insight, problem-solving capabilities, and motivation
3. Overall physical assessment, including the musculoskeletal and nervous systems, the cardiovascular and pulmonary systems, and the urogenital system
4. Family, caregiving, and economic support systems.

A poor prognosis for the return of functional independence has been associated with cognitive impairment, perceptual impairment, advanced age, comorbidity, and depression.[8–11] However, the associations are not so explicit that they should be permitted to bias individual goal setting. These predictive associations give us guidelines for individual evaluations and may focus our treatment planning so that we can preempt wherever possible the development of adverse conditions. Some predictive factors with which we can intervene include contacting the social worker or physician when we observe the development of depression; setting the environmental stage for optimum early independence, even if only in minor tasks; communicating with psychologists, occupational therapists, and speech pathologists to optimize the client's cognitive and perceptual abilities; and referring clients for extended home services or suggesting support groups for clients (and their families) with limited personal resources for independent community living. Studies have shown the importance of independent personal care and mobility in keeping individuals in the community.[10] Therefore, it is extremely important that our treatments address realistic community living goals, if appropriate, and not merely basic closed-environment tasks that limit the demands on the neuromuscular system.

CASE PRESENTATIONS

Four client cases will apply the information about how to plan and progress a treatment program using the taxonomy. The cases were selected because they represent the types of clients frequently seen by a home health therapist. The four cases range from severe impairment with poor prognosis to minimal impairment with good prognosis. Readers can apply information from the chapter to clients treated in a normal home health case load.

CASE 1: 50-YEAR-OLD MAN WITH ENCEPHALOPATHY

Mr. S. has a diagnosis of encephalopathy secondary to a myocardial infarction. Mr. S. is 50, 6 feet 3 in tall, weighs 265 pounds, worked for 30 years as a mechanic, has a 70-pack-year smoking history (2 packs a day for 35 years), has had mild hypertension (160/105 mmHg) for 20 years, had a laminectomy and fusion for an L-4–L-5 disc in 1975, and leads a sedentary life-style. Mr. S. is currently at home in the care of his family after having discharged himself, against physician's advice, after 5 weeks of treatment at a rehabilitation hospital. Contrary to all medical prognosis, the family and Mr. S. remain firmly convinced that he will learn to walk again "no matter what it takes." Key evaluation findings:

1. Alert and oriented to person, place, and condition and follows two-step commands consistently
2. Severe spastic dystonia of both lower extremities (extensor synergy, right much greater than left) and in the right upper extremity (flexor synergy)
3. Passive range of motion of all three extremities approximately 20 percent of normal secondary to hypertonia and no functional voluntary use of these extremities
4. Equinovarus deformity of the right ankle secondary to extensor hypertonia
5. Minimal voluntary use of the left upper extremity
6. Bowel and bladder incontinence
7. Moderate orthostatic hypotension
8. Functional mobility:
    a. Bed mobility with maximum assist by one person
    b. Transfers with total assist (wheelchair to bed and back)/by one or two people
    c. Nonambulatory
    d. Erect sitting posture (4 minutes).

Discussion

Given his functional level at 2 months postinjury with 6 weeks of therapy, the prognosis for Mr. S is poor. The problems were:

1. Unrealistic expectations by Mr. S. and his family of the ultimate functional recovery
2. Extreme hypertonia in three extremities with associated deformity and problems associated with prolonged immobility
3. Difficulty of delivering care given the client's size and mobility limitations
4. Community access

The strengths were:

1. Mr. S's determination and willingness to work toward functional recovery
2. Family support
3. Willingness of private insurance to pay for physical and occupational therapy 5 days per week as long as progress continues

Mobility Goals

Through discussion with Mr. S. and the family, five mobility goals were identified (Fig. 6–4). These goals were directed at four major objectives:

1. Maximizing mobility to help client assist with personal care
2. Instructing caregivers in positioning to inhibit hypertonia
3. Instructing caregivers in proper lifting and transfer techniques
4. Pregait activities

With a primary goal of teaching the patient to maximize the assistance he can offer in his own care, a first decision in planning the treatment program is to reduce task difficulty by focusing exclusively on treatment activities in a closed environment with no intertrial variability, that is, activities in the bed as well as transfers to and from the wheelchair. Treatment ac-

		BODY STABLE		BODY TRANSPORT	
		without manipulation	with manipulation	without manipulation	with manipulation
CLOSED	without intertrial variability	Optimal W/C sitting balance x 5 min Static standing balance x 1 min		Bed mobility with min assist Transfers <=> bed with mod assist Fwd and bwd weight shifts in standing	
	with intertrial variability				
OPEN	without intertrial variability	ACTIVITIES IN THE OPEN ENVIRONMENT ARE NOT APPLICABLE			
	with intertrial variability				

Figure 6–4. Goals for Mr. S.

tivities to facilitate bed mobility come from the body transport without manipulation in a closed environment without intertrial variability cell. Because the environment is closed and unchanging, the client is free to focus on selecting and executing the intended movement pattern.

Activities within this cell appropriate to the goal include rolling in bed, bridging, coming to sit at bedside, sitting balance, sit to stand from the bed, bed-to-wheelchair transfers, and sit to stand from the wheelchair. A key to maximizing initial success under these performance conditions is to minimize intertrial variability. That is, the client should always attempt the same movement pattern if it is working and the therapist should always cue the same critical components using the same simple instructions. Initial success and consistency are based on repetition of the same successful strategy. After initial strategies have been mastered consistently, the client's movement repertoire can be expanded by introducing intertrial variability in a closed environment without manipulation, for example, transferring from the wheelchair to other seats, such as dining room chairs or couches, and then working on sit to stand from these variable surfaces.

A common mobility problem experienced by clients who function primarily from a wheelchair and bed is pelvic control. Even with the best wheelchair seating systems, slump-sitting on a posteriorly rotated pelvis is a consistent problem. A physical therapist assistant[12] developed a novel activity for relearning pelvic mobility and control. Placing a 6-in diameter rubber ball under the sacrum of a supine client creates a fulcrum. By rolling the ball from side to side as well as toward the head and feet, the client rotates the pelvis independently of the trunk and establishes better pelvic and trunk control (Fig. 6–5). Only after overcoming posterior pelvic rotation can

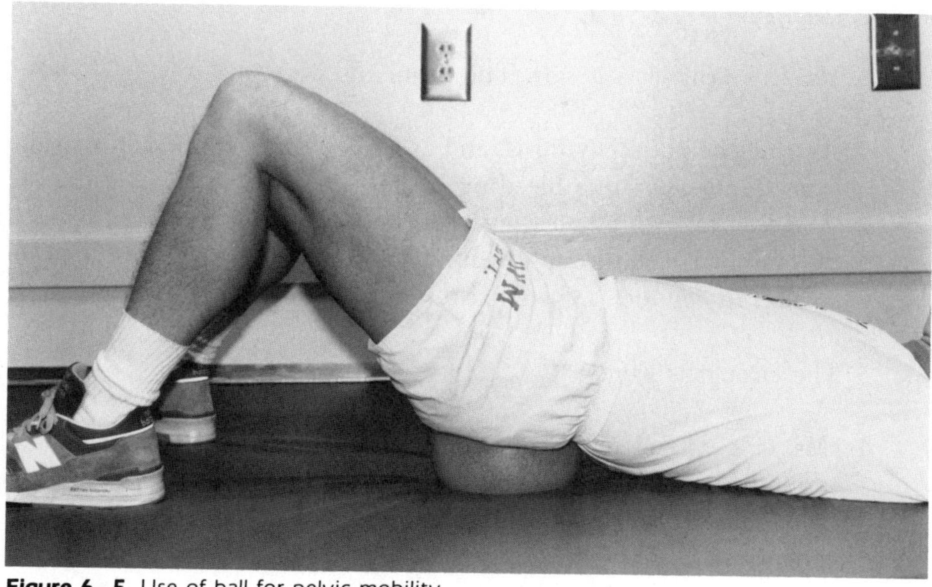

Figure 6–5. Use of ball for pelvic mobility.

clients shift enough weight forward to stand from a sitting position using a normal movement pattern.

An additional concern in managing the care for Mr. S. was his equipment needs. He required a hospital bed with an electric head lift; a wide, tall reclining wheelchair, and right ankle and bilateral hand splints. A Hoyer lift was ordered for the therapeutic pool that the family had installed. With this equipment and a final briefing on the home program, Mr. S. and his family were discharged from home health care. The final resolution of this case was determined by the third-party payer's unwillingness to continue payment because of the client's lack of progress. In spite of the physician's opinion and the therapist's best efforts to explain the situation, the family members never changed their unrealistic expectations that Mr. S. would walk again.

CASE 2: 63-YEAR-OLD WOMAN WITH A TOTAL HIP ARTHROPLASTY

Ms. C. received a right total hip arthroplasty 2 weeks ago. Following surgery, Ms. C. had significant bleeding into the soft tissue surrounding the joint; this extended her hospital stay to 10 days. Ms. C. is 63 years old. Other medical problems include hypertension and chronic obstructive pulmonary disease. She receives aid for families with dependent children (AFDC) and currently lives at home with her two daughters and their four young children. The house is one story with steep stairs to the front and back doors. Neither set of stairs has a hand railing.

DISCUSSION

Ms. C.'s prognosis is fair. The problems were:

1. Pitting edema, ecchymosis, and extremely limited range of motion due to postoperative bleeding
2. Concern for compliance with the home exercise program
3. A cramped, chaotic home situation—a difficult environment in which to conduct a systematic rehabilitation program

The strengths were:

1. Ms. C.'s expressed willingness to work to become an independent ambulator
2. A daughter's expressed willingness to help with the home exercise program.

Mobility Goals

In discussions with Ms. C. and the family, mobility goals were selected (Fig. 6–6). Ms. C.'s long-term goal was to become an independent community ambulator. To acquire the necessary skills, she had to begin with increasing weight bearing and maintaining good standing posture (body stability in a closed environment). We began with standing at the bedside using a walker for assistance (no intertrial variability). Transfers progressed from sit to stand through standing pivot. The use of assistive devices progressed from walker to single-point cane as ability permitted.

Use of an assistive device does not constitute independent limb manipulation. Because safe ambulation requires an assistive device, the motor problem being solved by the client is how to incorporate the assistive device as part of the gait pattern. Because the upper extremities are responsible for controlling the assistive device, they are not free to engage in a manipulative task independent of the gait pattern. In Ms. C.'s case, she had to progress to a cane before one of her upper extremities could be free for independent manipulation.

To ambulate independently in the community, Ms. C. had to be safe in variable environments. The introduction of variable surfaces began early in the rehabilitation program starting in the closed environment while Ms.

		BODY STABLE		BODY TRANSPORT	
		without manipulation	with manipulation	without manipulation	with manipulation
CLOSED	without intertrial variability	Maintain good standing posture with walker/ cane	Maintain stability at kitchen counter and get cup from cupboard	Transfers and ambulation inside with assistance as necessary	
CLOSED	with intertrial variability		Dressing, personal hygiene, housework and ADLs with assistance as necessary	Transfers and ambulation, over all surfaces, in and outside	Transport cups of coffee or glasses of water from kitchen counter to table
OPEN	without intertrial variability				(I) take a seat at dining table as family convenes for meals
OPEN	with intertrial variability				(I) shop in a crowded grocery store

Figure 6–6. Goals for Ms. C.

C. was mastering advanced transfers and walking with a walker. Intertrial variability in a closed environment was achieved by transferring from variable surfaces (variable shapes, textures, and heights). While the physical therapist (PT) worked on bed mobility, transfers and ambulation, the occupational therapist (OT) worked on personal hygiene, dressing, and housework activities of daily living (ADLs). Treatment activities began in a closed environment with body stability; Ms. C. worked on dressing, hygiene, and housework activities. Intertrial variability was introduced by dressing with different types of clothes (blouse, dresses, skirts, underwear); personal hygiene, with toothbrushes, combs, and hair brushes; and housework activities like cooking and cleaning.

To create an open environment in the home we chose to work during meals. Everyone's converging on the kitchen to find a seat at the table, get seated and served, and eat provided a *very* open environment. Asking Ms. C. to get to the table, take a seat, and eat required her to anticipate and respond adaptively to the movements of others. Successful completion of the meal required her to achieve body stability as well as body transport, including independent limb manipulation, in both closed and open environments.

The steep stairs in and out of the house were an obstacle for re-entry into the community. No railing was present and no resources were available to have one built. Therefore, Ms. C. was taught to turn her walker sideways. Using a quad cane in her right hand, together with the assistance of a family member stabilizing the walker, she was able to negotiate the front steps safely (Figs. 6–7 and 6–8). Only after progressing to the use of a quad cane would she become independent in entering and leaving the house. An alternative method was to turn the walker sideways, and with the stability imposed by the family member, Ms. C. could then walk sideways down the steps. Both methods were taught; Ms. C. preferred the first.

Finally, the goal of shopping in a crowded grocery store required transport plus independent limb manipulation (moving from aisle to aisle and retrieving products from the shelves) in an open environment with intertrial variability (other people and their carts moving in the aisles plus the different configurations of packages and shelving in the produce, frozen food, and dairy sections). Direct participation in these activities is outside the scope of home health care. Lead-up activities that we did practice at home included asking Ms. C. and her daughters to work together washing and returning the dishes, pots, and pans to the cabinets.

CASE 3: 78-YEAR-OLD WOMAN WITH RHEUMATOID ARTHRITIS

Ms. R. has a diagnosis of rheumatoid arthritis. Prior to hospital admission for "painful spasms in her left hamstrings," she had been

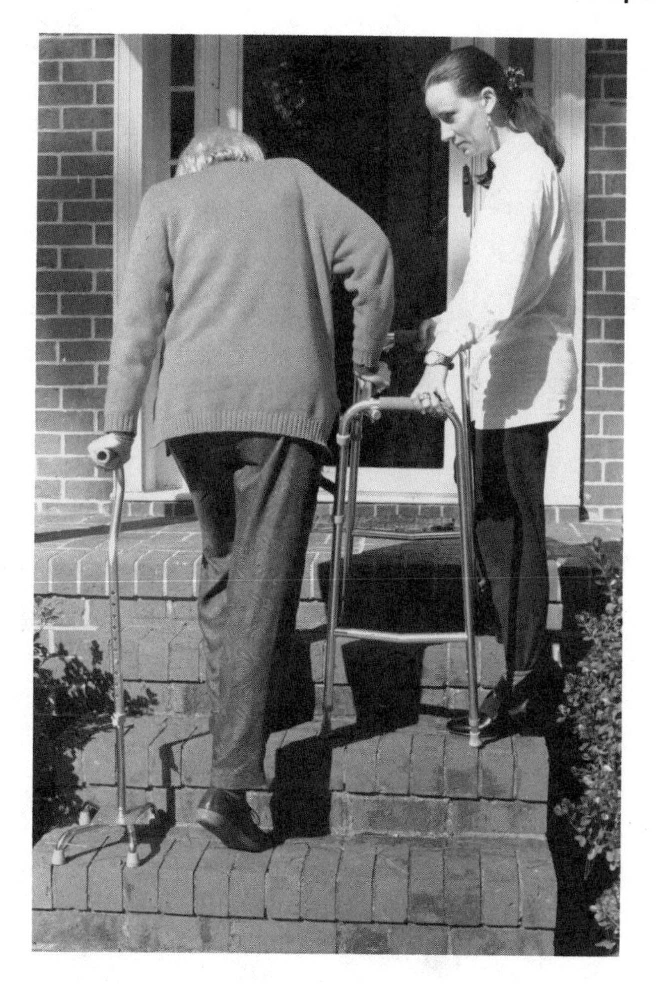

Figure 6–7. Turning a walker sideways for ascending and descending steps: forward progression.

living alone in her own house with support from family and neighbors. She was discharged into the care of her daughter. At initial interview Ms. R.'s daughter indicated that the family was concerned that Ms. R. would never be able to walk again and that they did not know how to handle the situation, since they have four children (age range 16–8) and she had given up part-time employment to look after her mother. For the past 12 months the family has become increasingly concerned about Ms. R.'s deteriorating condition. Although she was able to use a walker, it took her 30 minutes to walk from her bedroom to the kitchen, with frequent rests on strategically placed chairs. She was sometimes confused, was "probably not eating well," and, other than being able to prepare simple meals, relied on the family and neighbors for washing, housecleaning, and shopping. She managed her personal hygiene with a sponge bath in the kitchen. She had been troubled for some time with urinary incontinence and, unable to walk quickly to the

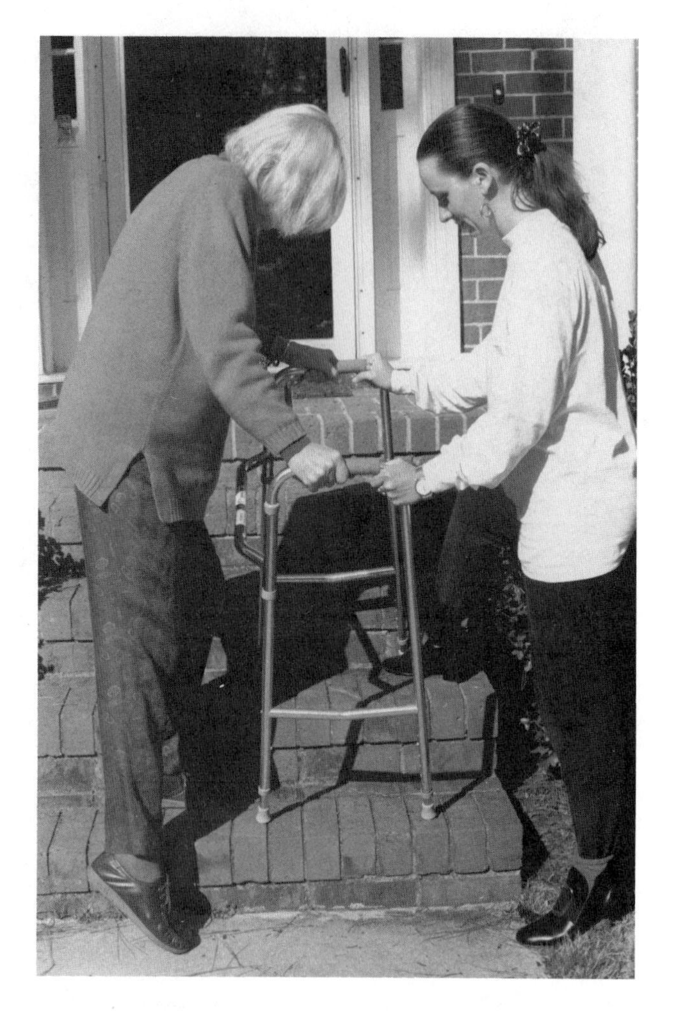

Figure 6–8. Turning a walker sideways for ascending and descending steps: sideward progression.

bathroom, had placed potties in each room. Key evaluation findings:

1. 78-year-old woman who is oriented and expresses the wish to walk again and return to her own house. She sees no problems because she managed before "just fine."
2. Physical findings: Knee flexion contractures 20 degrees both sides; tight heel cords but plantargrade both sides; hip flexion contractures 10 degrees flexion both sides; kyphosis, scoliosis, forward head. Strength in both lower extremities grossly grade 3+; upper extremities, 4+; arthritic changes in feet, knees, elbows, shoulders, and spine
3. Independent mobility in bed—rolling, bridging to facilitate changing of diapers. Moderate assist by one person for supine-to-bedside sit; maximum assist by one person for wheelchair transfers. Dependent in wheelchair mobility.

4. Durable medical equipment: Wheelchair, too large, fixed arms. Hospital bed. Walker, Commode.
5. Family concerns for future.
6. Prior "confusion."

Discussion

Overall assessment of the situation is not favorable for a return to independent living in her home environment, on the basis of her physical status, reports of previous mental confusion, and lack of insight into the difficulties associated with returning home. Ms. R.'s capacity for self-care had been deteriorating. The option for living with the family depended on how well Ms. R. could learn to be safe and independent in her daughter's home. If she remained dependent and unsafe, it was unlikely that her daughter could manage, since she needed to resume part-time work to help with the family finances. However, she expressed reluctance to admit her mother to a nursing home. The problems were:

1. The ability of the family to care for Ms. R. at home
2. Ms. R.'s lack of insight into the difficulties associated with returning home
3. Physical limitations

The strengths were:

1. Considerable network of local support
2. Daughter's willingness to give the situation a trial

Mobility Goals

Through discussion with the client and her daughter some basic mobility goals were identified (Fig. 6–9). These focused on independent mobility within the safety of a closed environment. We chose consistency of context and task instructions to facilitate Ms. R.'s learning because her previous confusion and current lack of insight suggested that learning new skills might present difficulties.

When training mobility skills under these circumstances, it is very important to convey precise instructions to the caregiver. If consistency is not maintained, the client is less likely to learn the new skill effectively. Accurate feedback is important. Caregivers must not merely know the instructions, but must understand the basic components of the movement so that they can provide accurate performance feedback in the early stages of learning. The PT can emphasize the value of training the client in independence, thus avoiding dependency relationships ("She won't do it for me"). Caregivers need to understand that caregiving in haste, with added assistance,

		BODY STABLE		BODY TRANSPORT	
		without manipulation	with manipulation	without manipulation	with manipulation
CLOSED	without intertrial variability	Maintain correct posture and balance in W/C Bridge to facilitate diaper change	[I] bathing in bed of 50% of body [I] W/C propulsion in set pathways within house	[I] bed transfers: scoot up and down, & sideways. Roll. [I] tranfers: W/C<=>bed & car	
	with intertrial variability		Maintain correct posture & balance in W/C while performing household tasks e.g., fold laundry	Ambulation with SBA for 30 ft from ≠bedroom to kitchen over carpet and hardwood floors	
OPEN	without intertrial variability				
	with intertrial variability				

Figure 6–9. Goals for Ms. R.

teaches dependency, but that initial extra training time promotes independence.

Ms. R.'s wheelchair mobility within the house was hampered by environmental and equipment problems. There were wooden thresholds on the floor between rooms and large pieces of furniture or kitchen equipment were found near doorways, reducing the maneuvering space. Ms. R. was very small, but the chair was large with fixed arms; this needed to be changed before wheelchair mobility training could begin. The dealer exchanged her chair for a smaller one that fitted her appropriately and was more easily maneuvered through the narrow doorways; removable arms facilitated transfers. The client was schooled in wheelchair mobility using both hands and feet, at first with straight-forward progression in a short corridor, and later with circular turns. The thresholds in the doorways were difficult for Ms. R. to push across, and the family removed them to permit better access between rooms. It was not possible to move furniture or kitchen equipment, and it proved challenging for Ms. R. to achieve full independent mobility to tight spaces.

Motor learning was the cornerstone of Ms. R.'s treatment and was applied to bed mobility and transfers. Initial transfers were taught as modified sliding board transfers, padding the space between the bed and the wheelchair with blankets because Ms. R.'s hands were unable to manage the sliding board. Concomitant practice of sit to stand resulted in the transfer changing from a sliding board pattern to standing pivot transfers. This method enabled Ms. R. to transfer without having to remove the arm of the chair, which was a challenging task for her upper extremities. She had difficulty remembering to brake the chair and had one fall as a result. Her son-in-law, a handyman, created some brightly colored brake extensions, which did not get in the way of the transfer and reminded her that the brakes needed attention. They also gave better leverage for correct braking, since Ms. R. had decreased strength in her upper extremities secondary to her arthritis. Mental practice and verbal rehearsal were used extensively in teaching the transfer and Ms. R learned to repeat the following critical performance elements in the task: Scoot close to the wheelchair, scoot to the edge of the bed, check the brakes. After that process she learned a set of instructions to rehearse involving the transfer. We tried to limit verbal rehearsal to three or at the most four critical performance cues, but for the transfer we used six, repeated together until the performance was learned. These were: Lean forward, stand, (reach for the) outside armrest, walk (your feet) around, head forward, sit. She mastered the sit to stand early, but stand to sit remained uncontrolled, so the cues were changed to place more emphasis on controlled sitting. The critical cues became: stand, walk (the feet) around, head forward, sit slowly. As training progressed we stopped using the verbal cues and after each transfer would ask Ms. R. whether she had transferred well or not. If not, we asked what was wrong. Soon she was able to analyze her performance, and her skill increased until she was able to transfer 100 percent safely and without verbal cueing.

Walking was not stated in the original goals because we felt that the wheelchair would be the primary method of mobility, given Ms. R.'s deformities, poor strength in lower extremities, and pain. As she gained independence, however, she became motivated to try walking again using a standard walker. She achieved 60 ft independently using the same motor learning approach as with transfer training. However, with increased walking she experienced increased joint pain, and the walking was limited to a small walk once daily if her arthritic pain permitted. Her motivation was also linked to unrealistic hopes of independent living; at about this time the decision was made to sell her house, which depressed Ms. R. so that she became less motivated to walk or even get out of bed.

Stress incontinence of urine remained a major problem. She was unable to transfer without losing urine and wore diapers at all times. She was able to tell when she needed to use the bathroom but had insufficient standing balance without support to perform the manipulation skills needed in letting down the diaper before transferring to the commode. Her daughter was reluctant to try her without diapers and this issue remained unresolved at discharge.

Community access was not addressed. The daughter's house did not offer easy community access, since the only means of getting in and out of the house was a steeply graded ramp. The family was unwilling to put money into a less steep ramp until a decision was made about Ms. R.'s future. At time of discharge from home health care this decision had not been made.

CASE 4: 69-YEAR-OLD WOMAN WITH A BELOW-KNEE AMPUTATION

Ms. P. is a 69-year-old client with a history of Raynaud's syndrome, hypertension, and hypovolemia. She underwent left below-knee amputation about 4 weeks before referral. On initial evaluation she was found to be independent in wheelchair transfers and had independent mobility in the wheelchair but was not ambulatory and did not know how to wrap her residual limb. She had a 10-degree knee flexion contracture, 3+ to 4− strength in her right lower extremity and left hip, and 3+ strength in the left quadriceps and hamstrings. She was not independent with a walker. Her mental status was clear, and she was oriented, well educated, and realistic. Ms. P. was sharing a home with her sister. The house was a three-bedroom, one-story home with three steps up to the front door (no guardrail) and a steep ramp up to the back door from the garage. On initial evaluation, standing balance was good but walking balance was only fair; Ms. P. was afraid of falling and needed close supervision to walk with a walker. Her goals were to be fitted with a prosthesis and become independent, although she verbalized fears that she would not be able to achieve this. She stated that she and her sister had been planning a 2-week cruise to the Bahamas before she hurt her foot; the foot did not heal and this led to the amputation. She stated that she would still like to take the cruise; she selected this activity as her long-term goal.

DISCUSSION

Given Ms. P.'s long-term goal of rescheduling her cruise to the Bahamas, she must be independent in an open environment with her prosthesis. A cruise liner represents an open environment because the movement of the liner in the water creates demands on balance that are not predictable. Moreover, walking on deck or to meals would involve making adjustments for constantly changing configurations of people in her immediate path. Before these high-level goals were addressed, some basic mobility tasks had to be achieved. Figures 6–10 and 6–11 outline some of the major goals addressed during the preprosthetic and later the prosthetic phase for Ms. P.

		BODY STABLE		BODY TRANSPORT	
		without manipulation	with manipulation	without manipulation	with manipulation
CLOSED	without intertrial variability		Residual limb wrapping in sitting		
CLOSED	with intertrial variability	Standing balance activities on different surfaces: soft, hard, even, and uneven	Wheelchair locking in many different environments Self care & ADLs from wheelchair		
OPEN	without intertrial variability				
OPEN	with intertrial variability			[I] ambulation with walker in home over different surfaces, taking different routes through the house	

Figure 6–10. Preprosthetic goals for Ms. P.

		BODY STABLE		BODY TRANSPORT	
		without manipulation	with manipulation	without manipulation	with manipulation
CLOSED	without intertrial variability		[I] personal care - able to take tub/shower		
CLOSED	with intertrial variability		Weeding and planting while seated on a low stool in yard	Manage steps of different heights and surfaces	
OPEN	without intertrial variability				
OPEN	with intertrial variability	Maintain balance in unpredictable environment		[I] ambulation in the community using a cane.	

Figure 6–11. Prosthetic goals for Ms. P.

Mobility Goals

Preprosthetic Stage

The first activities that needed to be addressed were Ms. P.'s basic ADLs involving the residual limb. She needed to learn to wrap the residual in sitting, which is a closed-environment task with a stable body and manipulation. The task in itself involves some balance activity, but this would not challenge her in the way she needed to be challenged to achieve her long-term goals. Balance activities were added in standing. This was done on different surfaces in preparation for using the walker and later for gait training with the prosthesis on different surfaces. We achieved this with her shoe on in the kitchen on vinyl flooring, in the bathroom on a tiled surface, in the bedroom on a carpeted surface, and in the hallway on a hardwood floor. Later we added standing on a pillow with her shoe off. Single-legged standing balance is not an easy task, and we added double-legged balance activities by having her kneel on a low, padded chair with the residual limb so that she could bear weight through both sides.

Despite her desire to reschedule her cruise, Ms. P. was very fearful of her condition and somewhat unsure about the wheelchair and its handling. Although she was independent on initial evaluation she was not judged to be very safe. She was observed to be negligent in braking the chair before transferring. To train safety in her wheelchair she did wheelchair obstacle courses within the house with transfers on and off different chairs as she passed them. This reinforced the need for braking as well as practicing transfers under variable conditions. One of her most frequent episodes of forgetfulness about braking the wheelchair was associated with helping herself to a snack from the refrigerator. She would wheel up to the refrigerator door, open it, stand up pulling onto the refrigerator, and, when she had selected her snack, sit back down too quickly.

While the PT worked in activities of this kind, the OT was working on ADLs from the wheelchair. Ms. P. learned tub transfers and independent bathing using a stool and hand-held shower; she learned to dress herself while on the chair and used her standing balance skills to complete dressing tasks, such as putting on underpants and doing up her skirt.

She began walking with a walker. This too was practiced over different surfaces, at different speeds, and in different directions—forwards, sideways, and backward. Standing tasks were added to her obstacle course. Outside walking was introduced as she became comfortable with the indoor environment.

Learning to get in and out of the house with a single guardrail is often challenging. Initially we turned her walker sideways (Fig. 6–7) and had her use the guardrail for support on one side and the walker for support on the other while her sister stabilized the walker.

Unlike Ms. R., Ms. P. needed constant challenge to her abilities. The variety of different surfaces was one of the main ways of achieving this during the preprosthetic phase. If we wait until the client has a prosthesis before walking her inside over different surfaces and outside over uneven surfaces, she develops an additional fear of the changed terrain as well as that of the new prosthesis.

Prosthetic Stage

Before she could walk independently using a cane, Ms. P. needed to become comfortable with her prosthesis in the home environment (Fig. 6–11). Initial balance exercises outside the walker needed to be introduced in a safe situation. We had her set the table for dinner, which involves sideways walking around the table with reaching activities. First, her sister would place all the items in the center of the table, and Ms. P. would reach forward for the items and then set them down in the places as required. The table was always in front of her for support should she need it, but she was discouraged from leaning against it as she reached to the center for each item.

For community access she needed to manage intertrial variability, so we introduced step training on a variety of steps—different heights, different surfaces, and so forth. (We carry some steps designed for this purpose in our cars. Some have wooden surfaces and other carpet. We use the home environment, which often offers quite hostile steps, such as those having narrow surfaces with cracks and high risers.) Going up steps, Ms. P. used a sound-leg lead pattern and learned to negotiate the steep ramp by walking up it sideways. Going down the ramp was accomplished by leading with the prosthesis.

If she was to go on her cruise, Ms. P. needed to be able to maintain balance with external perturbations such as happen with normal motion on the cruise ship. We used a balance and proprioception surface (baps)/rocker board for this purpose. These can be easily constructed for the home therapist on a low budget by sawing a croquet ball in half and screwing it to the bottom of an 18-inch diameter circle of 1-inch plywood (Figs. 6–12 and 6–13).

Ms. P. liked gardening and was eager to return to this activity. She did gait training over outside surfaces, which provided a closed environment with a great deal of intertrial variability. She walked over grass, pebbles, and concrete and brick surfaces, both wet and dry so we could evaluate her safety under different conditions. Because she did not like to kneel she was advised to use a low chair in the yard. This necessitated learning sit to stand from surfaces of different heights.

At discharge Ms. P. had rescheduled her cruise to take place in 3 months and was independent in and out of the house. She was ready to resume driving, having practiced backing up and driving forward within her driveway. She was referred to a local handicapped driver program. She was ready and confident about resuming community activities such as shopping.

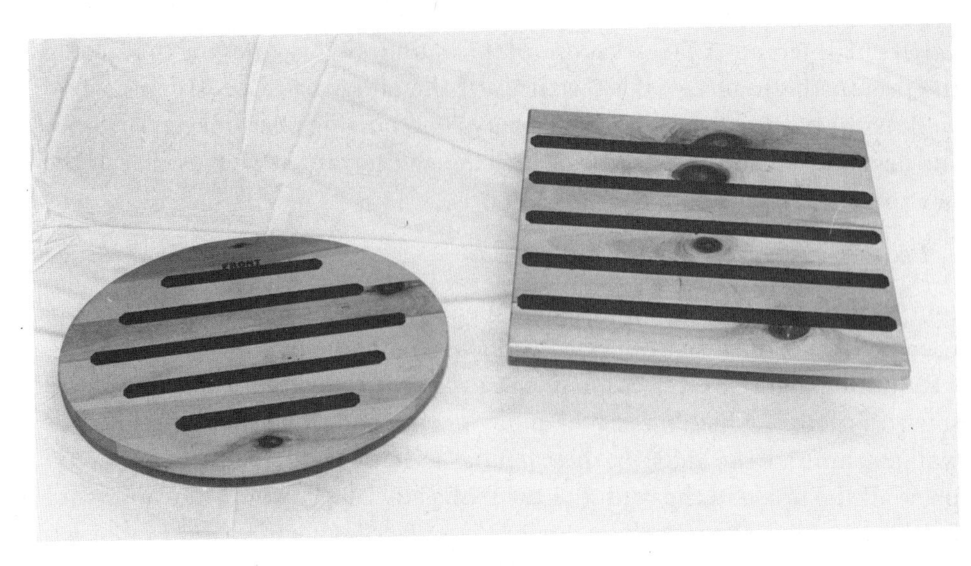

Figure 6–12. Home constructed baps and rocker boards.

SUMMARY

This chapter has stressed the importance of setting appropriate mobility goals and gearing mobility training to meet those goals. Within the case studies we have demonstrated the importance of involving the client and the family in the goal-setting process. While a rehabilitation program must often begin in a closed environment, to achieve maximum rehabilitation potential the program must progress to include performance in an open environment where appropriate. A home health therapist planning a treatment session in the home to include an open environment usually integrates the client's performance with the movement of others. In this setting the client must work at performing treatment activity while responding adaptively to the movement of others.

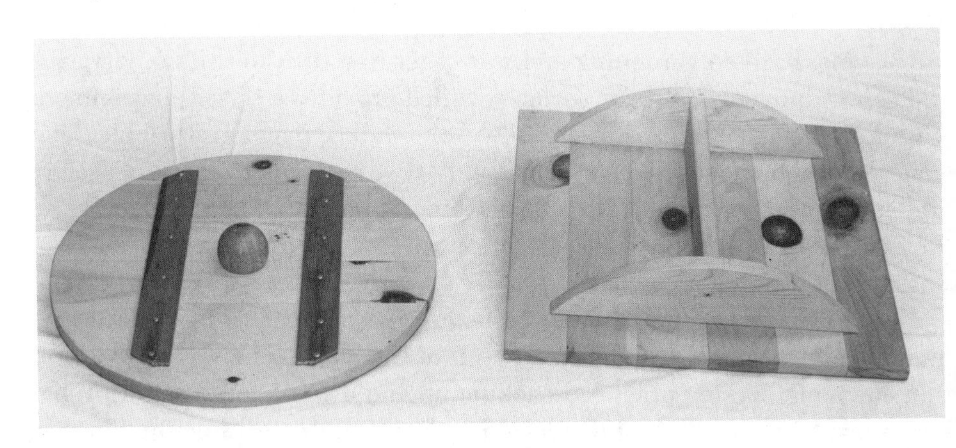

Figure 6–13. Underside of baps and rocker boards.

Teaching a client to perform in the community is complicated by the regulations governing home health care reimbursement from third-party payers. In general, coverage of home health treatment ends when the client can ambulate independently in and out of the house. Unfortunately, taking independent control of one's life involves transportation on busy streets and shopping in busy stores. To assist a client in achieving this level of independence, the home health therapist will probably need to refer the client to an outpatient rehabilitation program with a progressive community-based program.

REFERENCES

1. Gentile, AM: A working model of skill acquisition with application of teaching. Quest 27:3, 1972.
2. Schmidt, RA: Motor Control and Learning: A Behavioral Emphasis. Human Kinetics Publishers, Champaign, IL, 1982.
3. Gentile, AM: Skill acquisition: Action movement and neuromotor processes. In Carr, J and Shepherd, R (eds): Movement Sciences Foundations for Physical Therapy in Rehabilitation. Aspen, Rockville, 1987.
4. Poulton, EC: On prediction in skilled movements. Psychol Bull 54:467, 1957.
5. Foundation for Physical Therapy, Proceedings of the II Step conference, 1991, Alexandria, VA.
6. Fitts, PN and Posner, MI: Human Performance. Brooks/Cole, Delmont, CA, 1967.
7. Maring, JR: Effects of mental practice on rate of skill acquisition. Phys Ther 70:165, 1990.
8. Bonar, SK, et al: Factors associated with short- versus long-term skilled nursing facility placement among community-living hip fracture patients. J Am Geriatr Soc 38:1139, 1990.
9. Coughlin, TA, McBride, TD, and Liu, K: Determinants of transitory and permanent nursing home admissions. Med Car 28:616, 1990.
10. Magaziner, J, et al: Predictors of functional recovery one year following hospital discharge for hip fracture: A prospective study. J Gerontol 45:101, 1990.
11. Mayo, NE, Korner-Bitensky, NA, and Becker, R: Recovery time of independent function post-stroke. Am J Phys Med Rehabil 70:5, 1991.
12. Griffen, A: Personal communication.

Chapter 7

The Home Environment

BELLA J. MAY

Home health therapists function within the client's environment and are acutely aware of the influence of that environment on function. Reading the address, the therapist forms a mental image of the community in which the home is located. On arrival, the therapist becomes acutely cognizant of that environment and of areas that may either enhance or limit independent function. In a study of the effects of the environment on function, Lawton[1] suggests that an individual's behavior capabilities are affected by the personal, social, and physical environment as well as the biologic health, sensory-perceptual, motor skills, and cognitive capabilities and ego strength. Kahana[2] has developed a theoretic model to study the degree of compatibility between a person and the environment necessary for effective function. She suggests that the more congruence exists between individual needs and environmental factors, the more likely a person is able to function effectively. For example, an individual with a strong need for privacy would have difficulty living with the large family of a relative. Pastalan[3] theorizes on the effect of the shrinking environment of the elderly, suggesting that theory and research should focus on specific environmental needs. Faletti[4] reviews human factor research and recommends the study of specific task analysis in relation to environmental demands as a precursor to engineering and design changes.

CONTROL OF THE ENVIRONMENT

Control of one's environment, particularly if capabilities diminish with normal aging or disability, is a critical component of life satisfaction.[5–8] To what extent can the individual make and carry out the many decisions that are part of everyday living? To what extent does the client perceive the environment as supportive? The ultimate goal of our intervention is to help clients regain the highest possible level of independent function. Being able to control one's environment is critical to maintaining a sense of self-worth and independence. Helplessness in one area of function may spread to other areas. Most home health therapists have encountered the client with the physical capabilities for independent self-care who would not assume responsibility for such function while living in the home of a relative.

In a study of 280 elderly individuals 74 years of age or more, Wister[9] found that people tended to adapt psychologically to the situation in which they were rather than try to make major alterations or change their environment. Individuals living with a relative, for example, would indicate dissatisfaction with the living arrangement but would not attempt to investigate a change in domicile. Research further indicates that individuals may not be accurate in evaluating the physical conditions of their homes objectively and may not "see" such problems as peeling paint, cracks in linoleum, or broken furniture.[10,11] A review of all the research in human behavior and the environment is well beyond the scope of this chapter. However, expanding study in this area may help guide the home health therapist to better match individual client limitations with practical suggestions for environmental change.

THE IDEAL ENVIRONMENT

The ideal environment supports rather than restricts a person's daily life. It facilitates competence and satisfaction while allowing individuals to meet physical, psychological, and social needs. The ideal environment is safe, provides needed resources in close proximity, and meets the esthetic needs of each person.[12,13]

Safety

The safety dimension includes security of person, family, and belongings both in and out of the home. Personal safety in the neighborhood has been found to be positively related to life satisfaction.[7,12–17] An increasing number of elderly individuals are currently moving to metropolitan areas and experience safety concerns related to fast-paced city life and increased crime.[18] Others are remaining in older neighborhoods with changing socioeconomic conditions. Safety is an important consideration for the elderly, who are more vulnerable to falls and other environmental hazards. The National Safety Council estimates that 82 percent of fatal home falls happen to elderly people. Many physical therapists have treated individuals who broke their hips getting up in the middle of the night.[19] Recognizing and reducing environmental hazards is an integral part of the therapeutic process.

Resource Proximity

Proximity of resources includes the accessibility of services such as food and drug stores, banks, health care services, shops, restaurants, entertainment, and social supports.[12,13] Is the client able to function in the external environment and obtain necessary items independently? Are the resources within walking distance? Is there public transportation? Can the client use available transportation?

Esthetics

Esthetics refers to beauty, quietness, space, lack of pollution, and a desirable, pleasant atmosphere. Jirovec, Jirovec, and Bosse[16] report a direct relationship between the neighborhood and life satisfaction. In a study of elderly women living alone in San Francisco, Carp and Carp[13] report that esthetics was ranked higher in value than resource proximity as important to the ideal environment. Esthetics is a personal dimension and involves social, psychological, and cultural elements. While not directly amenable to intervention by the home health therapist, awareness of degree of satisfaction with neighborhood esthetics can be helpful in seeing the environment from the client's point of view.

ENVIRONMENTAL ASSESSMENT

Home health therapists are directly concerned with areas both inside and outside the domicile. Individual therapeutic goals affect the scope of the assessment as well as the recommendations. Is full recovery expected? Is balance expected to remain at least somewhat impaired? Has the client lost bilateral hand function? In all instances, the therapists considers safety, function, and practicality in assessing the environment and making recommendations for change. Environmental assessment is continuous process. The initial focus may be limited to those areas where the client is currently functioning, such as the home entrance, the bedroom, or the bathroom. Getting to and from the physician for recheck appointments may be a major hurdle in the early recovery period. As function improves, areas the client has learned to use, such as the kitchen, workroom, porch, or garage, must be assessed. Prior to discharge, assessment of any remaining internal areas and all external areas is necessary to ensure as full and normal function as possible. An environmental checklist can be a useful guide to ensure that nothing important is overlooked while providing a written record of problems and recommendations. Involving the client and family in the assessment is essential. Because no single environmental checklist will be equally applicable to all situations, different forms have been published.[20-23] I have adapted a sample environmental checklist from several sources (see Appendix 7–1); the checklist allows description of critical problems as related to the client's individual needs. The client's interaction with the environment is the focus of the home assessment so that the client's functional capabilities become an integral part of the total home assessment. Functional assessment is explored in detail in Chapter 4. The client and caregiver can often provide valuable information regarding areas of difficulty and potential hazards.

THE EXTERNAL ENVIRONMENT

The immediate external environment includes the entrances and exits in the home, the yard and parking areas if appropriate, and the immediately adjacent walking area such as a front sidewalk, driveway, or path. The focus of the assessment and related recommendations will differ if the home is located in a rural, suburban, or urban area, and if it is a freestanding house, an apartment, a single, or a multistory dwelling.

Assessing

Transportation

Considerations must be made for the type of usual transportation to and from the home. Is the automobile the main form of transportation in the community? If so, the assessment must include the client's ability to get in and out of a car, to drive or be driven, and to get to and from the car and the house. On the other hand, if public transportation is to be used, assessment will focus on the client's ability to get to and from the closest public transportation and get in and out of the conveyance. In situations in which the usual mode of transportation is no longer feasible, other arrangements may be necessary. In some communities limited transportation services are available for the elderly. The home health therapist must be aware of local community resources.

Around the Home

The home health therapist will check the accessibility and safety of the pathways around the major entrance to be used by the client. The assessment includes the type and condition of the surface, the distance from the arrival point, and the lighting. If the path and entrance to the home are not owned by the client and family, as with apartments, condominiums, and rented homes, making necessary changes may be more difficult.

Home Entrances

One entrance must be accessible to the client using whatever form of mobility aid is appropriate. Doors must open easily and smoothly and stay open until the client has entered safely. Elevator doors must allow the client time to enter, and adequate lighting is necessary. Clients must be able to lock and unlock doors without loss of balance. Assessment of the entrance itself includes the weight of the door, the width of the opening, the type and height of threshold, and the ease of keeping the door open while the client passes through it. A screen or storm door in front of the regular door (particularly if kept locked) creates an additional hazard to be overcome. Entrance steps, handrails, and the size of the porch are other considerations. Many recently built structures have handrails by the steps, but many older buildings, particularly in large cities, may not. The number and height of steps, their condition, and the presence or absence of a porch is assessed. The client may be able to get to the door but not have enough space to open the door after reaching the top step.

Adapting

Around the Home

Individuals living in rural areas face different problems from those living in urban areas. Parking areas, entrances, or walkways may not be paved or well graded. Pathways in and out of the home can often be made safer with some maintenance. Weeds can be removed from between paving stones, holes in dirt paths can be filled, some hilly paths can be graded down to a desired eight-percent level, and lighting can be installed if it is not already present. Paving stones can be purchased at most home repair stores and installed over dirt, gravel, or grass pathways. Paving stones must be close enough for easy stride lengths. Impediments such as trash cans, potted plants, or lawn furniture must be moved from direct pathways. Cleaning street debris may be necessary in city areas. Welcome mats may need to be removed from in front of doors.

Home Entrances

If the client is permanently limited in mobility, uses some form of external support or a wheelchair, or has impaired balance, a direct entrance from the path, garage or parking area is desirable. The most accessible entrance steps need at least one handrail with steps of no more than moderate height (6 in). In some instances a walker, stabilized by a family member, can serve as a temporary handrail (Chapter 6, Figs. 6–7 and 6–8), but in other instances solutions may be harder to find. Having one accessible entrance may pose major difficulties in rented homes or apartments.

Ramps are necessary for wheelchair access. Ramps must be sturdily built, with a grade of no more than 1 ft per 10 ft and preferably 1 ft per 12 ft, that is, 1 ft of height for every 10 or 12 ft of length. Figure 7–1 illustrates a

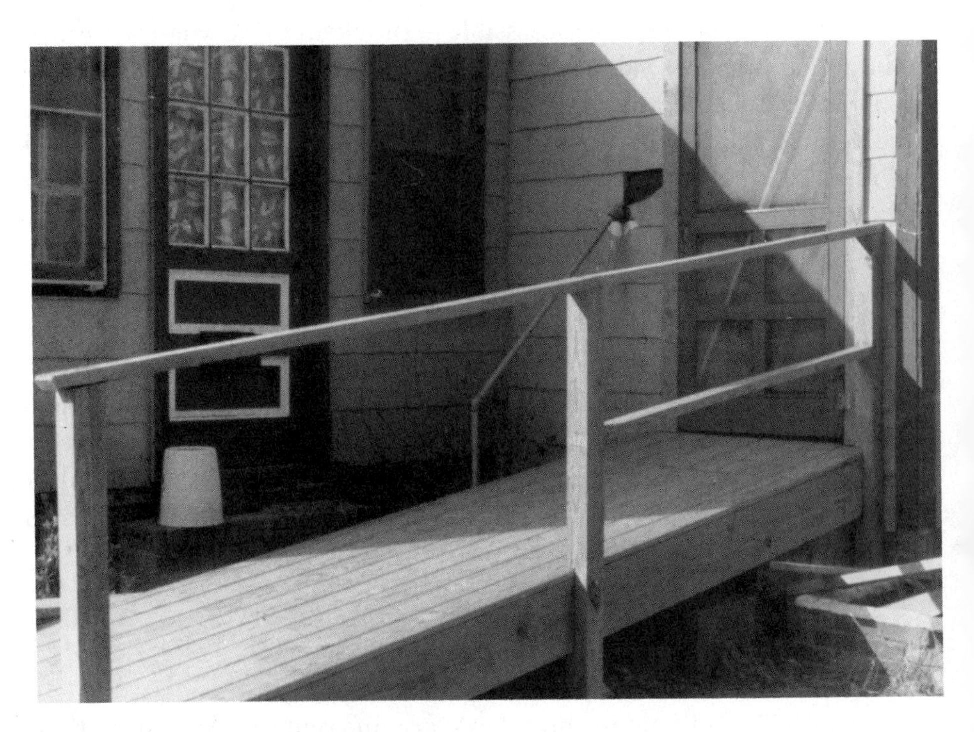

Figure 7–1. Family-built long ramp with one handrail.

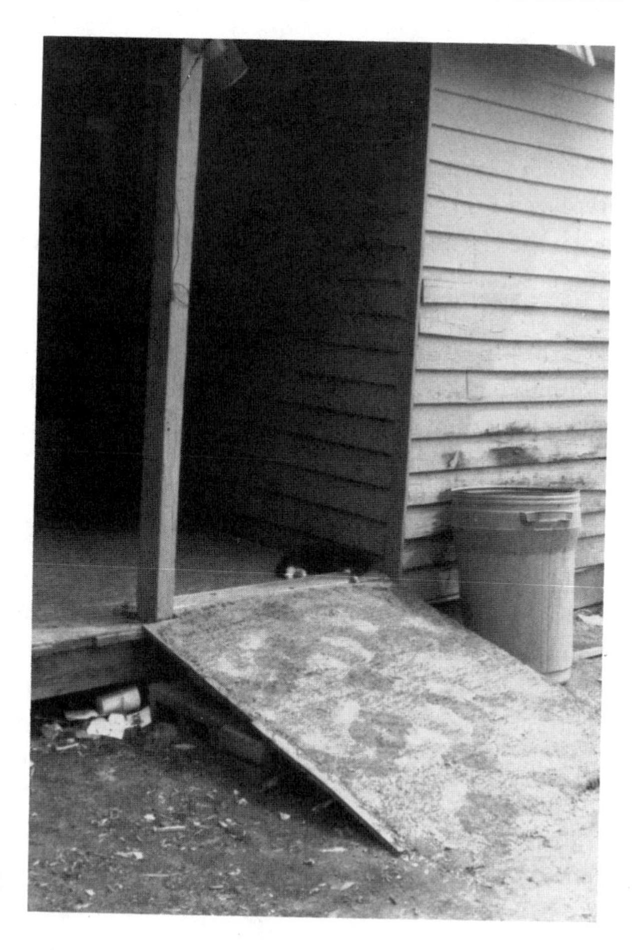

Figure 7–2. Family-built short ramp covered with carpeting.

family-built ramp of appropriate rise that would benefit from a second handrail and the addition of nonskid material on the surface. Figure 7–2 depicts another homemade rail with carpeting tacked on to provide a nonskid surface. Handrails on at least one side would make this ramp safer. Ramps take considerable space, which may not always be available. In such instances other alternatives may need to be found; this is not always easy. Portable ramps are helpful to wheelchair-bound individuals but may create as much of a hazard as steps do for ambulatory persons. Ambulatory individuals may need a handrail on one or both sides to safely maneuver up and down steps. In many communities, social organizations or church groups assist families in building a ramp or adding a handrail.

THE INTERNAL ENVIRONMENT

Assessing

Clients and families, particularly those who have been living in the same environment for a long time, like their homes as they are organized. The type and placement of furniture, locations of lights, and presence of scatter rugs are as much part of the esthetic quality of the home as the pictures on the walls and the presence or absence of plants. The therapist may find it difficult to dictate change. It is not unusual for a home health therapist to remove a scatter rug from the client's doorway on one visit just to find it replaced on the return visit. The therapist may be more successful working with the client and family to make the home safer and more functional rather than dictating changes. The therapist can highlight the difficulties and facilitate the client's or family's finding appropriate solutions. In some cases, the lack of physical or financial assistance may prevent implementation of recommendations. However, the therapist, consulting with the social worker, can often find resources to make the home more functional.

Furniture

Once inside, the client needs enough space to be able to move safely from one area to the other, using assistive devices if indicated. The family is the best source of information regarding usual pathways through the house. Crowding is often a problem, particularly when individuals have moved from larger to smaller residences, or when medical equipment such as a hospital bed and a commode have been added. Furniture may have sharp edges and there may be low tables with many objects (Fig. 7–3). Chairs may be too low or shaky and swivel rockers are unstable. The client may not be able to transfer from available furniture unaided. The type of seating may be important depending on the specific disability. Soft armchairs or recliners may

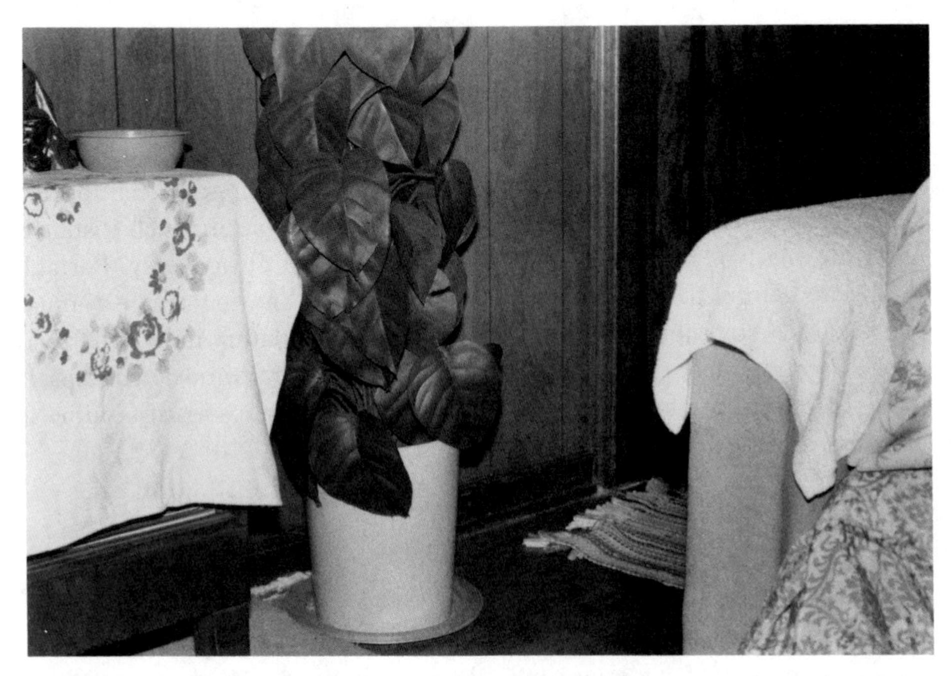

Figure 7–3. In this home, crowded with furniture, there is little room for a wheelchair or walker.

place individuals who have had a total hip replacement or hip fractures in a poor anatomic position. Clients who have sustained a stroke may be placed in a posteriorly rotated pelvic position. Clients with terminal bone cancer or osteoporotic compression fractures may not find adequate trunk support in their chairs.

Electrical Appliances and Outlets and Lighting

Many homes are dark; good lighting is necessary, particularly for older individuals who may have diminished vision. Note the clarity of lighting as well as the location of light switches and the number and placement of nightlights. The presence of smoke alarms and their functionality must be noted. Clients without smoke alarms should be advised to obtain them although finances may be a limiting factor in some instances.

Floors

Scatter rugs are a known hazard and therapists routinely request their removals (Fig. 7–4). Large area rugs can also cause a hazard because the client may catch a toe on the edge. The type of floor covering and its condi-

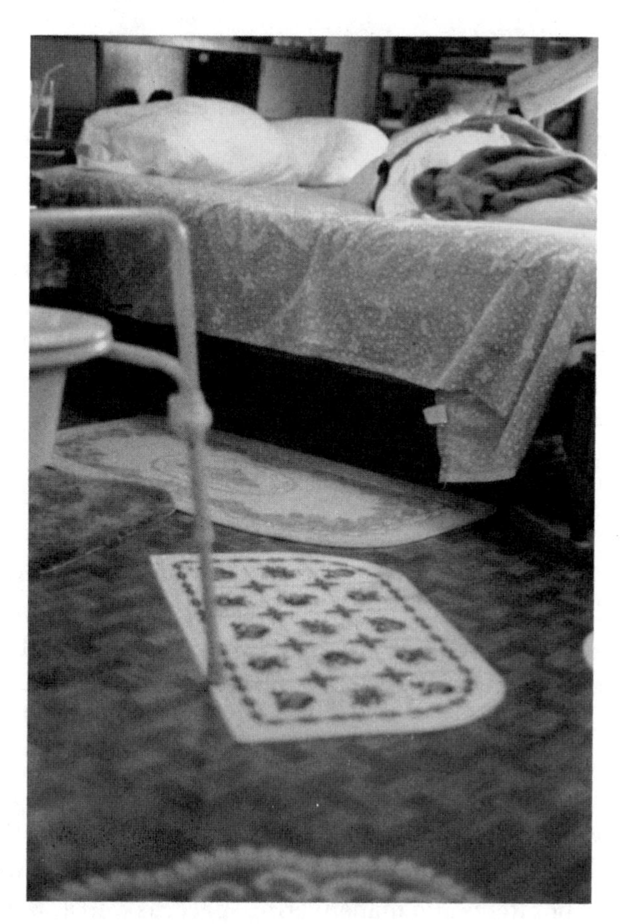

Figure 7–4. Scatter rugs pose a hazard.

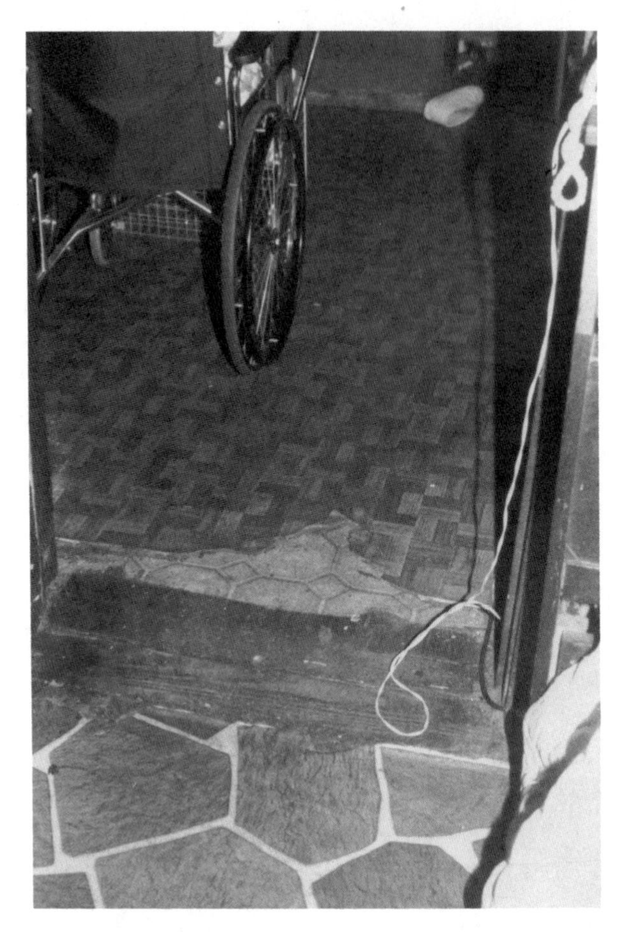

Figure 7–5. Electric cords and broken floor tiles present hazards to mobility.

tion is noted for each room. Carpeting may cause a problem if worn or too thick for safe walking or wheeling of a chair. Noncarpeted surfaces may create a hazard if slippery from waxing or wet or if tiles are broken (Fig. 7–5). Thresholds or small steps between rooms may be another hazard for clients with impaired balance or for those who may not lift the foot high enough or see well enough for safety.

Kitchen

Kitchens may present several difficulties, from high storage cupboards to low ovens. The assessment includes noting the type of stove (gas or electric), the location of the knobs, the accessibility of major appliances, and any restrictions to independent function.

Bathroom

The bathroom is traditionally poorly accessible to handicapped clients. The doors are usually not wide enough for wheelchairs or walkers, the tub is slippery and hard to enter, and the commode is low. Usability of major items and maneuvering space, as well as the presence of safety bars and the availability of special equipment, are noted in the assessment. It is also helpful to note the location and construction of towel racks, which clients often use for support. It is very important for clients to understand that most towel racks are not secure enough to be used for support.

Other Concerns

To achieve independence, clients must be able to go from one area of the home to another without difficulty. Note the width of hallways, the presence of stairs or single steps, any sharp corners, and clutter such as piles of newspapers or excess furniture narrowing passageways and creating hazards. The client's usual attire (e.g., shoes, long robes) and the presence or absence of obstructions on the floor (e.g., toys, electrical or phone cords, pets) must be noted. Clothing can create its own hazard—the long sleeve of a gown can catch fire dangling over a gas stove burner and house slippers may not provide adequate foot support. The regular availability of assistance in meeting daily needs, the client's premorbid independence level, and the anticipated recovery of function all contribute to the assessment formula. If the client lived alone before onset of disability and is expected to regain independent function, the home must support all required daily activities. If the client lived with a caregiver who usually did the cooking and cleaning, the assessment will focus on the client's usual activities. The home health therapist can often enhance the function of the caregiver as well as the client by sharing specialized knowledge in areas identified as problems.

Adapting

It is beyond the scope of this chapter to explore all possible environmental situations and provide suggestions for adaptions; rather, the reader can use general concepts and some examples for individual clients as desired. Environmental alterations and selection of adapted equipment are greatly influenced by the scope of the disability and by whether changes in function are expected to be temporary or permanent. Financial considerations are always a factor, since few pieces of adapted equipment and no home renovations are reimbursable under Medicare, Medicaid, and many private insurances. Knowledge of community resources, civic organizations, or church groups available to provide assistance is valuable information. Throughout the process, the home health therapist works closely with client, family, or significant others to help make the environment as functional as possible in as practical a manner as feasible.

If a major change in the home environment or a change of domicile is necessary, preparing the client gradually for the change and providing opportunities to investigate the new environment and alleviate anxieties will increase the likelihood of a successful outcome.[3] It will be easier for the client and family to consider environmental changes if some triage is done. Some changes can be considered critical to the client's basic ability to function safely in the home environment and rate the highest priority. Other changes may be necessary for independence in mobility and self-care but may not be critical to safety. Finally, some changes make everyday life easier but are not required for safety or basic independence.[22,23] The home health therapist may help the family set priorities for needed environmental changes, focusing initial activities on the most critical. It is recognized that not all environmental problems can be solved either through construction or through a change in the home. Conversely, the client or family may not choose to solve certain environmental problems for esthetic or economic reasons. Finally, the home health therapist must recognize that clients and families may not perceive environmental hazards as the therapist does. In such instances, the therapist can only advise and provide alternatives, documenting the recommendations.

Furniture

Too much furniture or clutter in rooms or major pathways is often a problem. Habit and esthetics as well as function must be considered when the therapist guides the family in rearranging the furniture. Wheelchairs and walkers require more room for maneuverability, which must be considered when rearranging furniture. The wheelchair or walker user needs approximately 3 ft of space to approach chairs or commodes or to turn in a semicircle. Sharp edges can be covered and small unstable pieces can be moved. Many chairs are too low for ease in rising and sitting. A pedestal can be built for the client's favorite chair at a height that will allow easier movement (Figs. 7–6A and B). Electrically operated chairs can raise the client to the

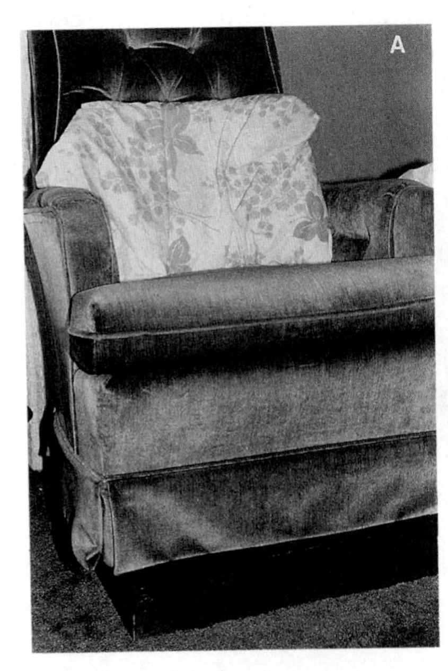

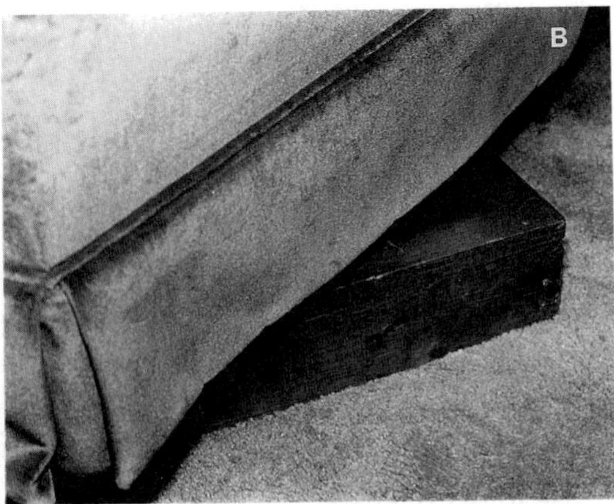

Figure 7–6A and B. A wooden pedestal raises the height of an armchair to permit easier rising and sitting.

standing position; but they are expensive and third-party payers may not reimburse for all diagnoses. Frequently chairs will need to be adapted with padding, pillows, or cushions for the individual client.

Beds may be too high or too low. A high bed may be cut to a more functional height; a low bed can sometimes be raised by placing bricks or paving stones under the feet. An electric hospital bed can be helpful, even on a temporary basis, for client and caregiver alike. Beds on wheels must be locked or stabilized against the wall. Sometimes the bedroom must be rearranged to allow easy access. Two-story houses or apartments may have all the bedrooms upstairs. If the client is unable to climb the stairs, a downstairs room will have to be adapted into a bedroom. If mobility is permanently impaired other living arrangements may be necessary. For the individual using a walker, steps present a considerable challenge. Inside the home the client may be able to obtain the necessary support with a cane and a handrail.

Electrical Appliances and Outlets and Lighting

Inadequate lighting, particularly for an elderly person whose vision may be impaired, is a major safety hazard. Not enough lamps and too low–wattage light bulbs contribute to the lack of adequate light. Night lights in bedrooms and hallways are a necessity; clients must be reminded to leave the lights on and replace the bulbs when they burn out. Sixty-watt bulbs are needed in most lights, with multiple-bulb lights for large areas. High-intensity lights are often useful for reading or close work. Make sure that the client is willing to use available lights and understands the importance of adequate lighting for safety reasons. Some individuals keep areas dark for economic reasons; other may not be able to tolerate bright light. Naturally, all electrical outlets, cords, and electrical equipment must be checked. Clients may overload outlets by plugging in too many cords. The local fire department is often willing to check a home for fire safety, and some social agencies will help elderly or handicapped persons make necessary changes. Lamp and appliance placement may lead to cords crossing pathways; electrical cords that cannot be moved can be covered with colorful tape to secure them and make their presence known. A cordless telephone can resolve the problem of telephone cords on the floor and provide easy accessibility to the client.

Floors

Floor coverings can present major safety problems. Scatter rugs are a disaster waiting to happen and must be removed; larger area rugs can sometimes be anchored securely with two-sided tape. It is a good idea to check the security of the tape regularly, since it may wear out over time. Thick plush carpets are an obstacle for both wheelchair-bound or limited-ambulatory individuals. Elderly clients do not always lift their feet high enough to clear a high pile or may feel unsteady on a plush surface. Sculptured carpeting, which is uneven, can also be a hazard. Sometimes plastic runners, well tacked down, can be used to cover thick carpeting, providing a better surface for wheelchair or ambulation. Linoleum or tile floors must be smooth and unbroken, but care must be taken on floors that become slippery when wet. Resolving floor covering problems is often very difficult because recarpeting a house can be expensive and individuals have strong opinions regarding what is esthetically pleasing. The bathroom is often a particular problem area because little bathmats are slippery and few people carpet their bathroom from wall to wall. However, a removable wall-to-wall bathroom carpet may be the answer to safety problems. The carpeting is large enough to be secure yet can be removed for cleaning.

Kitchen

Reachability and movability are the major problems in the kitchen. They can often be alleviated by appropriate adapted devices. A high stool is useful for helping a client sit while working at the kitchen counter. A wheeled cart helps move items from one part of the kitchen to another. Placing frequently used items in low cupboards or leaving them on the counter limits excessive reaching. Reachers and other adapted devices for the kitchen may help the client regain independence (see Chapter 8).

Bathroom

Rebuilding a bathroom is very expensive and usually not practical. Adapted equipment for the bathroom is discussed in Chapter 8.

Doorways

Most houses are not built for wheelchair access; doorways are often too narrow and maneuvering room is limited (Fig. 7–7). It is sometimes helpful to remove a door to provide additional space for wheelchair access. Equipment companies traditionally rent standard-sized wheelchairs with fixed arms; these are wider than narrow adult chairs with removable arms. Many clients can use the narrower chairs and need removable arms for safe transfers. The home health therapist must work with medical supply companies to obtain wheelchairs suitable for the particular home environment.

Other Concerns

A cluttered house can create a delicate situation. The home health therapist must find a way to suggest diplomatically that, for safety or ease of movement, the client get rid of items that may have accumulated over the years. Clients who live alone may not physically be able to clean house, get rid of clutter, or even move furniture. In some instances the home health therapist may have to guide the client to finding assistance with home chores or make a referral to a social worker. Some safety hazards can be created by the requirements of caring for a disabled individual, whether temporarily or not. The addition of a hospital bed can require moving of furniture and crowding of pathways. Sometimes bed linens are draped over the end of the

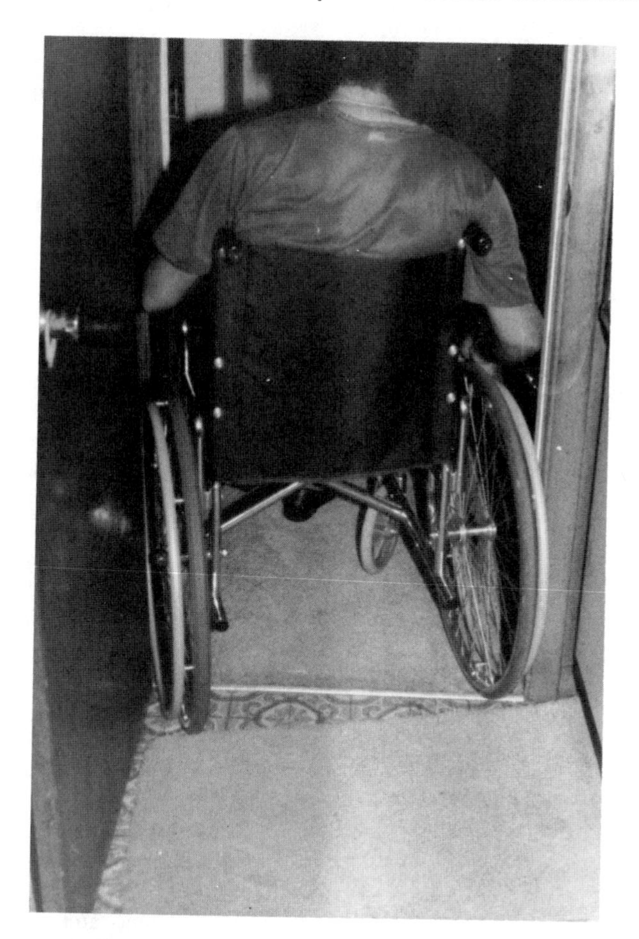

Figure 7–7. Small doorways limit wheelchair maneuverability.

bed onto the floor, creating a hazard for walkers and feet. Clients often prefer wearing house slippers, which are easy to put on, rather than well-fitting, supportive low-heeled shoes. Most third-party payers do not reimburse for shoes, and many home health clients do not have the resources to buy appropriate footwear. The advent of relatively inexpensive sports-type shoes has relieved the problem somewhat, but the client and family must be counseled about the functional value of obtaining properly fitted shoes. Often the home health therapist is the source of information regarding types of shoes and where they may be obtained.

SUMMARY

Home health therapists work within the client's functional environment, providing the opportunity to design the rehabilitative program around the client's specific needs. The environment is often not supportive and may actually deter functional independence. The home health therapist must be able to assess the environment, recognizing safety hazards and functional barriers and discriminating between possible and impossible changes.

Many factors affect clients ability to change their environment. Financial considerations, esthetics, resistance to change, and availability of assistance may all limit the possibility of change. The home health therapist needs flexibility and understanding to work with the client and family and to help them maintain cultural and esthetic satisfaction while reducing hazards and enhancing function.

REFERENCES

1. Lawton, MP: Competence, environmental press, and the adaptation of older people. In Lawton, MP, Windley, PG, and Byerts, TO (eds): Aging and the Environment: Theoretical Approaches. Springer-Verlag, New York, 1982.
2. Kahana, E: A congruence model of person–environment interaction. In Lawton, MP, Windley, PG, and Byerts, TO (eds): Aging and the Environment: Theoretical Approaches. Springer-Verlag, New York, 1982.
3. Pastalan, L: Research in environment and aging: an alternative to theory. In Lawton, MP, Windley, PG, and Byerts, TO (eds): Aging and the Environment: Theoretical Approaches. Springer-Verlag, New York, 1982.
4. Faletti, MV: Human factor research and functional environments. In Altman, I, Lawton, MP, and Wohlwill JF: Elderly People and the Environment. Plenum Press, New York, 1984.
5. Carp, FM and Christensen, DL: Technical environmental assessment predictors of residential satisfaction: A study of elderly women living alone. Research on Aging 8:269, 1986.
6. Langer, E and Rodin, J: The effects of choice and enhanced personal responsibility for the aged: A field experiment in an institutional setting. J Pers Soc Psychol 34:191, 1976.
7. Kiernat, JM: Promoting independence and autonomy through environmental approaches. Topics in Geriatric Rehabilitation 3:1, 1987.
8. Vallerand, RJ, O'Connor, BP, and Blais, MR: Life satisfaction of elderly individuals in regular community housing, in low-cost community housing, and high and low self determination nursing homes. Int J Aging Hum Dev 28:277, 1989.
9. Wister, A: Environmental adaptation by persons in their later life: Research on Aging 11:267, 1989.
10. Chen, A and Newman, S: Validity of older homeowners' housing evaluations. The Gerontologist 27:309, 1987.
11. Golant, S: Subjective housing assessments by the elderly: a critical information source for planning and program evaluation. The Gerontologist 26:122, 1986.
12. Yerxa, EJ and Baum, S: Environmental theories and the older person: Topics Geriatric Rehabilitation 3:7, 1987.
13. Carp, FM and Carp, A: The ideal residential area. Research on Aging 4:411, 1982.
14. Lawton, MP: Environment and other determinants of well-being in older people. The Gerontologist 23:349, 1983.
15. Ebersole, P and Hess, P: Mediators of personal security. In Ebersole, P(ed):Toward Healthy Aging: Human needs and nursing response. CV Mosby, St Louis, 1990.
16. Jirovec RL, Jirovec, MM, and Bosse, R: Environmental determinants of neighborhood satisfaction among urban elderly men. The Gerontologist 24:261, 1984.

17. Chapman, NJ and Beaudet, M: Environmental predictors of well-being for at-risk older adults in a midsized city. J Gerontol 38:237, 1983.
18. Golant, SM: The metropolitanization and suburbanization of the U.S. elderly population: 1970–1988. The Gerontologist 30:80, 1990.
19. National Safety Council. Accident Facts. Author, Chicago, 1983.
20. US Administration on Aging, Office of Human Developing Services, US Department of Health and Human Services. Home Safety Checklist for Older Consumers. US #475-981:32202, Government Printing Office, Washington, DC, 1985.
21. Tideiksaar, R: Falling in Old Age: Its prevention and treatment. Springer series on Adulthood and Aging. Vol 22. Springer-Verlag, New York, 1989.
22. Van Iderstine, C: Home environment analysis. In Scully, R and Barnes, ML: Physical Therapy. JB Lippincott, Philadelphia, 1989.
23. Schmitz, TJ: Environmental Assessment. In O'Sullivant, SB and Schmitz, TJ: Physical Rehabilitation: Assessment and Treatment, ed 2. FA Davis, Philadelphia, 1988.

Appendix 7–1

Home Safety Checklist

Type of home

House: Apartment: Single-level: Multilevel (elevator):

Multilevel (no elevator):

Urban: Surburban: Rural:

Outside the home

Pathway to client's primary entrance (describe key elements):

Outside steps: Handrail (Yes/no/side going up/down):

Entrance porch (yes:no): Describe entrance in relation to client needs:

Door(s) (describe lock, type and weight of door, presence of screen or storm door, height of doorsill in relation to client needs):

Other (describe any other critical items that may affect client independence):

Inside the home

Lighting:

Adequacy of overall lighting (describe):

Light switches easily accessible near all room entrances (list exceptions):

Nightlights in bedroom: Bathroom: Hallway:

Pathways:

Width of hallways: Bathroom door: Bedroom door:

Special problems (describe any hazards or specific needs):

Living areas:

Accessibility of chair or sofa (describe):

Accessibility of telephone: Television: Radio: Side table:

Special problems (describe any hazards or specific needs):

Dining area:

Space for client to get to and from table: Seating arrangements:

Kitchen:

Accessibility and usability (comment):

Stove: Refrigerator:

Sink: Cupboards:

Countertop: Table:

Floor covering (describe):

Special problems (describe any hazards or specific needs)

Laundry:

Laundry facilities in home (yes/no): Accessibility:

Bathroom:

Accessibility and usability (comment):

Bathtub:

Shower:

Toilet:

Sink:

Floor covering (describe):

Presence or absence of grab bars:

Special equipment:

Bedroom:

Accessibility and usability (comment):

Bed: Night table: Dresser:

Closet:

Special problems (describe any hazards or specific needs)

General Considerations:

Describe the floor covering in the various rooms noting problems or hazards (deep pile, scatter rugs, etc):

Describe any safety hazards in the home (frayed electrical cords, rough flooring, sharp furniture edges, crowded conditions):

Is the telephone accessible to the client for emergencies?

Can the client leave the home in an emergency?

Other:

Recommendations:

Please list any specific recommendations or suggestions discussed with the client and family:

Chapter 8

Adaptive Equipment for the Home

REBECCA AUSTILL-CLAUSEN

EQUIPMENT FOR THE BATHROOM
- Free-Standing Commodes
- Raised Toilet Seats
- Grab Bars for Toilet and Bath
- Bathtub and Shower Benches
- Hand-Held Showers
- Bathing Accessories

EQUIPMENT FOR THE KITCHEN
- Meal Preparation
- Utensils and Eating Implements
- Cooking and Dishwashing

EQUIPMENT FOR SELF-HELP
- Dressing and Grooming Accessories
- Household Cleaning
- Environmental Control Units

ADAPTING HOME FURNITURE

TELEPHONE, EMERGENCY SAFETY ALERT SYSTEMS, AND CALL BELLS
- Telephone
- Emergency Safety Alert Systems
- Call Bells

The home health therapist often uses a wide variety of equipment that is portable, lightweight, and typically inexpensive. Therapists frequently bring a sturdy bag or container filled with evaluation and treatment supplies into each client's home. Often items for treatment are obtained directly from the home environment, facilitating use due to the client's familiarity with the objects. There are thousands of commercially available therapeutic devices commonly obtained from medical equipment catalogues and/or the local home medical equipment (HME) store. The home health therapist can also become quite creative and make or instruct the family in designing homemade adaptive equipment.

The use of adaptive equipment should improve a client's functional ability in the performance of daily living activities. The physical characteristics of the client's disability must be considered along with the client's psychological, emotional, vocational, and cultural conditions, when the therapist recommends adaptive equipment. There must be mutual collaboration among the therapist, the client, and the client's family for equipment in the home to be used effectively.

Often the client is sent home with adaptive equipment from the hospital or rehabilitation center. The home health therapist's job is to evaluate the adaptive equipment within the home for appropriate use, care, and safety as well as to determine the need for other equipment. Hospital-based therapists usually do not have the advantage of visiting the client's home prior to discharge. Familiarity with the wide selection of adaptive devices is paramount to effective home health services.

This chapter provides an overview, rather than an extensive listing, of potential adaptive equipment for the home health therapist. Environmental control units and home safety are examined. Energy conservation issues are considered. There follows a section on obtaining adaptive equipment from HME stores, home health agencies, computerized information retrieval networks, and professional and disability-oriented associations. The chapter closes with a discussion of how to obtain reimbursement for adaptive equipment.

EQUIPMENT FOR THE BATHROOM

The bathroom is probably the most important area to assess during the therapist's initial visit.[1] Bathrooms can be filled with safety hazards. The use of appropriate equipment can reduce falls, facilitate safe transfers, and maximize independence.[2] A wide variety of tasks can be observed by asking the client to walk into the bathroom. Functional ambulation can be assessed along with the need for supervision, mobility devices, dressing and undressing instruction, architectural barriers, and bathroom equipment.

Free-Standing Commodes

Several issues are involved in choosing the correct commode. First, the home health therapist must determine that the client is unable to ambulate into the bathroom safely or fast enough to prevent "accidents." This situation could indicate the use of a freestanding commode. Next the therapist must determine the safety and independent maneuverability of the client's transfer onto a commode. If the client is unable to complete the transfer independently, a system must be immediately arranged for the client to contact the caregiver to facilitate the transfer. If the client can ambulate into the bathroom, a bedside commode may still be needed for nighttime. Positioning the commode to allow maximal transfer safety, especially in the dim nighttime light, is critical to the successful use of a freestanding commode. A freestanding commode should include a removable pail, a hinged cover, and adjustable-height legs positioned to fit the client's seat and leg length. A major problem for the home health client when using a free standing commode is ensuring that the commode pail is emptied. Determining who is to empty the pail (preferably not the client) and how the pail is to be removed (by lifting the pail up and sliding it to the side or rear of the commode) all must be considered when the commode is positioned. Emptying the pail at least once every 24 hours is highly recommended for sanitary reasons, but often elderly spouses or caregivers cannot safely lift a used commode pail due to its weight.

Families appreciate advice on reducing the bedside commode odor. Common all-purpose cleaners or baking soda can be placed inside the pail with a small amount of water to help mask the scent. There are also new disposable commode bag liners on the market called CareMate[3,4] that absorb urine by immediately forming it into a gel along with holding bowel movements. These bags can be easily removed from the commode, sealed shut, and thrown away in the trash. CareMate disposable liners eliminate the need for daily commode pail lifting and emptying, but cost becomes an issue since they are not usually covered by Medicare or insurance carriers.

Accessories for the commode include swing-away arms, drop arms, and a toilet paper holder that clamps onto the side of the commode legs. If esthetics are important or if there is limited space in the bedroom, furniture-style commodes are available. these look like a regular chair but have a seat that lifts up, exposing the commode pail.

Rolling commodes with four small wheels are useful if the commode must be frequently moved or used as a rolling chair. Self-propelled commodes with the large wheels in back can usually double as shower chairs (frequently called "wet wheelchairs") and are often used by clients with spinal cord injuries. Clients, families, and caregivers should *always* be encouraged to use the brakes when operating any rolling commode.

The "3 in 1" commode, sometimes known as the backless commode, can be extremely helpful for the home health therapist. Its three primary features include use as a commode, a bathtub seat, and a raised toilet set with arms. This portable commode fits directly over the toilet, has no back, and is often a very convenient way to raise the height of the toilet and include toilet arms without permanent installation (Fig. 8–1).

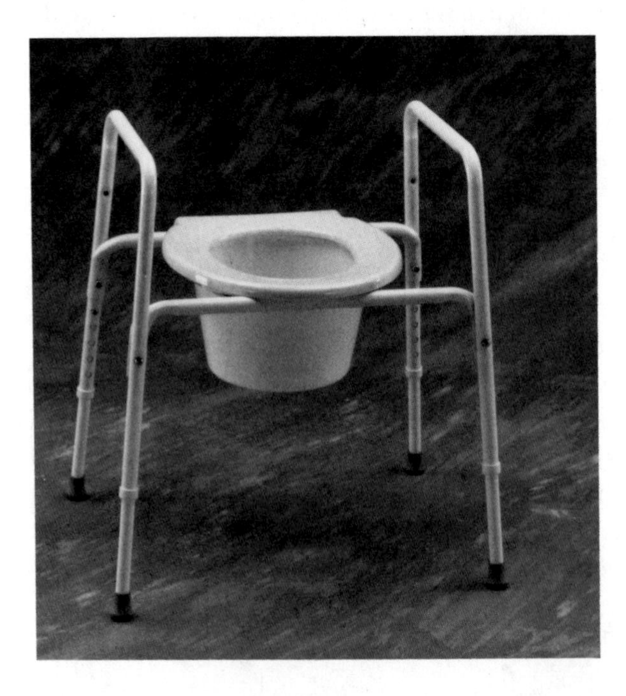

Figure 8–1. "3 in 1" commode. (Model #6476. Courtesy of Invacare Corp., Elyria, OH.)

Raised Toilet Seats

Clamp-on raised toilet seats are frequently used, especially during the first few months of a client's arrival home from the hospital or rehabilitation center. They are easy to install but, due to liability, it is highly recommended that the medical equipment dealer or family carpenter rather than the therapist install them. Padded seats are more comfortable, but overweight individuals often stick to the seat padding, possibly causing an unsafe rise from the commode. The firm seats are most commonly used and usually mimic the size and shape of a regular toilet seat. Raised toilet seat height varies between manufacturers. Therefore, the therapist must be aware of the ideal height for toilet use prior to ordering the raised seat, or, order an adjustable-height raised seat. Portable raised toilet seats are not usually recommended for daily use due to their light weight and instability, although they have been found to benefit frail elderly clients with arthritis. The portable raised seats are helpful for clients who travel (carrying cases are available) or for clients with only one bathroom, where the use of a clamp-on raised toilet seat would cause difficulty for other family members. Contoured portable seats are another possibility and are usually more comfortable than the portable flat commode seat. One of the main problems with using clamp-on raised toilet seats is that the cover of the toilet cannot be lowered. Esthetically, some families object to this "open air" concept. Another issue is that they are not easily removable. Raised toilet seats usually come with a splash guard inner liner that helps to keep excretions inside the toilet bowl. Separate raised splash guards that attach to the front of the toilet are particularly beneficial for male clients who must sit down to urinate.

Grab Bars for Toilet and Bath

Clamp-on raised toilet seats (Fig. 8–2) with safety rails attached are available. These seats are particularly useful for smaller-framed clients due to their narrow width. Otherwise, toilet safety rails can be mounted relatively easily to the rear of the toilet by sliding the rails through the back of the toilet seat cover hinge. Occasionally the hinges may need to be removed and replaced depending on the type of safety rail obtained. Clients should be instructed in the appropriate use of toilet seat rear-mounted grab rails because the rails are not attached to the floor and can lift up; clients must be advised to exert firm *downward* pressure when using them. Again, to avoid liability problems installation should be by the HME dealer or family carpenter rather than the therapist.

Grab rails can be permanently mounted to the wall beside the toilet or on the bathtub wall. Often grab rails with a knurled surface provide a more supportive handgrip, particularly when hands are wet from a bath or shower. Grab rails come in various lengths (some adjustable) and can be placed horizontally, vertically, or in an L shape. The therapist should instruct the in-

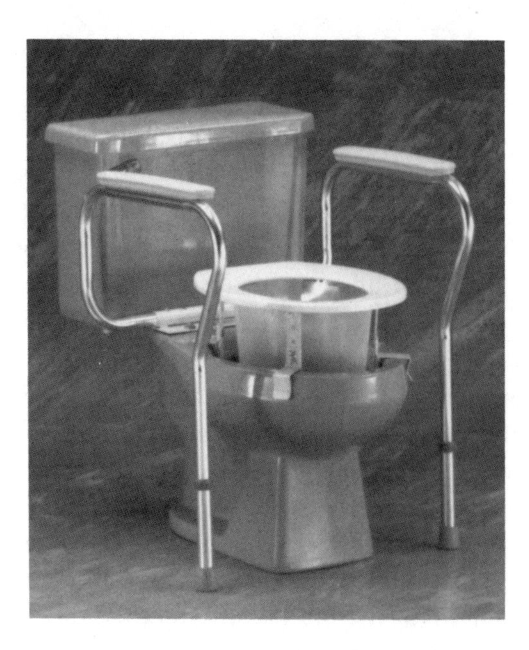

Figure 8–2. Clamp-on raised toilet seat (Model #1396) and toilet safety rails (Model #1392). (Courtesy of Invacare Corp., Elyria, OH.)

staller clearly regarding the exact height and location for the rails, and may even want to draw a diagram on the wall so that placement can be exact. If a client lives in a rental property, wall-mounted grab bars may not be feasible. Approval from the property owner is required before a permanent attachment can be installed. Some homes have preformed fiberglass bathtub frame walls; grab rails cannot be easily attached to these walls because they will crack the fiberglass. Using floor-to-ceiling poles, with a horizontal or triangular bar for grasping, is often an appropriate substitute. Mounting grab bars onto the bathtub is another option. Easily installed, tool-free grab bar tub clamps are available (Fig. 8–3). Home health therapists should impress on client and family that towel rails are *never* to be used for transfer assistance due to their instability.

Bathtub and Shower Benches

A wide variety of bathtub benches are available. One of the most common is made from lightweight plastic, has a seat with small perforations to assist drainage, offers adjustable height legs (ranging from 14 in to 21 in), and comes with a seat back option (Fig. 8–4). The seat back is often indicated for safety reasons, although overweight people tend to be pushed too far forward when using the bench back.

Transfer tub benches assist the client who must sit down to transfer into the bathtub. The benches have either a padded or a smooth seat. Padded benches (Fig. 8–5) are comfortable but large and bulky. Both seat benches provide a firm and safe surface for the client to sit down outside the tub before sliding over to the middle of the tub. Clients must be able to lift their legs over the tub wall (or have someone assist them) when using the transfer tub

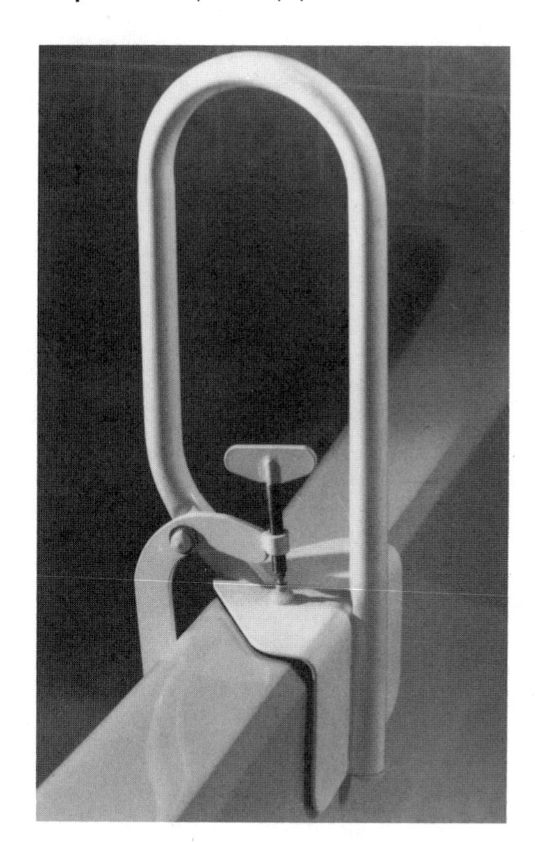

Figure 8–3. Easy-on bathtub safety rail (Model #6961). (Courtesy of Lumex, Inc., Bay Shore, NY.)

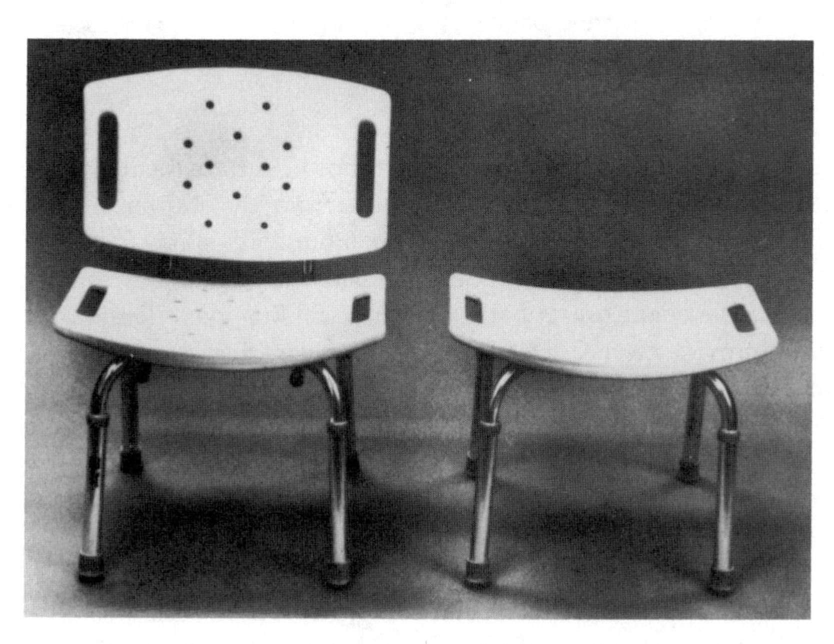

Figure 8–4. Adjustable height bathtub bench (Model #32-GF-1993). (Courtesy of Temco Health Care, a Graham-Field Company, Hauppague, NY.)

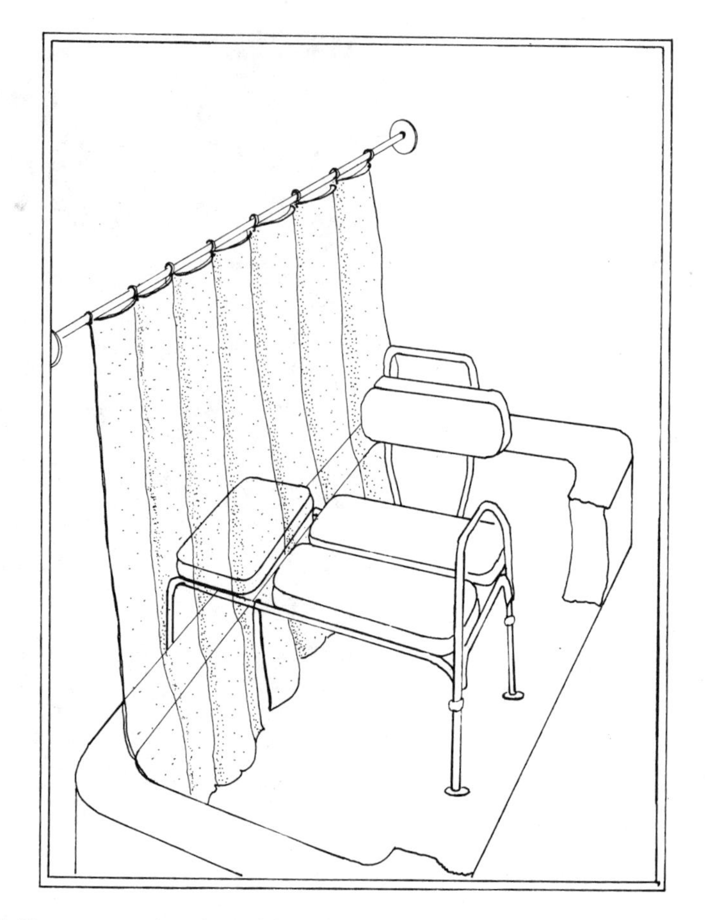

Figure 8–5. Shower curtain adapted for use with a transfer bathtub bench. Two slits in the curtain at the points where the seat rails cross the tub wall allow the closed curtain to remain completely inside the tub. The padded transfer bench, which has suction cup footpieces, is Model #98014, available from Guardian Products, Inc., Arleta, CA. (Illustration by Marina Gresham, Phoenixville, PA.)

benches. Two small slits can be made in a shower curtain to allow the bench legs to be placed through the curtain; otherwise the shower curtain goes around the outside of the tub and water often spills out.

Tub showers that have sliding glass doors are often problematic, particularly if the client uses a bathtub bench. Sliding glass doors can be removed to provide more space for transfers or a caregiver's assistance. Installation of a wall-mounted grab bar to facilitate a safe transfer is usually necessary. If it is not agreeable or practical to remove the shower door, it may be necessary to cover the water spout with a heat-resistant rubber cover (frequently obtainable in the children's section of department stores) because limited space is available for transferring between the sliding glass door and the wall faucet. Adhesive safety treads on the bottom of the tub help reduce slippage. Many apartment and rental complexes will not allow safety treads to be affixed due to the difficulty of removal. In these cases, use a long rubber mat. Mats should be replaced every 1 to 2 years because the adhesive quali-

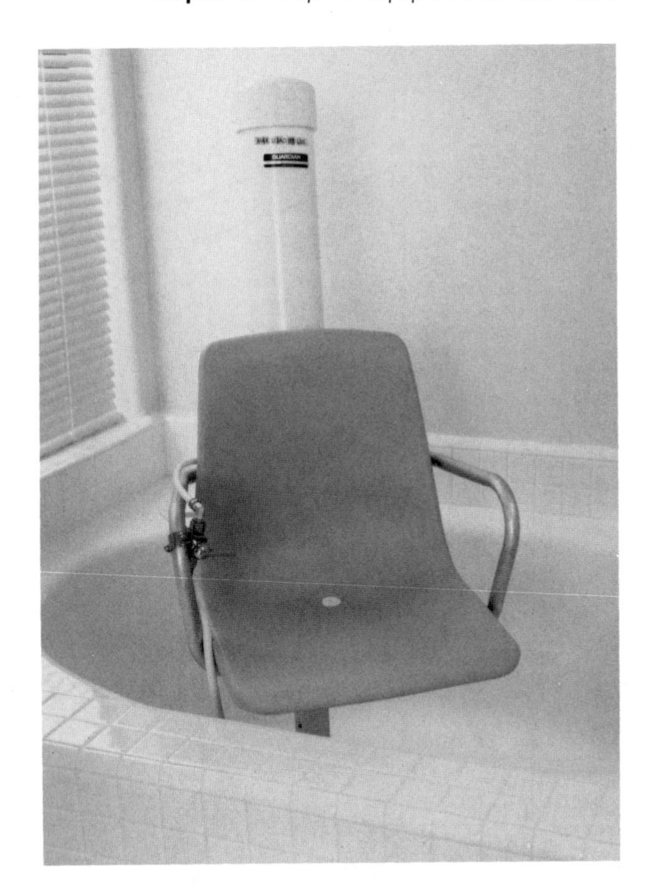

Figure 8–6. Bathtub hydraulic lift seat (Model #040-0117 AC). (Courtesy of Guardian Products Co., Inc., Arleta, CA.)

ties diminish with age. For clients who want to sit down in the tub, a bathtub hydraulic lift seat, although costly, is very helpful (Fig. 8–6). The swivel seat option is highly recommended because it allows the client to swivel the seat perpendicular to the outside of the bathtub, sit down, and then swing the legs over into the bathtub. Without the swivel option, the client must climb into the tub first and then sit down on the hydraulic seat. The hydraulic lift enables the client to raise or lower the seat according to the amount of water in the tub.

Hand-Held Showers

Most individuals using a bathtub bench could benefit from a hand-held shower to facilitate independent showering skills. This portable aid is available from medical equipment companies, local retail shops, and hardware stores. There are three primary types of hand-held showers. One (usually made from rubber) attaches to the water faucet and can be easily removed. The second connects to the side of the shower head with a diverter valve, available from most hardware stores (Fig. 8–7). With the diverter valve other family members can use the regular shower head by turning a little switch on the valve. The third type uses a flexible extended cord, al-

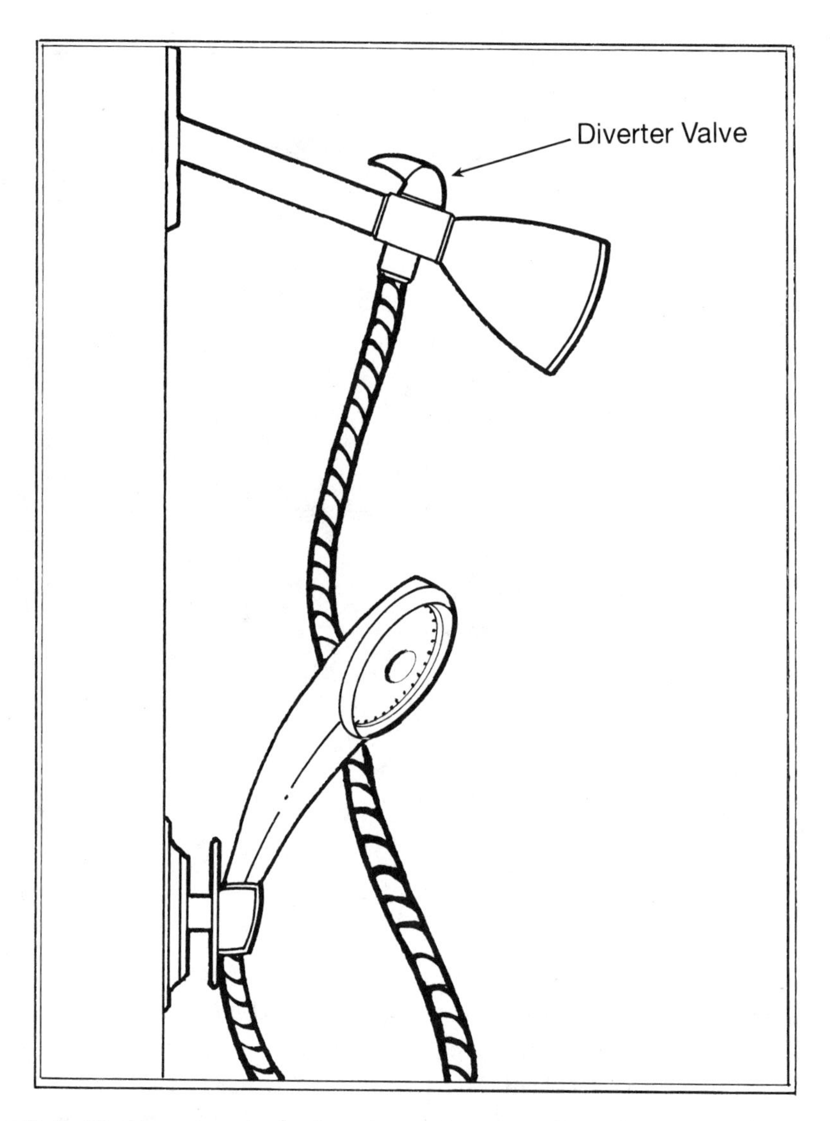

Figure 8–7. Diverter valve attached to shower head and hand-held shower hose. (Illustration by Marina Gresham, Phoenixville, PA.)

lowing the device to act as a regular shower head or be lifted out of its holder and used as a hand-held shower.

Therapists often recommend that a plumber or family member lower the client's water thermostat below 120° to prevent scalding, particularly if the client has sensory deprivation. It also may be advisable to cover the water faucet and handles with a non–heat-conducting substance, again, for clients who lack temperature sensitivity, particularly in older homes where the faucets heat up. Using a tap turner or reacher to turn on faucets can help, but these often are too clumsy or time-consuming for clients to use readily.

Bathing Accessories

Long-handled sponges, bath mitts, back brushes, reachers, and shoe horns covered with washcloths for toe cleaning can all be attached to the bathtub side walls with suction cups for easy accessibility. Clients unable to wash their hair in the bathtub or shower can use a wheelchair shampoo tray or inflatable shampoo basin, available from adaptive equipment catalogues[5-8] or local medical equipment suppliers.

EQUIPMENT FOR THE KITCHEN

Meal Preparation

Many disabled homemakers will require training in kitchen independence. Kitchen activities can be easily graded to allow for maximal independence in a safely adapted environment. Initially, a homemaker can be taught to sit in a chair at the kitchen table, slide the wheelchair under the kitchen table, or use the wheelchair lap tray. One of the most common and useful kitchen adapted devices is the cutting board (Fig. 8–8) with one to three galvanized (or aluminum) nails protruding from the middle of the board and an L-shaped plastic corner guard. One-handed homemakers use the galvanized nails, which do not rust, by placing vegetables (potatoes, carrots, cucumbers, etc.) on the nails to stabilize them for the one-handed cutting motion. The cutting board corner guard conveniently stabilizes bread for spreading butter or jam. These cutting boards can be homemade by the therapist or the client's family. Clients can purchase kits to use with their own cutting boards, or completely designed cutting boards can be purchased from adaptive equipment supply catalogues.[5-7] Suction cups placed under kitchen items, and Dycem[5-7] nonslip plastic mats, are excellent stabilizers for kitchen activities.

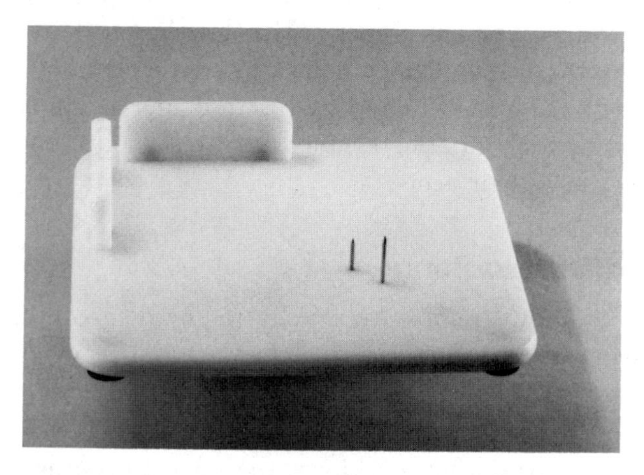

Figure 8–8. Adapted cutting board (Model #BK3099). (Courtesy of Fred Sammons Inc., Grand Rapids, MI.)

Many adapted kitchen tools are available. They include jar openers, one-handed electric can openers, lightweight plastic milk carton holders with a handle for easy carrying, and lightweight one-handed beaters. The list is almost endless. Each kitchen training session should include an evaluation of the basic kitchen skills. A client's inability to open the refrigerator door could necessitate the use of a door pulley system. Mixing bowls may need to be placed in an accessible open drawer that closes onto the bowl to allow stabilization. Clients can transport objects around the kitchen using aprons with pockets, walker baskets (be careful about overloading the baskets, thus tipping the walker forward), or sturdy rolling carts with a handle. Kitchen implements should be located in easily accessible drawers, and cabinets should be low enough for safe opening, reaching, and removal of articles.

Utensils and Eating Implements

Eating utensils can be quickly adapted by wrapping masking tape around the handles to increase their width, gradually reducing the size until the manipulation of a regular-width utensil is possible. The taped utensils can be washed and often last 7 to 10 days before requiring rewrapping. Commercially available black or white foam,[5-7] customarily in 36-in lengths, with various widths and a hole down the center, is also appropriate for expanding the width of kitchen utensils, pens, knives, and so forth. Hardware stores sell this foam for refrigerator coil covers. The foam part of old-fashioned hair rollers can be used easily and inexpensively to expand utensil width. Featherweight utensils with built-up handles are available from medical equipment catalogues along with swivel, weighted, offset, extended-length, and rubber-coated utensils. Handled cups, straws, rocker knives or pizza cutters, divided plates, scoop dishes, plate guards, and drinking straw holders can all be manipulated successfully by the homebound client. Often a wet towel or Dycem[5-7] can be placed under a plate to reduce slippage. High-technological equipment — such as the electric Winsford Feeder[9] (Fig. 8-9) with its automatic spoon movement, chin switch, remote-control hand and foot switch or headrest switch, plate rotation, and height adjustment is often prescribed by rehabilitation centers but can benefit home health care clients unable to use their arms.

Cooking and Dishwashing

Several therapy sessions are usually required to completely assess cooking and dishwashing safety in the kitchen. An important area to evaluate is oven and stove knob placement. If the knobs are not located at the front of the stove, the therapist *must* advise the client to wear close-fitting sleeves (not long, flowing sleeves) when working at the stove. Encourage the client to use primarily the front two burners for safety. Knob turners or reachers to turn on stove and oven knobs are difficult to manage but are a possibility.

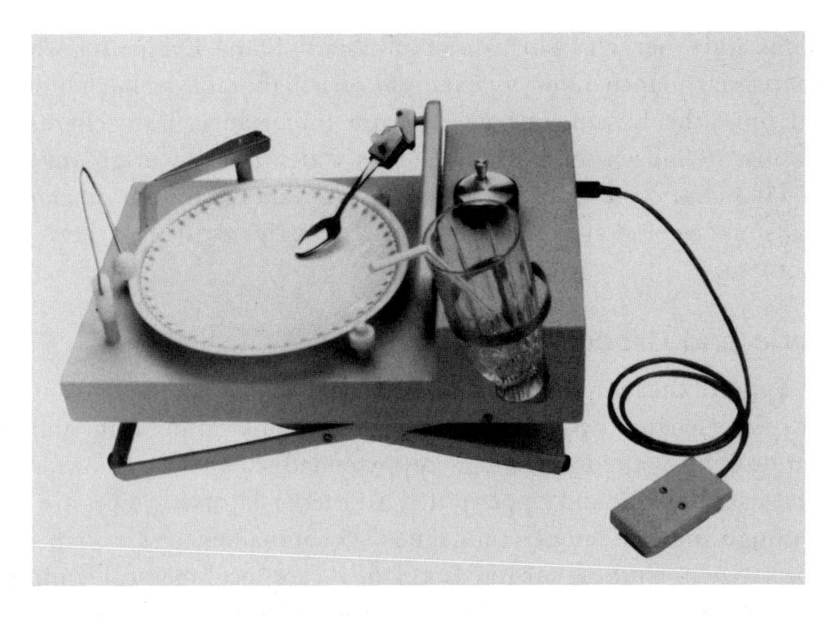

Figure 8–9. The Winsford feeder. (Courtesy of Winsford Products, Inc., Pennington, NJ.)

Placing "beads" of a substance called Hi-Marks[10] on the stove knobs can help the visually impaired client feel the knob gradations. Positioning an angled mirror strategically above the stove can help the client in a wheelchair see into the stovetop pans, although clients with perceptual impairments may have difficulty with this concept. Long-handled utensils are a safety feature appropriate for most disabled homemakers. Oven mitts are commonly recommended, but their bulkiness can detract from their effectiveness. Microwave ovens are helpful for many homebound clients. However, therapists should be very careful when assessing a clients's operating skill and ability to safely move items in and out of the microwave.

Washing dishes can often be easily accomplished by cutting out the area under the sink and padding the drainpipes with insulated covers, allowing the wheelchair user safe and close access to the sink. Other techniques include placing dishes on an overturned dishpan to raise the height of the washing surface, using bottle brushes for one-handed function, and using tap turners for the faucet. Round lazy susan shelves, particularly in corner cabinets, help with kitchen storage accessibility. One-handed jar openers can be fitted under a kitchen shelf, and a pegboard can be placed on an accessible wall to store kitchen utensils for clients with reaching problems.

EQUIPMENT FOR SELF-HELP

Most therapists are familiar with the adaptations available for self-help tasks such as dressing, grooming, and household cleaning. A main concern for the home health therapist is assessing the actual process of dressing, grooming, and other self-help tasks in the client's home. Evaluating where to place necessary adaptive aids, for example, on a night table stand, hanging by the bed, or on the dressing chair, is of prime importance. Many clients need specific instruction on the best location in which to dress or groom themselves. They may have learned the techniques in a rehabilitation center or hospital but need assistance individualizing the skills to their home environment.

Dressing and Grooming Accessories

Some of the more common dressing devices include the dressing stick with a rubber-coated hook and a small metal hook on opposite ends of a wooden dowel, sock aids; elastic laces; extended shoehorns; front fastened bras that use Velcro™; and zipper pulls. All these adaptive devices are available through medical supply catalogues,[5–8] companies, and organizations that specialize in clothing for the disabled,[11–13] or local medical equipment stores. Useful grooming devices include toothpaste tube squeezers, stabilized nail clippers, electric razors, and make-up kits with dividers and elevated sections. Universal cuffs[5–7] allow long-handled items such as toothbrushes, combs, or hair brushes to be placed in the palm cuff pocket, thus assisting clients without sufficient grasp. Mirror accessibility may require the placement of a portable mirror at a lower height in the bathroom. Usually wall-hung mirrors can be adapted easily for wheel-bound clients by lengthening a wire in the back of the mirror, allowing the top of the mirror to tilt downward. Clients can then look up into the mirror and see themselves. A portable lighted vanity mirror can also be used.

Household Cleaning

Long-handled dustpans, made by attaching a dowel to a dustpan handle, can assist with housecleaning chores. Long-handled brooms, mops, and dusters can effectively reduce the need to bend and assist the client in a wheelchair. Assessing the laundry system and recommending energy-saving techniques such as the appropriate-height shelves, handled soap containers, and front-loading washers and dryers can often be of major assistance to the disabled homemaker.

Environmental Control Units

Severely disabled clients often benefit from environmental control systems. These self-activated controls allow independent access to the telephone, television, radio, bed controls, lights, and other electrical appliances (Fig. 8–10). Control can be activated by the client's voice, a chin switch, a pneumatic sip and puff switch (Fig. 8–11), a light-touch switch, or one-step or two-step motion switches.[14–17] Less sophisticated environmental control units can be purchased from local electronic stores and allow independent

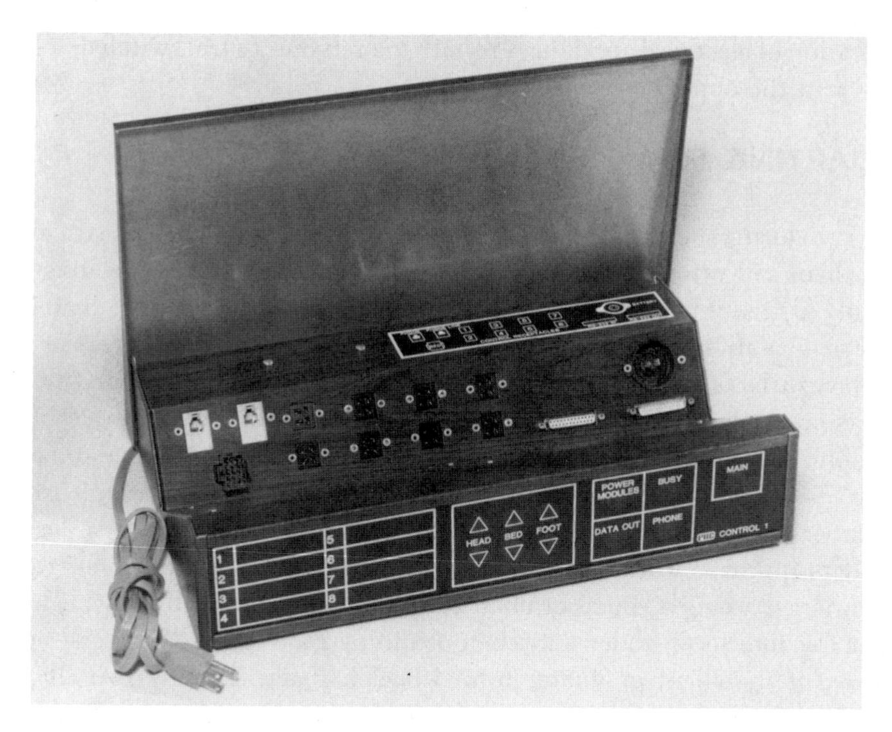

Figure 8–10. Environmental control unit (Model #CTRL-1 of CMS-2). (Courtesy of Prentke Romich Company, Wooster, OH.)

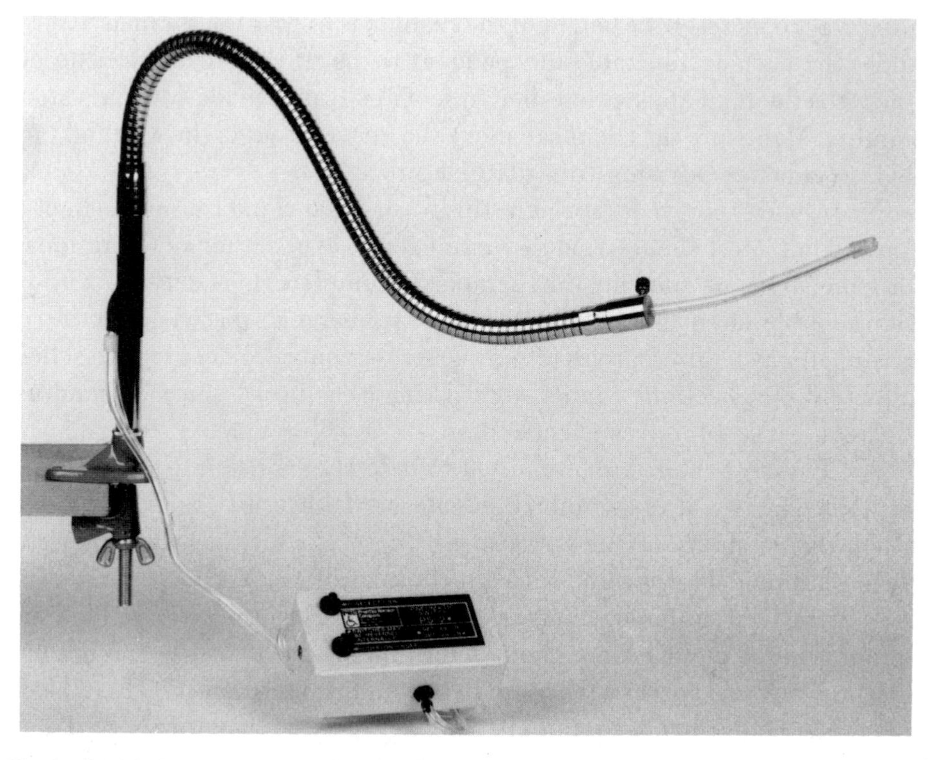

Figure 8–11. Pneumatic sip-puff switch (Model #PS-2) and Table Switch Mounting Kit (Model #SMT). (Courtesy of Prentke Romich Company, Wooster, OH.)

operation of electrical appliances by either a remote control switch or a light touch to the appliance.

ADAPTING HOME FURNITURE

During the initial therapy visit, it is extremely helpful to learn about the client's favorite sitting spots. If a couch or chair is too low, encourage the family to raise it by placing bricks or a wooden platform under the chair legs. A strong caution is needed here: the couch may slide if only bricks or flat-topped surfaces are used. It is safer to place sturdy molding around the leg risers or to place the legs in an appropriate-sized hole in a wooden block. Chapter 7 illustrates a pedestal for raising the height of a living room chair (Fig. 7–6). Commercially available chair leg extenders are available from a number of manufacturers and adaptive aid catalogues.[5-7] These leg extenders appear to work best with small-width kitchen-type table legs rather than larger wooden couch or chair legs. Extenders can allow a wheelchair user freedom to fit under a kitchen or dining room table. They can be removed if the client graduates from wheelchair use. Placing two chair or couch cushions under the client rather than only one can help a client who has difficulty rising from an overstuffed couch or chair. The bottom cushion may need a nonslip rug mat, available in local retail stores, placed on top to prevent the higher cushion from slipping as the client attempts to rise. Another way to increase the height of the cushion is to position a folded blanket under the cushion to enable independent rising. If the client's feet do not touch the floor, an appropriate-height footstool can provide adequate ankle stability. Make sure the client can move the footstool out of the way and then replace it before advising this adaptive procedure.

Always remove lightweight throw rugs that could cause the client to slip and fall. Most clients need a firm but gentle explanation of the rationale for removal before allowing the therapist to complete this safety precaution. Using double-faced adhesive carpet tape or rubber mats placed under the rug or runner may be alternatives to complete rug removal. Encourage the client and family to check the rubber rug backing periodically since constant use can reduce the adhesives effectiveness.

Easy-lift chairs are often used to help clients rise from their sitting position. The two most common types of electric easy-lift chairs are those in which the whole chair tilts forward and those in which just the chair seat rises. Both models also come with a reclining feature. Asking the manufacturer or medical equipment store representative to bring out a chair for a trial period prior to purchase may help determine if the client has enough balance, control, and space in the room to benefit from the easy-lift chair. However, these chairs do not commonly allow full knee flexion; therefore, a daily home exercise program with good knee flexion exercises is often indicated.

Doorknob extenders made out of rubber or lightweight metal are available for clients with limited wrist mobility, such as those with arthritis, or for clients in a wheelchair with limited reach. The doorknob extenders can be easily installed by a family member.

TELEPHONE, EMERGENCY SAFETY ALERT SYSTEMS, AND CALL BELLS

Telephone

During the first few days home, homebound clients are not often able to stay alone. Those who do live alone need an emergency safety system. The easiest, most accessible communication system is a telephone. The home health therapist must evaluate the location and accessibility of the telephone along with the client's ability to use it effectively. Often a telephone must be repositioned and placed directly beside the client's bed, with the therapist determining the more functional side for placement. After evaluating the client's ability to use the telephone, take care to place all telephone wires under rugs or beside walls, or tape them to the floor, to reduce the chance of a client or caregiver tripping over them.

The client or caregiver should complete a list of emergency and other important telephone numbers (police, fire, neighbor, family, poison control center) to place beside the telephone. The list should be printed in large letters in black ink on white, or preferably yellow, paper; visually impaired clients often see better the contrast between black ink and yellow background paper.[18] The list should be placed at all telephones and at an appropriate height for immediate use.

Replacing a rotary-dial with a pushbutton telephone helps with efficiency and assists the homebound client with energy conservation. A touch-dial telephone, commonly called a "memory phone," is an excellent safety idea. Usually a telephone with about nine numbers coded into memory is sufficient for the homebound client. The family members or caregivers will need to program the important numbers into the telephone, and the therapist can help teach the client how to access the numbers. Evaluating the client's ability to understand which button corresponds to each name coded into the memory is required before ordering memory phones. Often the space for writing the names beside the buttons is very small. The writing may need to be enlarged so that the elderly client can see readily. Again, using black ink on white or yellow paper helps with the visual contrast. Cordless memory phones that attach to a client's belt or can be placed in a pocket are often an efficient safety and communication system.

Emergency Safety Alert Systems

Emergency call systems are beneficial and usually are available through the social service departments at the local hospital or rehabilitation center. The user operates the emergency system wearing the alarm strap or button around the wrist or on a chain around the neck. Pressing the call button alerts the local hospital, police, ambulance, or whomever the call system designates to send help. It is most important for the client to wear the emergency call system at all times and to place it in an accessible location while bathing; otherwise effectiveness is negated.

Call Bells

For homebound clients who have a caregiver or family member living with them, a daily alert system should be established. Often small handbells or portable doorbell systems placed beside the bed can be rung when the client needs assistance. Other systems include portable electric or battery-operated nursery intercoms available at large toy or retail stores. The receiver is placed in the client's room and plugged into an electric socket. The portable monitor is then placed in any home location; the caregiver can move it readily. Any movement or sound that the client makes can be easily heard.

ENERGY CONSERVATION

Clients should always be evaluated during each of their daily living activities for ways to conserve energy. Worksheets and role-playing situations can be designed to assess and teach energy conservation techniques. Clients can be taught to plan household tasks to conserve energy. Shelves and closets can be rearranged for easy access to frequently used items. Using a lightweight electric broom instead of a heavy vacuum cleaner works well. An apron with many pockets is effective for the ambulatory or wheelchair-bound client. Often individuals disabled by spinal cord injuries are able to obtain commercial insurance coverage for a built-in vacuum cleaner system, which allows them to clean without pushing an electric broom or vacuum cleaner around.[19]

Energy conservation is paramount to the success of a homebound client. Occupational therapists are particularly skilled in recommending appropriate energy conservation techniques. Clients should be taught to think before acting, planning out their moves to maximize and conserve their endurance.

SOURCES OF ADAPTIVE EQUIPMENT

Home Medical Equipment Stores

The easiest way to obtain adaptive equipment is through a local HME dealer. These medical supply stores are often listed in the telephone directories under "Hospital Equipment and Supplies," "Rehabilitation Equipment," or "Physical Therapy Equipment." Most dealers are very cooperative and are interested in working with therapists. It is beneficial to visit one or several local HME stores and develop a relationship with the rehabilitation salesperson. Ask that person to stock your most commonly used items (splint supplies, reachers, dressing sticks, Velcro, Theraband, Theraplast, your preferred brand of walker, cane, crutches, wheelchair, etc). Dealers frequently allow therapists to borrow these items for individual client assessments. Holding a home health therapy workshop in a medical equipment store is an excellent way to become familiar with new home health equipment, develop a rapport with local dealers, and assist the salesperson in meeting more home health therapists.

Home Health Agencies

Many home health agencies have equipment loan closets and used equipment that can be either loaned or purchased at a nominal cost. Appropriate infection control procedures including sterilization, are recommended before loaned equipment is transferred to another client. Many home health agencies use preferred medical equipment dealers, who may offer volume discounts on smaller adaptive aids if they already provide the agency with larger items such as wheelchairs, hospital beds, nursing supplies, oxygen, and respiratory items. A relationship with your agency's preferred dealer can often allow you to borrow or receive trial equipment at no charge.

Computerized Information Retrieval Networks

Computerized information retrieval networks can be particularly beneficial for the therapist searching for a difficult-to-locate item, for the rural therapist without many resources or equipment stores, or for the therapist who wants to obtain a comprehensive list of the equipment types available. Some of the more common computerized information retrieval systems for medical equipment are listed below; this list is by no means exhaustive.

ABLEDATA[20] is a database of rehabilitation equipment and assistive technology products commonly used by occupational and physical therapists. It is housed at the Adaptive Equipment Center at Newington Children's Hospital in Newington, Connecticut. Each ABLEDATA product listing includes information on the manufacturer, common trade names, cost, availability, product description, subjective comments, and product evaluation. It is available by subscription for frequent users or by contacting the Adaptive Equipment Center at Newington Children's Hospital for information searches.[21] Hyper-ABLEDATA,[20,21] developed by the Trace Center at the University of Wisconsin at Madison,[22] is a microcomputer format for ABLEDATA that allows customized entries, enlarged print, and a simplified access system. At present it is only available for Macintosh users, but future plans include access for IBM and IBM-compatible computers.

NARIC,[23] the National Rehabilitation Information Center in Silver Spring, Maryland, is a federally funded library and information center that houses a support staff, information specialists, a REHAB-DATA bibliographic database, and information on assistive technology, medical conditions, and rehabilitation issues. NARIC can be accessed by a toll-free number and offers a variety of publications and individualized search systems.

The National Clearinghouse on Technology and Aging[24] is based in Athens, Ohio, and includes a database on both high-technological and low-technological equipment, sensory technology for the visually and hearing impaired, an expert network of people involved in technology and research, and technological publications.

One of the most useful organizations for those interested in adaptive equipment is *RESNA*,[25] an interdisciplinary association for the advancement of rehabilitation and assistive technologies. RESNA provides regular publications, strong technological interdisciplinary communication, and dynamic conventions. (Many other professional associations, including those that concentrate on a particular disability area, also have computerized information regarding their specialties.)

ECRI, the Emergency Care Research Institute[26], located in Plymouth Meeting, Pennsylvania, offers a profound awareness of equipment and testing techniques, and a willingness to help the home health therapist. ECRI, in this country and abroad, is commonly referred to as the "Consumer Reports" of healthcare technology because it does not accept advertisements and can in turn be objective about its information. Just as *Consumer Reports* studies cars and toasters, this nonprofit organization performs comparative technical evaluations of medical equipment and associated supplies. Medical equipment is extensively examined by a multidisciplinary team of engineers, chemists, physicists, clinical specialists, scientists, cost experts, and policy analysts. ECRI's research findings are available in print through its circulation department and, in many cases, in electronic formats that are accessed by thousands of healthcare organizations.

MEDLINE[27] is available in most city libraries, on medical campuses, and through many rehabilitation hospitals. Produced by the National Library of Medicine in Bethesda, Maryland, it provides a computerized analysis of medical literature. MEDLINE can be particularly useful for gathering information about medical conditions and unfamiliar equipment needs.

Often local libraries have computerized access to larger book collections, medical journals and computerized information retrieval systems. Spending a few moments with your research librarian can be of immense benefit when you are looking for technological information on a particularly frustrating or little-known medical condition or device.

Professional Associations

Networking with national and state occupational therapy and physical therapy association[28,29] members can help provide numerous professional contacts, equipment ideas, resources, and home health techniques. We have held many successful "show and tell" meetings in the Philadelphia region, inviting state therapy association members to bring their "bag of tricks" for home health practice. An amazing number of unique adaptive devices can be used in the home health field. Weights made from sand in plastic bags or vegetable cans, microwaveable moist heating pads, and frozen peas used as ice packs are all examples of low-cost creations available for the home health therapist.

Disability-Oriented Associations

Accessing information from national and state disability organizations can provide a wealth of disability-specific equipment needs. Some of these organizations have equipment loan closets or equipment funds earmarked for the particular individuals their association is dedicated to serving. (See Chapter 13, Appendix 13–1, for a list of associations.) The local senior citizens' center is often a valuable grassroots resource, eager to respond to community members' needs. The information section of the local telephone book can provide valuable information. The American Association of Retired Persons (AARP)[30] has excellent access to advocacy, legal, and funding strategies for the elderly. They have active state and local chapters, which provide both the therapist and the client with resource information and possibly with equipment ideas. Disability-oriented organizations are usually receptive to therapist input. Discussing equipment needs and ideas with the executive director or continuing education director can often lead to new referrals, funds for equipment, and equipment on loan.

REIMBURSEMENT FOR ADAPTIVE EQUIPMENT

Home Medical Equipment Store

The importance of developing rapport with local HME supply stores cannot be overstated. HME stores want the home health therapist's business. Most dealers provide a professional discount (usually 10% to 20% off retail price). It is appropriate to ask that this discount be extended to your clients. In addition, ask whether the HME dealer can be responsible for submitting *all* Medicare, Medicaid, or insurance carrier paperwork rather than having the client pay for the items initially. It is also beneficial to develop rapport with the rehabilitation salesperson or manager to learn of upcoming reimbursement trends and procedures.

Third-Party Reimbursement Specialist

The American Occupational Therapy Association (AOTA) has identified a Third-Party Reimbursement Specialist for each state. Often these people will have information regarding statewide medical equipment reimbursement practices for Medicaid and local insurance carriers. AOTA and the American Physical Therapy Association (APTA) both employ reimbursement specialists who have information on the federal Medicare system and national insurance policy plans. These individuals can help track reimbursement trends and suggest successful strategies for reimbursement in other parts of the country (see Chapter 14).

Home Health Equipment Reimbursement versus Acute or Rehabilitation Hospital Reimbursement

Usually, most adapted equipment ordered and received while the client is in the hospital can be reimbursed. Most adaptive equipment (except for the larger items such as wheelchairs, hospital beds, commodes, and splints) ordered while the client is at home is *not* reimbursed. Therefore, the home health therapist should develop a close working relationship with the hospital therapists and anticipate needs if possible.

Medical Equipment Catalogues

Hundreds of medical equipment companies distribute catalogues regularly to occupational therapists and physical therapists. Both AOTA[28] and APTA[29] produce a *Buyers' Guide* that lists their medical equipment advertisers. Some of the more common catalogues are cited in this chapter and listed as references. A successful technique for facilitating maximal daily living independence through the use of adaptive equipment is to give clients a copy of a consumer-oriented adaptive aid catalogue such as the BE OK! Sammons "Enrichments" catalogue,[31] "Comfortably Yours,"[32] or the "Accent on Living" publications.[33] The client can then begin to prioritize the need for different pieces of adaptive equipment. Having the client order equipment often generates more interest than having the therapist provide the equipment. Another reason for using the consumer-oriented catalogues is that often the therapists' professional catalogue is much more extensive and can overwhelm the novice consumer.

Billing the Client for Adaptive Equipment

Home health therapists should discuss the approximate cost of a piece of adapted equipment (and if possible, try it out) with the client and possibly the client's family *before* ordering. Ideally, the therapist can order the recommended equipment in the presence of the client or the family and have the bill sent directly to the client. Thus the therapist is not involved in any exchange of money between the client and the equipment representative. If the therapist pays for the equipment and then asks the client for reimbursement, it is always good policy to provide a written receipt, noting equipment, date, and amount received, with copies for both the client and the therapist. Many home health agencies have specific policies regarding the exchange of money between client and therapist. Check with the home health agency before ordering equipment.

SUMMARY

The use of adaptive equipment in the home health setting is a common and individualized practice. Therapists need to develop their own suppliers, keep abreast of new devices by visiting trade shows, regularly peruse numerous medical equipment catalogs, keep aware of reimbursement trends and procedures, and network with other home health therapists. Most importantly, home health therapists must strive to provide their clients with the most appropriate equipment recommendations possible, based on a comprehensive understanding of the adaptive equipment marketplace.

REFERENCES

1. Austill-Clausen, R: Bathroom Safety. Bathroom Aids, Universal Management System, Inc., Newtown Square, PA, 1989.
2. Austill-Clausen, R, et al: Guidelines for Occupational Therapy in Home Health. American Occupational Therapy Association, Inc., Rockville, 1987.
3. CareMate: Sunrise Medical. Guardian, 12800 Wentworth, Arleta, CA 91331, (800) 255-5022.
4. CareMate: Young's Medical Equipment. North Penn Medical–Surgical Supply, Inc., 711 West Main St., Lansdale, PA 19446, (215) 855-3545.
5. Sammons Catalog 1991: Be OK! Fred Sammons Inc., A Bissell Healthcare Company, PO Box 32, Brookfield, IL 60513, (800) 323-5547.
6. Cleo, Inc., 3957 Mayfield Road, Cleveland, OH 44121, (216) 382-9700.
7. ADL Catalog 1991. North Coast Medical, Inc., 187 Stauffer Blvd., San Jose, CA 95125-1042, (408) 283-1900, (800) 821-9319.
8. JA Preston Corporation: A Bissell Healthcare Corporation, 60 Page Rd., Clifton, NJ 07012, (800) 631-7277.
9. The Winsford Feeder. Winsford Products, Inc., 179 Pennington-Harbourton Rd., Pennington, NJ 08534, (609) 737-3297.
10. Hi-Marks, Part 85311. Maxi Aids, 42 Executive Blvd., PO Box 3209, Farmingdale, NY 11735, (800) 522-6294, (516) 752-0521.
11. FashionAble. Support Plus Catalogue, Surgical Products, Inc., 99 West St., Medfield, MA 02052, (508) 359-2910.
12. Techni-Flair: Designers and Manufacturers of Adaptive Clothing, White River Industries, 2nd and Dalton, PO Box 40, Cotter, AK 72626, (501) 435-2000.

13. PRIDE: A National Organization Dedicated to Solving Clothing Problems, 71 Plaza Court, Groton, CT 06340, (203) 445-1448.

14. Prentke Romich Company, 1022 Heyl Rd., Wooster, OH 44691, (216) 262-1984.

15. DU-IT Control Systems Group, 8765 Township Road 513, Shreve, OH 44676, (216) 567-2906.

16. Butler-in-a-Box. Master Voice, 10523 Humbolt St., Las Alamitos, CA 90720, (213) 594-6581.

17. TASH, Inc., 70 Gibson Drive, Unit 12, Markham, Ontario, Canada L3R4C2, (416) 475-2212.

18. Pennsylvania Association for the Blind, Chester County Branch, Inc., 71 South First Ave., Coatesville, PA 19320, (215) 384-2767.

19. National Spinal Cord Injury Association, 600 West Cummings Park, Suite 2000, Woburn, MA 01801, (617) 935-2722.

20. Hall, M, Vanderheiden, G, and Thompson, C: ABLEDATA and Hyper-ABLEDATA. Assistive Technology 1:4, 1989.

21. ABLEDATA. Adaptive Equipment Center, Newington Children's Hospital, 181 E. Cedar St., Newington, CT 06111, (203) 667-5405, (800) 344-5405.

22. Hyper-ABLEDATA. Trace Center, University of Wisconsin at Madison, S-151 Waisman Center, 1500 Highland Ave., Madison, WI 53705-2280, (608) 262-6966.

23. NARIC: National Rehabilitation Information Center, 8455 Colesville Rd., Suite 935, Silver Spring, MD 20910-3319, (800) 346-2742, (301) 588-9284.

24. National Clearinghouse on Technology and Aging, College of Health and Human Services, Ohio University, Athens, OH 45701, (614) 448-2804.

25. RESNA, 1101 Connecticut Ave. NW, Suite 700, Washington, DC 20036, (202) 857-1199.

26. ECRI, 5200 Butler Pike, Plymouth Meeting, PA 19462, (215) 825-6000.

27. MEDLINE, US National Library of Medicine, 8600 Rockville Pike, Bethesda, MD 20894, (800) 638-8480.

28. American Occupational Therapy Association, Inc., 1383 Piccard Dr., PO Box 1725, Rockville, MD 20850-4375, (301) 948-9626.

29. American Physical Therapy Association, 1111 N. Fairfax St., Alexandria, VA 22314, (703) 684-2782.

30. American Association of Retired Persons, 1909 K Street, NW, Washington, DC 20049, (202) 872-4700.

31. "Enrichments for Better Living," 145 Tower Drive, PO Box 579, Hinsdale, IL 60521, (800) 323-5547.

32. Comfortably Yours. Aids for Easier Living, 2515 E. 43rd St., Chattanooga, TN 37422, (201) 368-0400.

33. "Accent on Living," PO Box 700, Bloomington, IL 61702, (309) 378-2961.

Chapter 9

Medication Management

Barbara W.K. Yee & Betty J. Williams

Serious health and sometimes life threatening concerns about improper medication management have been expressed for the elderly.[1,2] Home health care providers can and frequently do play a critical role in drug education, compliance, and enhancement of health promotion for their elderly clients. Although there is considerable debate about the relative risk of illicit drug use, stronger concerns are expressed about hidden alcohol abuse among the elderly. Improper management of medications or substance abuse often goes undetected by primary health care providers, but is often identified by those in frequent contact with the elderly person such as family members, friends, or home health care providers. The home health care provider plays a pivotal role in proper medication management and detection of substance abuse. This chapter highlights the major issues in drug management and substance abuse.

MANAGING PRESCRIBED MEDICATIONS

Elderly Americans make up approximately 10 percent of the US population, but they are prescribed approximately 25 percent of the prescription drugs dispensed each year. It has been projected that, by the beginning of the next century, persons in this age group will be taking nearly half of all prescribed medications.[3] The Commissioner of Food and Drugs of the Food and Drug Administration has estimated that as many as 50 percent of the prescribed drugs fail to produce their desired result because they have been used improperly.[3] The seriousness of this problem is illustrated by studies suggesting that almost 20 percent of the hospitalizations on the geriatric service of any general hospital can be attributed to drug toxicities.[4]

Risk Factors for Developing Medication Problems

Several factors contribute to the vulnerability to medication problems of persons (particularly elderly persons) who are receiving home health care.[5-9]

1. Physiological changes in elderly adults may alter how the body handles a drug and how a drug behaves at its sites of action.
2. The interaction of primary and secondary changes in elderly adults causes unpredictable responses to drugs.
3. Complicated drug regimens that require taking several drugs at different times of the day increase self-administration errors.
4. Self-medication with over-the-counter (OTC) drugs, folk medicines, and home or quack remedies may interfere with efficacy of prescription medicines or create serious drug interactions.
5. Commonly used drugs often have a smaller margin of safety between therapeutic and toxic doses for the elderly than for younger adults.

6. Conditions common in elderly people influence the body's reaction to drugs. These conditions include bed rest, dietary changes, malnutrition, dehydration, altered body temperature, stress, congestive heart failure, and thyroid disease.
7. Elderly patients may have difficulty remembering and comprehending complex instructions.

The Impact of Aging and Disease Processes on Medication Management

The changes that occur in bodily function with advancing age, disease, or both present significant problems. There is a common myth that the elderly are more sensitive to the effects of drugs than are younger adults. In fact, the elderly are more sensitive to some drugs but are less sensitive to others and may react more or less vigorously than younger individuals. Physiological changes due to aging processes influence the way a person handles a drug. For instance, gradual reductions in liver and kidney function can influence considerably the length of time the drug stays in the body, and also the magnitude of the effect.

The process of producing a drug effect consists of several steps: absorption (e.g., from the stomach after swallowing a tablet), distribution throughout the body, and interaction with tissues to actually cause the effect. The rates at which these steps occur determine not only how fast a drug works and how long the effect lasts, but also the blood concentration that will be reached and, therefore, the magnitude of the therapeutic or toxic effect. Physiological changes that influence metabolism and excretion processes, as well as drug absorption and distribution coupled with homeostatic mechanisms, may be important in specific situations.

There is little evidence that aging alters the rate of drug absorption from the gastrointestinal tract. Absorption may, however, be altered by some conditions associated with aging. Poor nutrition may increase drug absorption, whereas excessive laxative or antacid use may retard it.

The distribution of a drug depends on its chemical composition. Some drugs are water soluble and distribute themselves primarily in the water compartments of the body: blood, extracellular fluid, and so forth. Other drugs are fat soluble and may concentrate in adipose tissue. Still others have a particular affinity for protein and may bind to protein in muscle or serum. The elderly have a reduced lean body mass, reduced body water, and an increase in fat as a percentage of total body mass. Because of the relative alterations in the size of body compartments, a drug dose calculated on the basis of a patient's body weight may produce an unexpectedly high blood concentration and a toxic effect. Dehydration can complicate the situation further. Drugs that accumulate in body fat may linger in the body longer than expected when therapy is terminated. In the elderly, a small miscalculation in dosage or a self-administration error may cause a toxic reaction and, because a large amount of the drug is stored in fat, it may take a long time to rid the body of enough drug to eliminate the toxicity.

Metabolism of drugs takes place to some small extent in virtually every tissue of the body, but by far the greatest amount occurs in the liver. While aging may impair the liver's ability to metabolize some drugs, a decreased liver blood flow or a decline in the ability of the liver to recover from disease or injury, such as that caused by alcohol or hepatitis, is probably more important in determining liver function. Reduction in liver blood flow decreases the liver's extraction of drugs from the blood; injury reduces all liver function. Additionally, congestive heart failure or severe nutritional deficiencies reduce liver function and the rate of drug metabolism.

While some drugs are excreted in the feces, and to a very minor extent in sweat, in tears, and via the lungs, the kidney is the major organ of drug excretion. Renal function declines with age, reducing the excretion rate of drugs and their metabolites. Reduced excretion allows drugs and their metabolites to accumulate in the body, possibly causing toxicity and undoubtedly increasing the duration of action. Of equal importance are diseases common in the elderly that impair renal function. In congestive heart failure, cardiac output is reduced and the kidney is less effective in clearing foreign material from the blood. The elevated renal pressure seen in hypertension can, if left untreated, produce irreversible damage to the kidney and thereby reduce the kidney's ability to deal with drugs and their metabolites.

Many drugs, especially those affecting the cardiovascular system, are administered with the full expectation that compensatory reflexes will occur and participate in the overall effect. The compensatory reflexes, like all homeostatic mechanisms, become blunted with age. Drugs that normally evoke compensatory changes, therefore are overly effective in the elderly. For example, if a vasodilator drug is given in an emergency situation in which rapid reduction of blood pressure is needed (e.g., hypertensive crisis), a young adult responds with compensatory reflexes that modulate the fall in blood pressure. In an elderly person, however, these reflexes do not operate as briskly, and the blood pressure may drop to a dangerously low level with the same drug dose.

Similarly, an elderly diabetic person may experience a hypoglycemic attack if he or she does not eat within a short time after taking medication, because the body does not respond with sufficient speed to the lowering of blood sugar. Exercise also tends to reduce blood sugar and can be dangerous in elderly diabetics unless care is taken to ensure that medication and food are taken on schedule.

It is not uncommon for elderly persons to suffer from more than one disease at the same time. Depending on the organs involved, one disease may affect the way the body handles the drug or drugs given for other conditions. Additionally, one disease may distort the response to a drug given for another condition; for example, a drug given for hypertension normally elicits a compensatory response from the heart. A diseased heart may not be able to provide this response.

Common Health Problems and Their Associated Drug Therapies

The most common chronic conditions in the elderly for which drug therapy is prescribed include arthritis, hypertension, heart disease (congestive heart failure, angina pectoris, cardiac arrhythmias and atherosclerosis), diabetes, depression (including insomnia and mental disorders), and dementia.[10] This section focuses on drugs used to treat these conditions.

Treatment of *arthritis* normally involves the group of drugs classed as nonsteroidal anti-inflammatory drugs (NSAIDs). Some of the NSAIDs are available as OTC preparations; these include aspirin and ibuprofen (marketed as Motrin IB, Nuprin, Advil, etc.). These drugs are commonly recommended as daily treatment for the pain and inflammation associated with rheumatoid arthritis. However, acetaminophen (Tylenol), another OTC agent used for the control of minor pain and fever, has no anti-inflammatory activity and should not be used to treat the inflammation of arthritis. Daily use of an NSAID carries the risk of some side effects. The most common is gastrointestinal upset, which in sensitive individuals may promote or exacerbate gastric ulcer. It now appears that there may be an additional benefit associated with daily NSAID use. In persons who have recovered from a heart attack or stroke, these agents have been shown to exert a protective effect against a second attack. Other NSAIDs, such as indomethacin (Indocin) and phenylbutazone (Butazolidin) are sometimes prescribed for arthritis. These agents have no advantage over aspirin and ibuprofen but may cause significantly more toxicities. In very severe arthritis, corticosteroids may be used. These powerful anti-inflammatory agents have some serious drawbacks including peptic ulcer, slowed wound healing, and, especially important in the elderly, increased rate of bone loss (osteoporosis).

Hypertension is a significant problem in the elderly, especially in Western cultures. While it is normal for the blood pressure to increase slightly with advancing age due to a gradual decrease in the elasticity of the blood vessels, extraordinary increases must be treated. Hypertension itself can be a virtually "silent," symptomless disease; its main danger is its possible sequelae: stroke, heart attack, and renal disease. Several different types of drugs are available to treat hypertension. These include diuretics such as hydrochlorothiazide (Hydrodiurel), beta-blockers such as propranolol, angiotensin converting enzyme (ACE) inhibitors such as enalapril, and calcium channel blockers such as verapamil (Calan), diltiazem (Cardizem), and nifedipine (Procardia). Each of these drug classes works through a different mechanism and has its own toxicities. For safety, many physicians will try nondrug therapy (weight reduction, salt restriction) initially. Thiazide diuretics (e.g., Hydrodiuril) are considered a reasonable first step in therapy, but these drugs are likely to produce some degree of hypokalemia, which may cause cardiac rhythm disturbances; hyperglycemia, which may complicate the treatment of diabetes; and hyperuricemia, which may provoke attacks of gout. These effects may be particularly problematic in the elderly. Much less serious but no less disturbing to the client is the urinary urgency and possible incontinence caused by these "water pills."

Calcium channel blockers and beta adrenergic blocking agents (beta-blockers) are both very effective in the general population. In older patients, calcium channel blockers are effective but beta-blockers seem less so. Either type of drug may have added benefit if the client has angina pectoris, since both can be effective in this condition, but both can slow and even stop the heart in overdose. Clients with congestive heart failure are particularly sensitive to this effect and should avoid the drugs. Nifedipine is a calcium channel blocker that differs from the rest of the group in that cardiac depression is not a prominent feature of its action. The beta-blockers also can cause some problems in asthmatics (can provoke attacks and reduce effectiveness of some drug treatments) and in diabetics (can reduce compensatory response to low blood sugar).

Congestive heat failure is a significant problem in the elderly, especially because some of the drugs used to treat this condition are extremely toxic. In congestive heart failure, the heart does not pump forcefully enough to supply blood to all of the body. The major symptoms are shortness of breath and fatigue. Congestive heart failure is treated either with cardiac glycosides (such as digoxin and digitoxin) or with vasodilators. The cardiac glycosides are plant alkaloids that have a powerful stimulant effect on the heart. Under the influence of the glycosides the weakened heart is able to pump more forcefully and to increase the cardiac output. These agents are not curative, and therefore must be given for life if they are used as the treatment modality.

Cardiac glycosides are very toxic compounds; the difference between the therapeutic and toxic doses is small. The dose is, therefore, crucial, and it is not unusual for small, seemingly insignificant changes in body function to allow enough drug accumulation to cause toxicity. The removal of digoxin from the body is slower in the geriatric population than in younger adults and is particularly slowed in the presence of renal disease. Early symptoms of toxicity — blurred vision, slowed heart rate — may not seem particularly severe, but may progress to significant cardiac rhythm disturbances and nausea and vomiting and indicate a life-threatening condition. Lowered body electrolytes, which result from diuretic use or diarrhea, increase the incidence of digitalis-induced arrhythmias. The elderly, unlike younger adults, may experience the earliest symptom of toxicity as confusion. Unfortunately this symptom can easily be mistaken for age-related forgetfulness. It is thus important for health care providers and family to be alert for changes in behavior that may signal drug toxicity.

Some physicians choose to treat congestive heart failure by administering vasodilators. These drugs are regarded as effective because they reduce the resistance of the vasculature, and thereby the pressure against which the weakened heart must pump; the heart can then pump more blood with each stroke. These drugs are certainly less toxic compounds than are the digitalis glycosides, but they may not be effective in all cases. Symptoms of vasodilator overdose, specifically fatigue and lack of energy, are somewhat similar to the symptoms of congestive heart failure.

Angina pectoris is a condition in which areas of the heart suffer from temporary oxygen lack, producing severe pain that radiates across the chest and down the arm. Clients often describe the pain as a crushing sensation. While angina has no single well-defined cause, it can be treated satisfactorily with vasodilator drugs, such as nitroglycerin and amyl nitrite. When these drugs are used, there is usually a need for a rapid drug effect; the route of administration of these agents is unique. Nitroglycerin is administered by putting a tablet under the tongue or through a skin patch. Blood vessels are very close to the surface in this area, and the drug can be absorbed quickly and travel to its site of action, the heart. Amyl nitrite is supplied in a crushable glass ampule, and the drug is inhaled as a vapor. Other drugs, such as the calcium channel blockers and beta-blockers, are useful when given routinely to prevent recurrences of anginal attacks.

Cardiac arrhythmias are disturbances in the normal rhythm of the heart. Beats may be abnormally slow, abnormally fast, or uncoordinated. Depending on the type of rhythm alteration, different drugs such as guinidine, procainamide, lidocaine, disopyramide and beta-blockers, are used for therapy. The rates of removal from the body of procainamide, quinidine, and lidocaine seem to be reduced in the elderly. Disopyramide affects bladder function, causing voiding problems, particularly in elderly men.

Atherosclerosis is a condition in which plaques of lipid material collect in the inner walls of blood vessels. When this condition becomes sufficiently advanced, blood flow to the affected area of the body can become seriously compromised. Blood vessel elasticity is reduced and blood pressure increases. The heart may also be affected, due either to atherosclerotic lesions in the vessels of the heart or to continued pumping against a high resistance. Once plaques have developed, there is no way short of surgery to eliminate them, so most therapy is aimed at preventing the development of plaques by reducing the blood levels of certain lipids, notably cholesterol. In the elderly, there seems little advantage in using drugs to lower serum lipids, rather than trying to decrease cholesterol by changes in diet.

Diabetes may be either insulin dependent or noninsulin dependent. Insulin-dependent diabetics cannot regulate their blood sugar or manage the transport of various nutrients into some tissues without insulin administration. Control of their disease requires careful scheduling of meals and insulin injections to prevent wide swings in their blood glucose levels. Even when blood glucose levels are closely controlled, the diabetic client is prone to many other health problems, including poor circulation, slow wound healing, and progressive vision loss. Poor circulation can make appropriate medication of any concomitant illness problematic because to be effective, any drug must be carried to its site of action by the circulation.

Diabetic clients who still have some pancreatic function can be treated with oral hypoglycemic agents such as tolbutamide (Orinase) and glyburide (Diabeta). Most clients who do well with this type of therapy can control blood sugar levels with only a change in diet. In all cases, when the same result can be obtained with drugs or by changing life-styles, a change in life-style is safer but may be more difficult to accomplish.

Insomnia is a frequently reported complaint among the elderly. Sedative-hypnotics such as the barbiturates and benzodiazepines (e.g., Valium) have variable effects in elderly persons, probably, in part, because the decline in liver and kidney functions causes the drugs to be retained in the body as much as three times longer than in younger clients. Sensitivity to these drugs also appears to increase with age. All the sedative-hypnotics can produce tolerance (a reduced effect in response to the same dose) and compulsive drug use. A particular problem in the elderly is drug "automatism," that is, forgetting whether or not the medication has been taken and automatically taking a second or third dose.

Depression in the elderly is often ignored, overlooked, or misdiagnosed as senile dementia and therefore may not be treated appropriately. The drugs used for this condition in younger individuals—tricyclics such as amitriptyline, and monoamine oxidase (MAO) inhibitors such as phenelzine, are effective in the elderly. Both agents are metabolized by the liver and excreted with their metabolites via the kidney, and thus may have a longer duration and greater incidence of toxicity in the elderly. Symptoms of toxicity may be hard to identify because they consist primarily of signs consistent with aging or with depression, for example, sedation, confusion, lassitude, tremor, and blurred vision, but may also include cardiac rhythm disturbances and difficulty in urinating. The MAO inhibitors may interfere with the metabolism of alcohol and other drugs, and thus may cause symptoms of toxicity from the other drug(s).

A variety of *psychiatric diseases* are treated in the elderly by the use of the antipsychotic drugs, the phenothiazines and the butyrophenones. These drugs are undoubtedly useful in managing schizophrenia of old age, as well as some of the symptoms associated with delirium or dementia, and agitation or combativeness. Much of the effectiveness of these drugs in agitated patients is probably due to their sedative effects. A phenothiazine, chlorpromazine (Thorazine), is frequently used in the elderly but may not be completely satisfactory in geriatric conditions. Unfortunately, increasing the effectiveness of the drug by simply increasing the dose is not advisable with the phenothiazines, since there is too great a possibility of producing toxic effects. Chlorpromazine may produce orthostatic hypotension, as well as movement disorders, pseudoparkinsonism, and tardive dyskinesia. Another phenothiazine, thioridazine, has effects very similar to those of chlorpromazine but produces less incidence of orthostatic hypotension. The butyrophenone, haloperidol (Haldol), has a less pronounced effect on blood pressure and produces less sedation than the phenothiazines, but is even more likely to produce movement disorders.

Alzheimer's disease, or *senile dementia*, seems to be associated with a profound and selective loss of cholinergic (acetylcholine-secreting) neurons in the central nervous system. Cholinergic neurons appear to play an important part in cognitive function, especially memory. Although the antipsychotic drugs (discussed above) may produce some symptomatic improvement in such disorders as disturbed behavior, emotional lability, and abnormal sleep-wake cycles, there is no improvement in the basic disorder. In addition, there is some indication that antipsychotic drugs may impair memory and intellectual function. Drugs currently under research hold some promise for more appropriate treatment of Alzheimer's disease.

Drug Interactions and Adverse Effects

Most elderly persons leave their physicians with one or more prescriptions. It has been estimated that the elderly may have 10 to 12 bottles of prescription medication in their possession at any one time.[10] Since the elderly, like much of the population, may visit several physicians for care of several problems, they may be taking four or more different prescription drugs at one time without any one physician's being aware of all the drugs being taken. Instead of visiting their physicians for diagnosis and treatment of new health problems, clients may try to diagnose on their own and may use old or expired medications from their or other people's medicine cabinets. Additionally, the patient may be taking OTC medications. The World Health Organization has estimated that 40 percent of people more than 60 use one or more OTC drugs on a regular basis.[4] It is important to recognize that drug interactions can occur not only between prescription medications, but also between prescription and nonprescription (OTC) drugs. Because elderly clients often take several different drugs at the same time, the risk for drug interaction with sometimes unpredictable adverse results is great among this group.

Whenever two or more drugs are taken at the same time, a client runs the risk of incurring a *drug interaction*. Drug interactions take one of two forms; either (1) one drug changes the way the body handles the other drug, or (2) one drug enhances or interferes with the action of the other. Of the two interactions, the former are the more prevalent and in some cases the more difficult to predict.

In the following discussion, no attempt is made to list drug interactions comprehensively. If drug interactions are suspected, several available books compile documented instances of drug interaction and discuss mechanisms (see bibliography). Pharmacists are also excellent sources of information on drug interactions.

Drug interactions can occur between any two drugs regardless of their chemical compositions. Interference with drug metabolism is probably the most common way in which one drug may alter the action of another. A drug that inhibits the metabolism of a second drug can cause the second drug to have an abnormally strong and long-lasting effect.

Enhancement of drug metabolism is usually accomplished by increasing the amount of enzyme in the specialized liver microsomal system. This enzyme induction may occur as a result of the action of several different types of chemicals. When drug metabolism is enhanced, a normally effective dose of drug will be metabolized so rapidly that its normal effect will not be seen. This enzyme induction is reversible, and when the effect of the inducer has abated, the concentrations of other drugs in the body can increase because their rate of metabolism drops back to normal.

Excretion of drugs occurs primarily via the kidneys but to a lesser extent through the gastrointestinal tract. Any drug that alters the function of either organ can alter the rate at which drug is excreted, and thereby the duration of an effective concentration in the body.

Interactions between drugs in which the action of one drug will interfere with the action of another are fairly easily predictable, and should be noted by the physician prescribing the drugs or by the pharmacist filling the prescriptions. The interaction can be eliminated only by changing one or both of the drugs. Another type of interaction occurs when two drugs produce similar effects individually, but together produce an effect greater than the sum of the individual effects. An example is a sedative such as diazepam (Valium) and alcohol taken simultaneously. Each agent produces sedation and central nervous system depression, and together the results can be deadly.

The presence of drug interactions does not mean that simultaneous therapy with the interacting drugs cannot be carried out, but it does mean that the dosage may have to be adjusted. Because elderly people commonly take many drugs, prescribed by different physicians, simultaneously, at least one responsible person must be aware of all the drugs being used and the forms of those drugs in use. A pharmacist is trained to recognize the risk for drug interactions and may serve in the coordinator role. For this reason, it is advisable to use a single pharmacy for all prescriptions if possible, so that a record may be maintained of all current medications. If it is not possible to use one pharmacy, medical records, especially medication records, should be transported with the elderly person. The pharmacist will work with any physicians involved to make sure that medication instructions are clear and as simple as possible.

Prescription Medications

While not all prescription medications have been shown to cause adverse interactions, many instances of interaction have been documented. The following are a few examples.

Sedative drugs such as phenobarbital and diazepam (Valium) increase drug metabolizing capacity and may therefore reduce the effectiveness of dicumarol, a drug used to slow blood clotting, and phenytoin (Dilantin), a drug used to treat epilepsy. In addition, these sedative drugs stimulate their own metabolism, so their effectiveness may decrease with chronic use. Cimetadine (Tagamet), a drug used to treat gastric ulcer, inhibits liver enzymes and thereby enhances the activity of a dose of dicumarol, dilantin, phenobarbital, or diazepam. Diuretics such as hydrochlorothiazide, which cause loss of potassium, enhance the toxic effects of digoxin. When these two drugs are given simultaneously, there is an increased risk that digoxin will cause a serious change in cardiac rhythm.

Prescription, Over-the-Counter, and Home Remedies

OTC antacids of various types (e.g., Tums, Di-Gel) can interfere with the action of many drugs because they decrease their absorption from the gastrointestinal tract. Among the drugs affected are such diverse agents as digoxin and tetracycline. Aspirin has a small effect of its own in slowing blood clotting. When taken along with a drug whose purpose is to slow clotting, aspirin increases the effect markedly. Aspirin can also displace penicillin from binding sites, which allows the penicillin to be excreted more rapidly, decreasing its effect. Acetaminophen (Tylenol) can also enhance the activity of anticoagulant drugs. An antihistamine, diphenhydramine (Benadryl), a component of many allergy and cold preparations, has a sedative effect and can increase markedly the effect produced by sedative drugs. Laxatives decrease gastric emptying time and for this reason can move drugs through the gastrointestinal tract so fast that absorption is not complete, and the expected effect is not achieved.

NSAIDs such as aspirin and ibuprofen (Advil, Nuprin) are frequently used for self-medication of headache and joint and muscle pain. Salves and ointments containing methyl salicylate (oil of wintergreen) and other aspirinlike compounds are available OTC for use in minor muscle strain or soreness. OTC cold preparations often contain one of these aspirinlike drugs for the relief of fever associated with a cold. Additionally, aspirin and similar drugs are prescribed in much higher doses for relief of the pain and inflammation associated with rheumatoid arthritis or osteoarthritis. The use of NSAIDs is, therefore, quite widespread and it is important to recognize toxicities associated with these agents, as well as the drug interactions that can occur.

It is well known that aspirin may cause or worsen gastric ulcers in many people. Therefore, the combination of aspirin with other ulcer-producing agents such as alcohol can produce severe problems. One of the ways in which aspirin produces ulcers is by delaying blood clotting. The action of anticoagulants, therefore, may be enhanced by aspirin. This property of aspirin is, coincidentally, the basis for the current suggestion that men over 40 take an aspirin a day to reduce the probability of heart attack. Aspirin and similar drugs also affect the kidney. If kidney function is already impaired, it may be further reduced by salicylate (aspirinlike) drugs. Additionally, drugs eliminated by the kidney may have a longer-lasting and stronger effect than normal. Because many drugs are eliminated by the kidney, it is prudent to be sensitive to changes in the subjective feelings of a client taking other drugs along with aspirin.

Health professionals should note a warning about drug interactions and their adverse effects. Although a large majority of home remedies are not harmful, some risk interacting or interfering with prescribed medications, decreasing the body's ability to absorb food and drugs in the normal manner, or delaying use of effective treatments. Home remedies may be substituted for the prescribed medication regimen, due to high costs or beliefs in the efficacy of traditional home remedies, or may be used simultaneously with the prescribed regimen.[11] The danger is the potential interference with the effectiveness of the drug in treating the condition for which it was prescribed or introduction of toxic substances present in some foreign medicines or in folk medicines made at home. For instance, alcohol-based medicines made at home for colds may produce the same drug interactions that drinking can produce with certain prescribed medications or OTC drugs.

Interactions Between Medications and Food

Some medications must be taken with meals to prevent gastrointestinal upset. Other drugs, however, can cause unwanted effects if taken with specific foods or can change the absorption of nutrients. For example, milk or milk products reduce the absorption of some antibiotics, such as tetracycline. Alcohol has numerous effects on drug action. For example, it increases the blood glucose–lowering effect of insulin, making diabetes even more difficult to control. Alcohol inhibits the metabolism of anticoagulant drugs, increasing their effect. One of the metabolites of acetaminophen is toxic to the liver. Normally, very little of this toxic metabolite is produced, but in the presence of alcohol its production increases. Some of the drugs used to treat depression, the MAO inhibitors, can cause a serious hypertensive reaction if cheese is eaten because of a reaction with a constituent of the cheese. Many other examples of food-drug interactions exist. If an unusual reaction to a drug occurs, interaction with food is a possibility that should not be overlooked.

Drug Use in Infants and Children

Drug use in children is governed by many of the principles that govern drug use in the elderly. Whereas aging decreases liver and kidney function, infants are born with immature liver and kidney functions. During the first year of life, the ability to metabolize and excrete drugs develops to near-adult levels. Development of these functions may be delayed in a sick child. Gastrointestinal function in infants may be quite variable, making it difficult to predict the extent of absorption of an oral drug dose. Distribution of drugs in infants differs from that in adults because infants have a higher percentage of body water and a smaller muscle mass, and they may have a higher percentage of fat. For these reasons, pediatric dosages of drugs cannot be determined as a simple fraction of the adult dosage, but must be calculated on the basis of the child's size and age.

Drug Use During Pregnancy and Lactation

Drugs taken by a pregnant woman cross the placenta and reach the fetus at rates that are related to the lipid solubility of the drug. Any drug that crosses the blood-brain barrier and acts on the brain will surely cross the placenta and affect the fetus. In addition to the risk of addicting the fetus if the mother is taking addictive drugs, there is also the possibility that prenatal development may be affected. Several drugs have been determined to cause fetal development problems such as those developed by "crack babies" or "fetal alcohol syndrome children." The effects of many other drugs are currently unknown. In absence of this information, by far the safest course is to use no drugs during pregnancy.

The possibility that a mother may pass drugs to her child does not end with delivery but continues throughout the nursing period. Many drugs are excreted into milk and can be found in concentrations sufficient to affect the infant. The health care provider should, therefore, be made aware when a nursing mother is taking drugs for any purpose.

Drug Education, Compliance, and Health Promotion Strategies

Adequate drug education for health professionals and their clients would enhance significantly the client's ability to practice effective medication management. Several proposed strategies exist, including:[5,9,12–14]

1. Improve geriatric training of physicians and other health care professionals.
2. Improve verbal instructions about prescriptions and self-medicating strategies of the elderly to address complex medication regimens, comprehension, and memory difficulties.

3. Develop new technologies to improve drug monitoring capacities of health care professionals caring for elderly clients.
4. Assist caregivers in helping their elderly relatives improve drug management.
5. Encourage use of generic drugs, if possible, at onset of therapy instead of switching from brand to generic drugs, which may affect bioequivalence after the client is stabilized on the brand medication.
6. Use form of medication that the client can most easily swallow.
7. Closely monitor fluid intake to promote easy swallowing of medication and maintain appropriate hydration.
8. Notice any changes in behavior soon after introduction of new medication and do not assume that even gradual changes are attributable to aging or disease processes. Many behavior difficulties can be attributed to adverse drug reactions that influence cognitive functioning, and many of these declines are reversible. Report these changes immediately to the physician or pharmacist for re-evaluation.
9. Encourage use of one pharmacy to improve monitoring of prescription and OTC medications and to establish familiarity with elderly clients and their needs by pharmacists.
10. Discourage sharing and swapping drugs with anyone.
11. Question the necessity of introducing one more drug into the treatment regimen of an elderly person without full evalaution of all medications taken.
12. Evaluate the utility of taking a drug on a long-term basis, especially if the drug is psychoactive or should be used short term.
13. Develop an effective strategy to organize medicines so that the client can follow the physician's orders regarding medication use:
    - **a.** Use pill boxes.
    - **b.** Use pill calendars.
    - **c.** List pill taken, time, and date.
    - **d.** Develop pill taking routines during the day.
    - **e.** Have someone else give the medicines if the client is unable to do so or unreliable.
14. Drug therapy review:
    - **a.** All prescription drugs and OTC drugs used regularly should be reviewed by the physician or pharmacist annually (e.g., bring drugs in brown bag or list all drugs used).
    - **b.** Whenever a new drug is introduced, the client should indicate which drugs are being currently taken—include OTC drugs in list.
    - **c.** Outdated drugs should be flushed down the toilet.
    - **d.** Hard-to-identify or unknown medications should be examined by the pharmacist.
    - **e.** Request that all medications be put in non–child-proof containers

if no small children are living in the household and if medications are not available when children visit.

15. Review the physician's instructions with the pharmacist to ensure that the client understands the instructions and ask additional questions regarding any unanswered questions in item 1 above.
16. The physician needs help in evaluating the effectiveness of the prescribed drug therapy. Tell the physician what other medications the client is taking; include OTC drugs. Even when taken as directed, some medications may produce adverse effects. Call the physician immediately for further instructions about drug use if the client experiences any side effects or has a problem taking the medication.

When to Panic

Many types of drug reactions or toxicities may occur quite suddenly. While sudden, severe, unexpected reactions are rare, it is important to recognize when the client "feels bad" for no apparent reason, or when observed behavior suddenly changes. These symptoms should be reported to the physician without undue delay but need not be considered emergencies unless the reaction is severe or life threatening. The following are examples of reactions that should be considered emergencies:

1. Difficulty in breathing
2. Crushing chest pain
3. Loss of consciousness
4. Seizures
5. Extreme, bizarre behavior

SUBSTANCE ABUSE

The targets of many substance abuse programs are the mobile and younger populations because the known prevalence of illegal drug abuse is substantially higher in younger populations than in middle-aged and elderly groups. The major problem with this notion is that it may significantly underestimate substance abuse among elderly people and other less visible members of our society.

Several factors are believed to increase the possibility of substance abuse.[10,15–19]

1. Poverty and emotional problems may encourage abuse of alcohol and other substances.
2. Genetic predisposition and environmental factors such as peer drinking or social isolation.
3. Stressful life transitions, such as retirement or death of significant

others, and increase or chronicity of physical and mental health problems.

4. Prescription of more psychoactive drugs to elderly people, especially women; and higher access of the elderly to potentially addictive drugs.
5. Stigmatization of elderly people who abuse alcohol or other substances. Relatives may treat abuse as a taboo subject or maintain silence, which is meant to protect the elderly abuser.
6. Lack of routine screening by primary care physicians for alcohol or substance abuse.
7. Primary diagnosis usually other than alcoholism or drug abuse.
8. Characteristics of alcoholism or drug abuse totally missed, attributed to aging or disease, or masked by other features of aging or disease processes. Presentation of alcoholism or substance abuse may be quite different in comparison with common patterns in younger populations.

Drug Misuse and Abuse

A review article[15] states that elderly persons have a higher use of psychoactive drugs such as tranquilizers, sedatives, and hypnotics than other age groups. A lower percentage of drug-related crises in emergency departments occurs for elderly persons than for younger persons, but when they do occur among the elderly, psychoactive drugs are frequently involved. Although past and current drug abuse among the elderly appears to be quite rare, this problem will grow larger in the future. For instance, as addicts who entered the drug culture during the 1960s get older and continue to survive, there will be a growing number of older addicts to be treated.

Chemically dependent elderly clients can be characterized by a positive history of drug use, positive blood and urine drug screens, and numerous signs and symptoms of autonomic hyperactivity.[14] When drug dependence is not promptly recognized, admission to intensive care units may be required to deal with the withdrawal symptoms. Withdrawal manifestations from nonopiate drugs include autonomic hyperactivity, irritability or depressed mood, anxiety, malaise or weakness, nausea, vomiting, and coarse tremors.

Alcoholism

Although the danger presented by medication mismanagement is greater, the dangers of long-term alcohol use or short binges cannot be discounted. For instance, getting drunk and falling down can have dire consequences for an elderly person — for example, a broken hip leading to secondary problems such as muscle atrophy or even death. The risk for alcohol and medication interaction presents a significant danger because of the sheer number and types of drugs taken by the average elderly person. Therefore, the Surgeon General's workshop on Health Promotion and Aging in Washington, DC, in March 1988 identified alcohol abuse among the elderly as a priority area in unmet needs.[20]

Our society, including health care providers, does not consider alcohol abuse among the elderly to be a serious problem and therefore overlooks telltale signs of alcohol abuse among elderly health care clients. Drinking can have dire consequences for the elderly. For instance, more than three drinks a day (13 g of absolute ethanol) increases the risk of disease in multiple organ systems for men. The level of safe drinking for women has yet to be determined.

As presented by Willenbring and Spring[18], common presentations of alcohol-related problems in the elderly include falling, confusion, memory deficits, anxiety, anemia, cardiac arrhythmias, gastrointestinal bleeding, weight loss, malnutrition, psychosis, poor balance, withdrawal or isolation, trauma, dementia, grief and depression, insomnia, hypertension, heart failure, fatigue, edema, osteoporosis, pain, numbness, difficulty in walking, and inability to perform self-care. Many of these common presentations of alcohol-related problems could be seen as symptoms of other disease processes, poor life-style habits, or several aging processes. The job of health care professionals is to determine the exact cause or causes of these symptoms and seek appropriate treatment. Alcoholism may be masked by other processes that occur with disease, aging, and reactions to life circumstances.

Willenbring and Spring[18] use a rapid, routine screening device called the HEAT with the elderly. If there is a positive response to one of four questions, a fuller history should be taken. The authors suggest that other substances can be substituted for alcohol in the following questions:

1. How do you use alcohol?
2. Have you ever thought you used to Excess?
3. Has Anyone else ever thought you used too much?
4. Have you ever had any Trouble resulting from your use?

The authors suggest that defensiveness, embarrassment, or discomfort provoked in the client may indicate a problem and that a more detailed history should be obtained.

Strategies for Treatment of Substance Abuse[19]

1. Increase methods for detection and treatment of alcohol and drug abuse, which is essential for the elderly population. Home health care providers can assist in detecting substance abuse problems in their elderly clients.
2. Improve treatment groups for elderly abusers, such as creation of age peer support groups at local chapters of Alcoholic Anonymous.

3. Increase awareness of signs for hidden alcoholism and substance abuse among the elderly by their peers, caregivers, and health professionals.

CREATE A DRUG DIARY (copy this page for each drug taken) (Adapted from Yee, Williams, and O'Hara[5])

Name of drug:
Dose:
Appearance (brand or generic):
Reason for use:
Expected action:
Quantity to be taken:
Frequency of administration:
Duration of therapy:
Adverse effects:
What to do if there are side effects:
Precautions:
Special instructions (foods, drinks, or other medicines):
What to do if a dose is missed:
Refill information:
Storage requirements:
Cost of medication:
Expiration dates:
Physician-ordered changes in drug regimen and their dates:

Show this diary to *all* of your physicians for review—especially when you get additional medications!

REFERENCES

1. Glantz, MD, Peterson, DM, and Whittington, FJ (eds): Research Issues 32: Drugs and the Elderly Adult. Publication (ADM) 83-1269, Department of Health and Human Services, Washington, DC, 1983.
2. Whittington, FJ (ed): Alcohol and drugs: abuse and misuse. Generations XII:4, Summer 1988.
3. Young, FE: Questions about your medicine? Go ahead—ask. FDA Consumer 21:23, 1987.
4. World Health Organization: Health care in the elderly: Report of the technical group on use of medicaments by the elderly. Drugs 22:279, 1981.
5. Yee, BWK, Williams, B, and O'Hara, N: Medication management and appropriate substance use for elderly persons. In Lewis, CB (ed): Aging: The Health Care Challenge, ed 2. FA Davis, Philadelphia, 1990, p 298.

6. Heckheimer, EF: Health Promotion of the Elderly in the Community. WB Saunders, Philadelphia, 1989.
7. Lamy, PP: Actions of alcohol and drugs in older people. Generations XII:9, Summer 1988.
8. Shimp, LA and Ascione, FJ: Causes of medication misuse and error. Generations XII:17, Summer 1988.
9. Morrell, RW, Park, DC, and Poon, LW: Effects of labeling techniques on memory and comprehension of prescription information in young and old adults. J Gerontol: Psychol Sci 45:166, 1990.
10. Council on Scientific Affairs: American Medical Association White Paper on Elderly Health. Arch Intern Med 150:2459, 1990.
11. Spector, RE: Cultural Diversity in Health and Illness, ed 2. Appleton-Century-Crofts, Norwalk, 1985.
12. Lesage, J and Zwygart-Stauffacher, M: Detection of medication misuse in elders. Generations XII:32, Summer 1988.
13. Eng, E and Emlet, CA: SRx: A regional approach to geriatric medication education. The Gerontologist 30:408, 1990.
14. Whitcup, SM and Miller, F: Unrecognized drug dependence in psychiatrically hospitalized elderly patients. J Am Geriatr Soc 35:297, 1987.
15. Gomberg, ESL: Drugs, alcohol, and aging. In Kozlowski, LT, et al (eds): Research Advances in Alcohol and Drug Problems, Vol 10. Plenum Press, New York, 1990, p 171.
16. Maddox, GL: Aging, drinking and alcohol abuse. Generations XII:14, Summer 1988.
17. Menninger, K: Man Against Himself. Harcourt-Brace-Jovanovich, New York, 1938.
18. Willenbring, M and Spring, WD: Evaluating alcohol use in elders. Generations XII:27, Summer 1988.
19. Schiff, SM: Treatment approaches for older alcoholics. Generations XII:41, Summer 1988.
20. Williams, EP: Health Promotion and Aging: Alcohol. In Abdellah, FG and Moore, SR (eds): Surgeon General's Workshop: Health Promotion and Aging Background Papers, DHHS/PHS, Rockville, MD, 1988, p A-1.

BIBLIOGRAPHY

Fillmore, KM: Critical explanations—biological, psychological, and social—of drinking patterns and problems from the alcohol-related longitudinal literature: Critiques and strategies for future analyses on behalf of the world health organization. In Kozlowski, LT, et al (eds): Research Advances on Alcohol and Drug Problems, Vol 10. Plenum Press, New York, 1990, p 15.

Gilman, AG, et al (eds): The Pharmacological Basis of Therapeutics, ed 8. Pergamon Press, New York, 1990.

Hansten, PD: Drug Interactions, ed 5. Lea & Febiger, Philadelphia, 1985.

Kalant, H and Roschlau, WHE (eds): Principles of Medical Pharmacology, ed 5. BC Decker, Toronto, 1989.

Katzung, BG (ed): Basic and Clinical Pharmacology, ed 4. Appleton and Lange, Norwalk, 1989.

Shinn, AF and Shrewsbury, RP: Evaluations of Drug Interactions, ed 3. CV Mosby, St Louis, 1985.

Appendix 9–1

Resources for Home Health Care Professionals Concerned with Managing Medications

A. GOVERNMENTAL AGENCIES AND ORGANIZATIONS

1. **The National Resource Center on Health Promotion and Aging American Association of Retired Persons (AARP)**
   601 E St. N.W., Fifth Floor–B
   Washington, DC 20049
   (202) 434-2200 or Fax (202) 434-6474
2. **National Institute on Aging (NIA)**
   Information Center
   P.O. Box 8057
   Gaithersburg, MD 20898-8057
   (301) 495-3455
3. **The National Council for Patient Information and Education (NCPIE)**
   666 Eleventh St. N.W., Suite 810
   Washington, DC 20001
   (202) 347-6711
4. **National Health Information Clearinghouse (NHIC)**
   P.O. Box 1133
   Washington, DC 20013-1133
   (800) 336-4797 or (703) 522-2590
5. **National Clearinghouse on Alcohol and Drug Abuse Information**
   P.O. Box 23245
   Rockville, MD 20852
   (800) 729-6686 or (301) 468-2600
6. **Administration on Aging (AOA)**
   US Department of Health and Human Services
   330 Independence Ave. S.W.
   Washington, DC 20201
   (202) 619-0441

B. RESOURCE MATERIALS FOR HEALTH PROFESSIONALS

1. **National Institute on Aging**
   Age Pages (1 sheet, large print information sheets, multiple copies, selected titles in Chinese or Spanish):
   Safe Use of Medicines by Older People
   Safe Use of Tranquilizers
   "Shots" for Safety
   Should You Take Estrogen?
   Aging and Alcohol Abuse

Health Quackery
Arthritis Medicine

2. **National Council on Aging**
   A Resource Guide for Drug Management for Older Persons ($5.00) (Order #2017)

3. **SRx, Central Office**
   1182 Market St, Rm. 204
   San Francisco, CA 94102
   (415) 558-3767
   See following reference for description of program:
   Eng, K and Emlet, CA: SRx: A Regional Approach to Geriatric Medication Education. Gerontologist 30: 408–410, 1990.
   a. 18 Medication Fact Sheets (in English, Chinese, Spanish, Vietnamese) about:
      Antidepressants, arthritis, antihypertensives, diabetes, diuretics, heart medications, potassium supplements, tranquilizers, neuroleptics, ulcer medications, alcohol, and sleeping medications
   b. 15 Mini-Class Guides (English only):
      From "Wise Use of Medicines, Folk Medicines" and "Home Remedies" to use of "Specific Medicines for Diseases and Health Conditions"
   c. Various other resources

4. **Department of Pharmacy Practice, College of Pharmacy**
   University of Rhode Island
   Kingston, RI 02881
   (401) 792-2734
   Brown Bag Prescription Evaluation Manual, ed 2
   (planning guide to conducting Brown Bag Program)

5. **Oregon State University**
   Extension Service
   a. Alcohol Problems in Later Life (PNW 342)
      Publication, 24 pp., $0.75/ea
      Publication Orders, Agricultural Communications
      Oregon State University, Administrative Services A422
      Corvallis, OR 97331-2119
      (503) 737-2513
   b. Winter Comforts
      20 min. slide/cassette program, transparencies, handouts, workshop guide ($67.50)
      ½-in VHS videotape (from slide or cassette)
      (17.00 with workshop guide purchase)

   Vicki L. Schmall
   Extension Gerontology Specialist
   Extension Home Economics
   Oregon State University
   Milam Hall 161
   Corvallis, OR 97331-5106
   (503) 737-1014

6. **Project TAP (Tenants Assistance Program)**
   Massachusetts Housing Finance Agency
   50 Milk St.
   Boston, MA 02109
   (617) 451-3480 ext. 399
   Anthony Flaherty, Director
   (Provides alcohol and drug abuse management training)

C. RESOURCE MATERIALS AND ORGANIZATIONS FOR ELDERS AND THEIR CAREGIVERS

1. **Worst Pills Best Pills: The Older Adult's Guide to Avoiding Drug-Induced Death or Illness ($12.00)**
   Sidney M. Wolfe, Lisa Fugate, Elizabeth P. Hulstrand, or Laurie E. Kamimoto
   Public Citizen Health Research Group
   Dept. HL, 2000 P Street, N.W., Suite 700
   Washington, DC 20036
2. **American Association of Retired Persons (AARP)**
   a. Using Your Medications Wisely: A Guide for the Elderly (D317)
   b. Getting the Most from Your Medications (D12083)
   c. Treating Yourself with Care (Slides and cassette, loan)
3. **AARP Pharmacy Service Prescription Drug Handbook**
   (color description of common medications taken by people over 50)
   AARP Medication Information Leaflets for Seniors
   (leaflets on specific medications ordered from AARP Pharmacy Service)
   AARP Pharmacy Service
   One Prince St.
   Alexandria, VA 22314
   (703) 684-0243
4. **National Council on Aging (NCOA)**
   Managing Medications (6 brochures, $3.00)
   NCOA Publications, Dept. 5087
   Washington, DC, 20041-5087
5. **Keeping on Schedule with Your Medications**
   Four-Week Medication Calendar
   American Heart Association
   Health Information Services
   Merck Sharp & Dohme
   West Point, PA 19486
   (see local phone directory for American Heart Association)
6. **AARP chapter (see local phone directory)**

7. **Alcoholics Anonymous chapter (see local phone directory)**

8. **National Council on Alcoholism chapter (see local phone directory)**

9. **Area-wide Agency on Aging for your county (see local phone directory)**

Appendix 9–2

Some Commonly Prescribed Drugs

DRUG	GENERIC NAME	USED FOR	CONTRAINDICATION	SIDE EFFECTS
Acromycin	Tetracycline	Urinary tract infections	Allergy to tetracyclines	Yeast infections, diarrhea
Aldomet	Methyldopa	Hypertension	Liver disease	Sedation, liver dysfunction, forgetfulness
Apresoline	Hydralazine	Hypertension	Severe heart disease, kidney disease	Blisters, chest pain, skin rash
Aristocort	Triamcinolone	Arthritis, severe allergy	Gastric ulcer, osteoporosis	Susceptibility to infection, odd behavior
Atarax	Hydroxyzine	Allergy, itching	Glaucoma, prostate enlargement	Disorientation, delirium, dry mouth, blurred vision
Ativan	Lorazepam	Anxiety, panic attacks	Liver disease	Confusion, delirium
Benadryl	Diphenhydramine	Allergy, coughing, sedation	Asthma, glaucoma	Dry mouth, constipation, confusion, delirium, problems with urination
Brethine	Terbutaline	Asthma, chronic bronchitis, emphysema	Diabetes, thyroid disease	Restlessness, confusion, nervousness
Calan	Verapamil	Hypertension, angina	Heart block, hypotension	Dizziness, headache, nausea
Carafate	Sucralfate	Gastric ulcer		Constipation, backache, lightheadedness
Cardizem	Diltiazem	Hypertension, angina	Hypotension	Dizziness, headache, nausea
Catapres	Clonidine	Hypertension	Heart block	Sedation, dry mouth, skin rash
Cleocin	Clindamycin	Severe bacterial infections	Allergy to aspirin, gastrointestinal disease	Diarrhea, weakness, weight loss, stomach cramps
Compazine	Prochlorperazine	Nausea, vomiting	Epilepsy, diabetes, glaucoma	Sweating, loss of bladder control, abnormal bruising
Cortef	Hydrocortisone	Allergy, arthritis	(for injection into joint) Infection at site of joint, osteoporosis	Pain, tingling at site of injection, skin rash or hives
Coumadin	Warfarin	Thrombophlebitis	Blood disorders, hypertension	Bleeding gums, nosebleed, unexplained bruising
Dalmane	Flurazepam	Sedation	Liver disease	Incoordination, dry mouth, confusion, drug dependency

(continued)

Drug	Generic Name	Used For	Contraindication	Side Effects
Diabeta	Glyburide	Non–insulin-dependent diabetes	Liver disease	Fruity breath, thirst, increased urination
Diamox	Acetazolamide	Glaucoma, altitude sickness	Diabetes, gout, heart disease	Tiredness, mood changes, dry mouth
Dilantin	Phenytoin	Seizures, irregular heartbeat	Heart disease	Blurred vision, slurred speech, dizziness, confusion
Dulcolax	Bisacodul	Constipation	Allergic reactions	Dehydration
Duraquin	Quinidine	Irregular heartbeat	Heart block	Ringing in ears, dizziness, palpitations
Elavil	Amitriptyline	Depression, migraine	Prostate enlargement	Confusion, delirium, disorientation, constipation
Feldene	Piroxicam	Arthritis	Hypersensitivity to NSAIDs	Gastrointestinal upset
Flexeril	Cyclobenzaprine	Muscle spasm, strains	Glaucoma, heart disease, prostate enlargement	Drowsiness, dry mouth, dizziness, weakness, blurred vision
Gantrisin	Sulfasoxazole	Urinary tract infections	Allergy to sulfa drugs	Skin rash, increased sensitivity to sun, aching joints
Haldol	Haloperidol	Psychosis, Huntington's chorea	Epilepsy, glaucoma, liver disease, prostate enlargement	Uncontrolled muscle movement, blurred vision, Parkinson's disease
Hydrodiurel	Hydrochloro-thiazide	Edema, hypertension	Allergy to sulfa drugs	Weakness, dry mouth, muscle cramps
Imodium	Loperamide	Diarrhea	Diarrhea caused by antibiotics	Dry mouth, rash, constipation
Inderal	Propranolol	Hypertension, angina, irregular heartbeat, migraine headaches	Congestive heart disease, diabetes, angina, asthma	Depression, slow pulse, confusion
Indocin	Indomethacin	Arthritis, gout	Gastric ulcer, sensitivity to aspirin	Confusion, depression, gastric ulcer
Isordil	Isosorbide	Angina	Glaucoma	Tiredness, dizziness, blurred vision
Keflex	Cephalexin	Bacterial infections	Allergy to any cephalosporin	Stomach cramps, diarrhea
Lanoxin	Digoxin	Congestive heart disease	Irregular heartbeat	Confusion, altered color vision, slow pulse
Laradopa	L-dopa	Parkinson's disease	Cardiovascular disease	Depression, mood changes, uncontrolled body movements
Lasix	Furosemide	Edema, kidney disease	Irregular heartbeat, gout	Dehydration, muscle cramps
Librium	Chlordiazepoxid	Sedation, muscle relaxation	Liver or kidney relaxation disease	Skin rash, vertigo, nausea, headache, depression
Lomotil	Diphenoxy-late/atro-pine	Diarrhea	Obstructive jaundice, some gastroinstestinal infections	Confusion, delirium, respiratory depression
Lopressor	Metoprolol	Hypertension, irregular heartbeat, angina, migraine headaches	Heart failure	Depression, confusion, slow pulse

(*continued*)

DRUG	GENERIC NAME	USED FOR	CONTRAINDICATION	SIDE EFFECTS
Luminal	Phenobarbital	Sedation, seizures	Porphyria	Confusion, difficulty breathing, slow pulse
Mellaril	Thioridazine	Psychosis	Epilepsy, glaucoma, liver disease	Dizziness, uncontrolled muscle movement, fever, breathing problems
Minipress	Prazosin	Hypertension	Acute heart failure, angina, kidney disease	Dizziness, chest pain, irregular heartbeat
Navane	Thiothixene	Psychosis	Epilepsy, glaucoma, lung disease	Dizziness, drowsiness, fever, seizures
Nembutol	Pentobarbital	Sedation, anxiety	Porphyria	Respiratory depression, addiction
Norpace	Disopyramide	Irregular heartbeat	Heart block	Chest pain, confusion, dizziness
Orinase	Tolbutamide	Non–insulin-dependent diabetes	Liver or kidney disease	Fruity breath, thirst, increased urination
Polycillin	Ampicillin	Bacterial infections	Allergy to penicillin	Trouble breathing
Procardia	Nifedipine	Hypertension	Hypotension	Dizziness, headache, difficulty breathing
Pronestyl	Procainamide	Irregular heartbeat	Heart block, digitalis toxicity	Dizziness, confusion, fever, chills, joint pain
Sinemet	Carbidopa/L-dopa	Parkinson's disease	Same as for Larodopa	Same as for Larodopa
Stelazine	Trifluoperazine	Psychosis	Epilepsy, glaucoma, prostate enlargement	Difficulty urinating, weakness, depression, chest pain, rapid pulse
Synthroid	Thyroxine	Replacement therapy	Heart disease	Chest pain, nervousness
Tagamet	Cimetidine	Gastric ulcer	Liver or kidney disease	Confusion, dizziness
Tegretol	Carbamazepine	Seizures, trigeminal neuralgia	Heart block, blood disorders	Dizziness, fast pulse, shallow breathing
Theolair	Theophylline	Chronic asthma, emphysema, bronchitis	Allergy to coffee or chocolate	Chest pain, dizziness, confusion
Thorazine	Chlorpromazine	Psychosis	Heart disease, liver disease	Hypotension, fainting, parkinsonism, fever
Timoptic	Timolol	Glaucoma	Heart block, asthma	Headache, eye irritation
Tofranil	Imipramine	Depression	Alcohol dependency, asthma, psychosis	Blurred vision, confusion, constipation
Valium	Diazepam	Insomnia, anxiety, muscle tension	Liver disease	Drug dependency, dizziness, confusion
V-Cillin-K	Penicillin V	Bacterial infection	Allergy to penicillin	Nausea, diarrhea
Vasotec	Enalapril	Hypertension	Renal stenosis	Cough, loss of sense of taste, skin rash
Vistaril	Hydroxyzine	Allergy	Early pregnancy	Confusion, delirium, dry mouth, constipation
Xanax	Alprazolam	Anxiety, sedation	Liver or kidney disease	Confusion, drowsiness, slurred speech
Zantac	Ranitidine	Gastric ulcer	Liver or kidney disease	Confusion, hallucinations, sore throat, fever

Chapter 10

Cultural Considerations

ELSA L. RAMSDEN

Home health professionals in our society have a unique opportunity to enter homes of strangers to give care. We are invited into the home as a guest might be and given permission to move about freely as we provide health care—in a manner that a guest would not. This is a special role with special responsibilities. We bring into the client's domain our skills and our personhood along with our values and beliefs. We are immersed in the arena of culture as we face the values and beliefs of the client.

This chapter focuses on some of the cultural issues related to the environment in which home health care is provided. Culture is briefly explained to provide a common ground of understanding on which the remaining discussion rests. Cues about culture are communicated in many ways, some of which are illustrated with examples. Finally some ways the health professional may learn about the client's beliefs and values are suggested, and some of the pitfalls are described.

A goal we all share is to provide optimal care to the client. Gaining an understanding and appreciation of the cultural components of the client's life informs our treatment planning and execution. When the values and beliefs of the client are different from our own it is sometimes difficult to plan treatment that meets the client's specific needs. Through careful observation and tactful questions we may identify an approach more acceptable than the "book" method or one that our own preferences would lead us to suggest.

CULTURE

A child is born, grows up, and learns to move, take nourishment, speak, play, work, marry, and raise a family following patterns established within a culture. Heredity gives us generic human capabilities. How we use those capabilities and how we live are determined in large measure by the rules of the culture into which we are born. One approach to culture is to consider it as a collection of ways to deal with the problems a group encounters. All people must develop ways of getting food and protecting themselves from the elements. All people must have ways of relating to one another. In all societies, individuals develop convictions about various aspects of their lives; we call them values. We have not found any society with strictly utilitarian goals; all have some form of aesthetic appreciation such as stories, music, art, dance, and song, as well as ceremonies and special rites that are broadly called "religious." The result of all these behaviors is a society with form and pattern, which we call "culture." The system has an order that provides a life-style for its people.

Communication of Culture

Attributes of culture are expressed in communication behavior that includes the words we use and how we use them, gestures and movements of all kinds, the choice of clothes and how we wear them, and the manner in which we live. Our dwelling is a reflection of cultural values through our choices of where to live, how we decorate, and material objects we select to have around us.

We may describe communication as all behavior perceived by another who encodes it or attaches meaning to it. If, when the therapist first visits the home of a new client she speaks with family members who do not make eye contact throughout the visit, the therapist may attach the meaning "He's shy" or "They haven't learned proper social behavior." The therapist may also infer that "These individuals are not listening to me" or "They are not interested in what I'm saying" or "The whole family is quite rude." However, the truth may be the opposite. The explanation may be attributed to cultural differences that require deference to authority in the form of downcast eyes.

Culture and communication are virtually impossible to separate. The rules within a culture govern who may speak to whom. An old rhyme well known in Boston speaks to this point: "And here's to dear old Boston, the land of the bean and the cod, where Lowells speak only to the Cabots, and the Cabots speak only to God."[1] Rules dictate what may be discussed and how the conversation proceeds, how messages are sent, and what meanings are assigned to messages received from others. It is not generally considered acceptable in our society to discuss intimate bodily functions with strangers. It is even difficult to do so with health professionals who may be able to help with a specific problem. Communication patterns rest on the foundation of culture. When the culture changes, the communication changes.

For most people the effect of culture is not recognized in day-to-day living. We hear reference to culture in phrases like "our throw-away society," referring to our preference for disposable items. We tend to assume that the way we do things is the way everybody does them or the way everyone should do them. Objectively we know that cannot be true, but our behavior suggests otherwise. The reputation of the "ugly American" is alive and well in countries all over the world. American visitors to countries abroad created and continue to nourish this "ugly" image when they expect everyone to speak English, want hamburgers, diet soda, and brewed decaffeinated coffee, and expect a private bathroom with all hotel accommodations.

Ethnicity

Most Americans do not expect to encounter cultural differences in our own country. Why this should be so is amazing when we look at the countries on all continents from which our citizens have come to settle in this land of opportunity. We are not a "melting pot," as early anthropologists would have had us believe, but rather a remarkable stew with identifiable ingredients and a wonderful gravy.

Members of various national groups who have immigrated to the United States, such as the Irish, Polish, German, Swedish, Chinese, or Armenian, are different from one another for several reasons in spite of living here for three generations or more. They come from different cultural backgrounds, came to the United States at different times, faced different conditions in American society when they arrived, settled in different parts of this country, and were treated differently after they settled. These many national groups also have varied in their determination to maintain their values and customs of the past. Of course, many Americans have suffered historical amnesia and claim no loyalty to national tradition. Close inspection of religious observances and holiday celebrations may divulge clear evidence of cultural heritage.

This country accords the same freedoms to all its citizens — to members of minority and majority groups alike. The result is a remarkable diversity, but not without tensions. Education and "Americanization" seem to be the responsibility of the schools, both public and private, while the family struggles to reinforce ethnic ties and national pride and individual identity.

Ethnic groups provide a resource for many aspects of life based on the perception of shared values and beliefs of a common origin. Greely[2] suggests that persons who have recently immigrated to this country first experience culture shock and then proceed through several stages in the process of adjustment. Since the 1970s, when Haley's book *Roots*[3] appeared, we have had a resurgence of ethnic group and national pride that legitimate and enhance the specialness of ethnic identity. However, the differences that exist among us produce stress and tension on public institutions. The "diversity" programs proliferating in higher education are an example of the tension within large institutions, in which large numbers of individuals gather to work toward personal and group goals.

So too in institutionalized health care, persons from many cultural backgrounds provide and receive care in a system that attempts, yet fails, to be egalitarian. The concept of uniformity fails to account for cultural differences in values and beliefs that exist among diverse people. The subculture of the hospital has developed in a structure dominated by physicians, nurses, and physical therapists from white middle-class and upper-class America. The implicit rules of that subculture govern relationships between health professionals and patients.[4] These unwritten rules are based on a set of assumptions that fail to account for cultural diversity within the patient population, not to mention the cultural differences that exist among the professional staff of today. How can a nurse, physician, or physical therapist from middle-class or upper-class America know the values and beliefs of a patient who is poor, or a recent arrival from Southeast Asia, or a Native American, or someone from Appalachia or Puerto Rico or Mexico? The list could go on and on. Without knowing what is important to the patient, how can the hospital possibly give treatment efficiently and effectively?

In the home health system of care, health professionals are not working under the direct aegis of the hospital subculture with its distinctive set of rules. Yet the socialization process inherent in becoming a health professional derives from that environment and strongly influences the role behavior. Hence it is easier for health professionals to behave in the community in a manner consistent with their behavior in the health care institution than to develop new guidelines independently.

When the caregiver enters the world of the client and becomes a guest in the client's culture, different behavior is needed. Careful observation will enhance a questioning mind that seeks to understand the world of the client. A specific act may be considered discourteous in one society, polite in another, and a serious moral offense in a third. An example is standing very close to a speaker who is not an intimate friend and touching that person's sleeve or lapel during conversation. Behavior, such as many hand gestures, that is considered quite ordinary in one culture may be considered unacceptably indecent or obscene by a second. The health professional is frequently in the difficult position of wanting to help and not offend, but not knowing the rules of conduct for the group.

Values

Every society has a system of beliefs and ideas that have strong feelings associated with them—a system of values. In general we may define a value as an idea or practice that is important to an individual. It endures over time and is expressed consistently in behavior. For ease of discussion we could divide these values into societal, family and personal, and professional levels. In reality we know the lines are not clear among these levels. The 1970s brought a new dimension to the public scene as health care was affirmed to be a right of all citizens, not merely those who could afford it. Our society believes today that everyone who lives in this country "should" have access to health care. Your family may hold this value as well. The family may even be willing to pay a little bit more in taxes, as recent surveys show, to make sure that 30 million Americans not now insured may receive basic health care. As a health care professional, you personally may hold this value but find yourself seriously stressed on occasion. With a full roster of patients and several new referrals, the decisions you make about who gets care right away and who has to wait make a statement of your values.

Americans have learned a collective expectation that positively values industriousness, thrift, and ambition. Competition, labor-saving gadgets, and fast cars are desirable. A common expectation is that young married couples will live in a place of their own and not move in with one spouse's parents. On the other hand, Hopi Indian children learn not to put themselves forward to win games or get ahead of playmates. The Hopi way teaches the cooperation of human and nature, and of human with human. North Alaskan Eskimos learn to excel, but in ways that do not disadvantage others.

Defining proper behavior depends on the cultural context. In the

Western mind, for example, an association exists between sexual and excretory functions. Exposure of certain parts of the body is considered sexually stimulating. The Americans in Japan after World War II experienced confusion when faced with public rather than private bathing traditions. The American practice of combining bath and toilet in one room was unheard of in Japan and much of Europe. Certain Muslim countries maintain rules that require women to cover themselves in garments from head to floor, remain separate from men except their husbands and closest relatives, and receive medical care from other women.

Europeans and Americans differ widely on swimming nude in public. This is a common practice in Scandinavia and Germany for example, but not in the United States. Kissing between husband and wife in public is unacceptable in Japan but common in the United States. Elimination of body wastes in public is repugnant to Americans but in many parts of the world is considered a casual act that does not require privacy.

Every society, including our own, has culturally defined behaviors that are required, permitted, and forbidden. Americans are shocked by some behavior allowed in other societies, and yet fail to realize that similar situations exist in our own society. For example, use of the left hand for eating is unacceptable in India because of its early association with personal hygiene functions.

Language

Through the use of language we may reach out to make contact with others. Use and *misuse* of words is a common experience for most of us in an average day. Linguists estimate that the 500 most frequently used words in English have over 14,000 meanings. The same word means different things to different people and in different contexts. When people from different cultural backgrounds converse, the possibilities for misunderstanding are great. Translation from a foreign language carries serious risk of error. At the end of World War II, the Japanese received an ultimatum from the Allied forces to surrender after Italy and Germany had surrendered. The premier of Japan used the word *mokusatsu* in announcing the receipt of the message. This word may be translated as *to consider* or *to take notice of*. The Premier apparently meant that the Japanese government would consider the surrender ultimatum. The English language translator in Japan's overseas broadcasting agency, however, used the other meaning of the word. The message was interpreted to the rest of the world as a rejection of the surrender ultimatum. The atomic bombs were dropped. Some historians now consider the message to have been mistranslated.

We do not have to go outside the boundaries of our own country to find words that are unfamiliar in the dominant culture. Special language has developed to allow conversation between individuals that excludes outsiders. This is a common use for Yiddish among European Jews in times of discrimination. The Amish and urban blacks have languages distinctive to their subcultures for similar reasons. The specialized languages of medicine and law set members apart from the lay public. If we want to learn about what matters to an individual, we must take account of the language that person uses. The language not only communicates the meanings of the culture but is shaped by the culture.

LEARNING ABOUT THE CLIENT

It is natural to have preconceived notions about the client based on very elementary information such as diagnosis, age, height and weight, name, address, and concomitant conditions. Consider the mental image that develops as you learn about a patient—diagnosis: arthritis; age: 70; height: 5′0″; weight: 170 lb; name: Maria DeAngelo; address: south Philadelphia (Italian section of the city); concomitant condition: hypertension. As we travel through the neighborhood, our observations inform us to make additional judgments. Some of our earlier notions may be confirmed and some may be replaced with more accurate information.

When we enter the home of the client our sensory systems are bombarded by data—we see, hear, smell, and feel the new environment. Those data are interpreted in the light of our own cultural mindset.

Two students went to the home of a client with a clinical instructor. Afterward the instructor asked the students to write down their first reactions after walking into the home. The first student, from an affluent suburb, stated that it looked a lot like her parents' home and felt comfortable and inviting. The second student, from a lower–middle-class urban community, wrote that she had never been in a house like that and it felt cold and unfriendly. The same home was perceived very differently because the two sets of eyes took in the same data but arrived at different judgments about it.

To become acquainted with the client and family we are accustomed to asking questions—many questions. In our culture direct questioning may be acceptable, but in many cultures it is considered impolite and may result in discomfort and even resistance. Frequently, information about a person's life is regarded as private. Navajo adults consider questions about spouse and children none of the Anglos' business, even when the intent is to be friendly. In other cultures questions asked by an outsider may be looked on with suspicion and accepted only when the motives are known to be friendly. Eye-to-eye contact is not acceptable to all people. Many clients cannot come directly to the point of the visit without a lengthy getting-acquainted conversation. If these clients perceive questions as inappropriate, they find evasive responses to signal their resistance and discomfort. Or, when the answer to a question is thought beyond the ability of the health professional to understand in its cultural context, the client may fabricate a "suitable" answer intended to please the questioner.

Careful initial observation of the people, the home, and the way language is used may provide guides to later interaction. The information gathered by eyes and ears will inform understanding of cultural components and should suggest several areas for questioning, when appropriate. A client in rural Appalachia may describe symptoms as "nerves" or "high blood." A client from southeast Asia may attribute problems to "wind" and "cold." Different generations in the same minority group may hold different values due to differences in life circumstances such as political, educational, or economic status. The behavior of the client and family provides the evidence needed to plan your own behavior carefully if the cultural context appears different from your own.

Orient yourself to the people. The following cultural characteristics are important to know before entering a home and trying to communicate:

Greetings gestures: How close together persons stand—with friends, elderly people, women, children, leaders in the group; use of family name or first name, use of titles; compliments with greetings: what to compliment, how and when to give and receive compliments.

Example **(Latin Americans in general):** *Men and new acquaintances generally shake hands. It is common among friends to greet with an embrace, or* abrazo, *perhaps also with backslapping. Women who are friends frequently greet one another with a kiss on both cheeks. Women generally do not talk to strangers in public until properly introduced. Deference is shown to the elderly, with use of the family name to show respect. Use of the first name suggests intimacy and would be rude in a stranger.*

Visiting: What should or should not occur when a visitor enters the home; compliments on decor, family members, or possessions; proper conduct; leaving the home; words to avoid.

Example **(Latin Americans in general):** *Visitors should wipe their feet and greet the family gathered at the door beginning with the head of the family. Enter after being invited to do so. A visitor should speak casually before discussing the purpose of the visit. Inquiry about the health of family members shows friendliness. Praise of good behavior and admirable personality traits is helpful to acceptance. Sincere compliments about home, children, and garden are appreciated. When leaving, wait for the "host" to open the door.*

Gestures: Motions of hands and feet that help convey a message and those that should be avoided; eye contact; crossing the legs when seated; use of feet to move objects; pointing at persons when seated; posture in standing and when seated; touching another person; smiling and laughing; calling someone with hand movements; handing objects to another.

Example (**Asian people in general**): *Avoid touching another person's head. It is permissible to cross legs with one knee over the other, but not with the toe directed toward any person. The feet are not used to move objects. It is very poor taste to hit the fist into the cupped hand. Do not use a finger to beckon another to you; instead, use the whole hand with the palm down. A slight bow is considered courteous when entering and leaving the home.*

Religion: General attitudes toward religion and predominant beliefs.

Example (**Koreans in general**): *Shamanism is the underlying ethos of Korea, but the people have been strongly influenced by Buddhism and Confucianism and well as Christianity, mostly Protestant.*

Example (**Chinese from Hong Kong in general**): *Chinese may observe more than one religion at the same time, with Buddhism having the largest number. Fewer than 20 percent are Christian of both Catholic and Protestant persuasions. Religious diversity may exist among members of the same family.*

Attitudes: A wide range, from people's role in nature, work, success and failure, and fate, to individual roles in society and family.

Example (**Koreans and many Asians in general**): *Asian philosophy views humanity as one with the universe. Social harmony and nonindividualism are basic attitudes. Protocol requires that social superiors be treated with respect regardless of any personal feelings toward them. Preserving the good feelings of others at all costs is stressed. Maintaining calm requires indirect rather than direct intervention, through private conversation with mutual friends, to avoid embarrassment to anyone. A severe breach of courtesy results from causing injury (embarrassment) to another in public.*

Common Problems

Developing trust is important in the relationship between health professional and patient or client. It is especially important when information from the client is needed for treatment. Many reasons exist for mistrust. As long as the health professional is considered a "stranger," trust will be difficult for the client. The professional may not have had enough time to demonstrate trustworthiness (the opportunity to do so will vary among subcultures). The client may have had unpleasant experiences with other health professionals and so may entertain a healthy distrust of all members of that group. Careful observation of nonverbal behavior may provide clues to the client's reaction, and may provide the opportunity to inquire about previous experiences with health care and health professionals.

Asking questions has many potential pitfalls. Some people will respond with what they think the questioner wants to hear, whether it is the truth or not. Members of some groups find it difficult to say no. In response to a query about doing exercises or taking a medication, the speaker may say yes when in fact he or she has no intention of doing the procedure but considers it discourteous to say no. The health professional may be asking the wrong question of the wrong person, at a bad time, or in a poor location. When a health professional asks questions about a specific behavior, it is possible that the client has not previously thought about it. Although the health professional may take such questions for granted, they may be too far beyond the client's experience to have been considered. In these circumstances the client will have difficulty dealing with the question, may need to have it repeated, and will need time to reflect.

The behavior or personality of the health professional may be offputting and influence the response of clients. A male health professional may meet embarrassment or resistance from a female client belonging to a subcultural group in which women are commonly segregated from men. Some clients do not divulge certain information, or even seek help from modern health care facilities, because they believe modern medicine cannot cure a particular ailment. They seek their own "healers" for these kinds of problems. Members of "establishment" western medicine are known to be skeptical of nontraditional health care practices such as religious healing and herbal treatments. Clients are guarded in the way they talk about these things until a certain level of trust develops. Even then the initial comments are careful tests of the health professional's acceptance of the concepts.

What Is Important

During conversation with the client, it is inevitable that important information will emerge about values and health care. We health professionals have a problem in listening to this spontaneous information. When it reflects values inconsistent with our own, we tend to discount the statement. It seems unimportant, when in fact it may be very important. Issues that may emerge include the status and roles of various family members, their relationship to the client, and their attitudes about the illness. Participation of family members in the care of the client may be rigidly set by cultural rules. The meaning of illness and how it should be handled by the client is determined in the culture. Suggestions that disregard these values and rules will appear insensitive and inappropriate, and the health professional will lose credibility as one who does not understand. To be effective, a problem-solving strategy must consider the cultural components to achieve the best outcome for the client. The obvious should not go unstated: The professional *should not* impose his or her own values on the client or family system.

The time of the visit may be important to some families, but not to others, for many reasons. Use of time is treated differently by different cultures. Hawaiians speak of "Hawaii time," meaning any time they get around to it. Americans of Northern European descent tend to value punctuality. Those from South America may not attend to appointments as seriously, and may miss an appointment altogether. The activity of the moment is more important than the future plans.[5]

The client may be too polite to tell the health professional to come back another time, but may harbor underlying hostility that will be counterproductive to the relationship and perhaps the treatment. Growing acquaintance with the family and culture will inform the health professional about many "special" times to avoid when making a home visit. Increased familiarity with the client will cue the professional to notice the subtle nonverbal evidence of discomfort when a nontypical event has occurred and the visit is inopportune.

SUMMARY

The objective of health care treatment in our society is to provide the best care possible under the specific circumstances. To do that most effectively, health care professionals must consider the beliefs and values of the client. This chapter links the culture of the client and the behavior of the home health professional in an interactive way. Responsibility for success of cross-cultural interaction rests with the health professional as the authority figure in the relationship.

The concepts of culture and ethnicity have been described and discussed. Values and beliefs have been explained as a function of the cultural and subcultural contexts in which they exist. The attributes of culture may be observed through a variety of communication behaviors. Language is an important clue to the fundamental issues of a culture such as orientation to nature, spirit, time, activity, and other humans. Finally, some potential problems have been identified that may occur when professionals work with clients of a cultural background different from their own.

REFERENCES

1. Bossidy, JC: Toast, Holy Cross alumni dinner (1910). In Beck, EM (ed): Bartlett's Familiar Quotations, ed. 14. Little, Brown & Co, Boston, 1968.
2. Greely, A: Why Can't They Be More Like Us? Institute of Human Relations, New York, 1969.
3. Haley A: Roots. Doubleday, Garden City, 1976.
4. Ramsden, E: Values in conflict: Hospital culture shock. JAPTA 60:289, 1980.
5. Gudykunst, WV and Ting-Toomey, S: Culture and Interpersonal Communication. Sage Publications, Newbury Park, 1988, p 53.

BIBLIOGRAPHY

Bauwens, EE: The Anthropology of Health. CV Mosby, St Louis, 1978.

Brown, IC: Understanding Other Cultures, Prentice-Hall, Englewood Cliffs, 1963.

Brownlee, AT: Community, Culture, and Care. CV Mosby, St Louis, 1978.

Chaffee, CC: Problems in Effective Cross-Cultural Interaction. Battelle Memorial Institute, Columbus, OH, 1971.

Department of the Navy: Overseas Diplomacy. US Government Printing Office, Washington, DC (in revision).

Falvo, DR: Effective Patient Education. Aspen, Rockville, 1985.

Gazda, GM, Childers, WC, and Walters, RP: Interpersonal Communication: A Handbook for Health Professionals. Aspen, Rockville, 1982.

Greeley, A: Why Can't They Be Like Us? Institute of Human Relations, New York, 1969.

Samovar, LA, Porter, RE, and Jain, NC: Understanding Intercultural Communication. Wadsworth, Belmont, CA, 1981.

Stewart, M and Roter, D: Communicating with Medical Patients, Sage Publications, Newbury Park, 1989.

Chapter 11

Psychological and Cognitive Considerations

CAROL SCHUNK

Cognitive and psychological considerations of client care are especially important for the home health therapist, given the intimate relationship that can evolve from treating people in their own environment. Because home health therapy is oriented toward obtaining the highest degree of independence in the home, issues of motivation, compliance, and cognition must be included in the treatment approach. If therapy is regarded from a purely physical dimension, treatment success is limited and accompanied by therapist and client frustration. The psychological aspect of care is also enhanced in home health therapy because the family is often an integral part of treatment. The therapist must consider family dynamics and the effect of family relationships on the client's health. Although home health care involves persons of all ages, most clients are elderly individuals, therefore, this chapter focuses on cognitive and psychological aspects more common in the elderly.

COGNITIVE CHANGES THAT OCCUR WITH AGING

Cognitive changes that are present with healthy aging are minimal. By definition, a person is not considered to experience cognitive dysfunction unless daily activity or social function is affected. Therapy challenges the client physically and mentally. Therefore, the therapist in the home may be the first person to recognize a significant decline in mental abilities. The therapist must understand the parameters of normal cognitive changes to establish a baseline from which to judge dysfunction.

Memory

One of the misunderstandings about growing old relates to memory. Many people believe that memory fails as the years advance. While lapses in memory occur, they usually do not interfere with personal or social activities in the healthy elderly person. Benign senescent forgetfulness (BSF) is the term often used to describe the memory factor associated with normal aging. Not severe enough to interfere with daily function, BSF is thought to be present in one third of persons more than 85.[1] If the memory lapse is progressive, with increasingly interfering dysfunction, BSF is most likely not an appropriate diagnosis. A diagnosis of dementia is then a consideration.

Home Health Issues

The therapist in the home can assist the elderly person with memory lapses by suggesting a system to minimize the inconvenience and frustration of forgetting. Techniques may include establishing a consistent place for commonly misplaced items such as glasses, and a cue system for doing exercises or making lists for shopping. Safety is a major concern. Ability to remain at home safely can be prolonged by alteration of activities, for example, using a microwave for cooking as opposed to a potentially more dangerous conventional stove.

Intelligence

As measured by the Wechsler Adult Intelligence Scale, intelligence peaks in verbal and performance scale scores by age 18 and remains stable until ages 55 to 60.[2] After 60, decline is more evident, primarily in performance scores, which are time related as well as being affected by reaction time. Because of this classic aging pattern, intelligence quotient (IQ) scores are age based.

Home Health Issues

Therapeutic activities should not present a problem to the elderly person given the minimal changes in intelligence with normal aging. The decline in performance scores can be attributed in part to sensory and motor alterations. Therefore, although the elderly person is able to learn, therapy instructions, which almost always have a performance component, may need to be modified slightly. Increasing the repetitions at a slower pace can compensate for slower reaction time. Most important to remember is that the ongoing ability to learn allows progress and success in therapy regardless of age.

Personality

Many of the numerous theories about personality composition have been studied in relation to aging. Although based on review of the research on trait theory, the conclusion of Hartke[2] basically summarizes the current view on possible changes in personality with aging, indicating that consistency in personality is more common than change with aging. Personality changes that may occur with aging are seen as ongoing demonstration of individuality rather than aging.

Home Health Issues

Because of the current lack of evidence documenting personality changes with healthy aging, personality changes that do occur should be considered as a possible symptom of a cognitive deficit. Given the therapist's limited exposure to the client and the lack of readily available history, family members and friends are often in the best position to assess personality changes. Observations by those familiar with the behavior of the client will be helpful. Practitioners should inform the family or caregiver of any ongoing variation in behavior that is interfering with function. The physician or nurse may also need to be notified. If the family members are not aware, they may ignore the change by attributing the new behavior to "just getting old." In turn, a reversible mental condition may be missed. The client may be the first to notice changes in cognitive function and react with symptoms of depression or anxiety. Consultation with the client and family about the individual's reaction can provide support for the client and decrease family anxiety.

Coping

Coping strategies vary with the individual. Mechanisms are developed during the lifespan and are fairly constant as a person ages. The differences probably depend on the types and frequency of stressors necessitating coping strategies. McCrae[3] describes coping in terms of exit versus entrance events, exit events happening with increasing frequency as the person ages. Exit events can be viewed as threats. They include impending illness resulting in decreased autonomy and dependence on others, financial hardship, and loss of family or friends. In contrast, entrance events such as marriage or children may be seen as challenges. While the focus of coping may vary, there is no validation of a declining ability to cope as people age. In the home, therapists may encounter individuals whose participation in therapy is jeopardized by the inability to cope with the stress of illness or decreased independence. It is probable that the person has never learned effective coping strategies or that usual strategies are not working. Part of therapy may involve suggestions on how to deal with a stressful situation. For example, a woman with arthritis may be unable to cook the traditional family holiday meal, a situation with which she is not able to cope. The therapist can minimize the stressful situation by helping the person devise alternative methods of preparing the dinner within her capabilities.

Coping strategies are sometimes categorized into problem-focused and emotion-focused coping. As defined by Lazarus and Folkman,[4] problem-focused coping is directed toward managing the stressor, whereas emotion-focused coping is directed toward regulating the emotional response to the stressor. According to the authors, emotion-focused coping is used when the individual perceives that nothing can be done to change the situation (e.g., the death of a spouse). When the situation (e.g., a job change) is viewed as changeable, problem-solving coping is used.

Manfredi and Pickett[5] designed a two-part study dealing with stress and coping in the elderly. The first part identified stressful events; the second identified coping strategies used with identified stressors. Results from the first part showed loss and conflict to be the two major categories of stressful events. Loss included loss of health, significant relationships, and economic resources. Conflict stresses revolved around both intrapersonal and interpersonal issues of control and power. Many coping strategies were identified, supporting the notion that the elderly use more than one coping style.[5] Likewise, coping mechanisms, regardless of age, included both emotion-focused and problem-oriented methods.

Keefe and Williams[6] compared coping strategies to deal with pain among different age groups. Results indicated that there was no difference among age groups in coping strategies used to manage the stress associated with pain. Middaugh and associates[7] also found that methods of coping with pain in different age groups were similar. They concluded that the elderly would benefit from chronic pain programs as much as younger persons.

Home Health Issues

Therapists who talk to their clients and, more important, listen will become aware of the clients' stressors. Knowing potential areas of stress allows the therapist to consider ineffective coping as a possible reason for lack of progress toward therapeutic goals. Progress toward goals, participation in the therapy program, and attentiveness provide the practitioner with clues about the effectiveness of the client's available coping mechanisms. If the client's ability to function is being jeopardized by the inability to cope, intervention is necessary. In some cases the therapist can facilitate coping methods by discussing the stressor with the client and exploring the emotional response or possible problem-solving alternatives. If the inability to cope is severe, referral to a social worker or other appropriate professional may be in order. In some cases the therapist can discuss the issue with the family or encourage the client to talk to the family to initiate support.

COGNITIVE DYSFUNCTION

The American Psychiatric Association Diagnostic and Statistical Manual[8] (DSM III) defines dementia as including mental symptoms severe enough to interfere significantly with work, social activities, or relationships with others and often resulting in an individual's inability to remain at home. While aging does cause some changes in mental capacity, the process is normally not severe enough to affect the ability to function at home.

Dementia

Dementia is the most common of the organic mental symptoms described by the DSM III.[8] Along with delirium, dementia impairment is global, with no specific pattern of symptoms or course of onset. Decline in intellectual function from a previous level is the essential clinical feature. The decline must be at a level sufficient to interfere with work, social activities, or relationships with others. According to the DSM III, the essential feature of intellectual decline is impairment in short-term and long-term memory with other characteristics including deterioration of abstract thinking, judgment, and additional higher cortical tasks.

Alzheimer's Disease

Sixty percent of those diagnosed with dementia have Primary Degenerative Dementia of the Alzheimer Type, or Alzheimer's disease, although the definitive diagnosis is post-mortem. McKhann and associates[9] have published widely accepted, diagnostic-oriented clinical criteria. The primary criterion is insidious onset of dementia not caused by any other disease known to produce memory loss and cognitive decline. Initially the individual may be able to continue socially, with forgetfulness as the primary symptom. As the disease progresses, acquisition of new information becomes difficult, impairing the ability to continue on the same level of independence. Depression may accompany the onset of symptoms as the individual becomes aware of the decline in cognition.

Although behavioral problems have not been empirically associated with the cognitive deficits of Alzheimer's disease, Teri and associates[10] studied the issue from the caregiver's perspective. Over 50 percent of those surveyed identified four behaviors as being the "biggest problem" in providing client care. These were memory disturbance, catastrophic reactions, suspiciousness, and accusations. Identification of the behavioral problems and the associated cognitive factors revealed that memory loss, confusion, and disorientation were the most common.

Cerebral Vascular Accident

Multi-infarct dementia is the organic mental disorder associated with cerebral vascular disease. The loss of brain tissue from infarcts produces select deficits that are difficult to predict even when the infarct has been located. This may be due to multiple strokes or to variation in the size of the insult. Although the clinical picture of impaired memory, judgment, and abstract thinking resembles that of Alzheimer's disease, distinct features include abrupt onset, step-by-step deterioration, and a fluctuating behavior pattern.

Depression

The essential feature for a clinical diagnosis of depression is either depressed mood or loss of interest or pleasure in almost all activities for a period of at least 2 weeks.[8] The depressed mood is established from subjective account or observation by others. In addition to one of the above, the person must display several of the following symptoms:

- Significant weight loss or gain
- Insomnia or hypersomnia
- Psychomotor retardation or agitation
- Fatigue or loss of energy
- Feelings of worthlessness or inappropriate guilt
- Diminished ability to concentrate or think
- Recurrent thoughts of death

All organic factors must have been ruled out prior to diagnosis. In addition, the symptoms must indicate a change from a previous level of function and be relatively persistent.

Pseudodementia

Pseudodementia occurs when dementialike behavior is the result of a depressive episode. While presenting symptoms may be similar to those of dementia (hence the label, dementia syndrome of depression) there is usually a definitive date of onset and rapid progression of clinical features.[8] Treatment with antidepressive medication often distinguishes between the two disorders. If symptoms are resolved and cognitive function returns to the prior level, dementia is ruled out, with the appropriate diagnosis being depression. Haggerty and associates[11] emphasize the possibility that the two conditions can coexist. They therefore discourage use of the term "pseudodementia," which implies the need to choose one condition or the other.

Reversible Dementia

While most cases are irreversible, 10 to 30 percent of individuals with symptoms of dementia have conditions that are reversible with proper diagnosis and treatment of the underlying cause. Conditions that can be reversed include those caused by drug interactions, infectious diseases, poor nutrition, psychiatric and metabolic disorders, and trauma. The most common drug complications result from self-medicating or inattentiveness by prescribing physicians to drug-drug combinations (see Chapter 9). Given the ease of reversing the cognitive deficits once the problem is addressed, it is essential that all possibly reversible conditions be investigated before a diagnosis of dementia.

COGNITIVE DYSFUNCTION AND HOME HEALTH CARE

Most of the cognitive deficits discussed are diagnosed in relation to a prior level of function. Symptoms become obvious when a person can no longer perform daily activities that were previously possible. The home health therapist is often in a position to initially identify this decline in function. Direct observation or a subjective report from the client or caregiver may lead to early identification of a cognitive decline not attributable to normal changes of aging. Two bedside tools for cognitive dysfunction—the Mini Mental Status Examintion and the Blessed Orientation Memory Test—have excellent test-retest reliability. The simplicity of the tools make them appropriate for the home health setting since extensive training is not necessary.[19] Although the tools do not provide detailed neurobehavioral descriptions, they do discriminate among levels of cognitive dysfunction on the basis of the severity and course of illness. It may be appropriate to recommend a formal assessment for diagnostic purposes if placement becomes an issue. Probably as important as the assessment are the modifications of the treatment plan, therapeutic approach, and treatment goals.

Although the rehabilitation potential for persons with cognitive dysfunction was once considered minimal, research now indicates that the severity of the deficit should not eliminate the individual from participating in a program.[12] Therapy must be modified according to the mental disability just as it must with a physical problem. Because memory loss is often a problem, the treatment approach may include verbal and visual cues, demonstration, simple consistent directions, and repetition. Involvement of the caregiver in the initial instructions is usually a positive factor in enhancing compliance.[13] The therapist's expectations in establishing goals may have to be appropriately scaled down when cognitive dysfunction is an issue. Reinforcement of small gains provides input to the client on the gradual progress that occurs. This includes praise for successive approximations of previous behaviors, even those the client may consider meaningless, that were part of the daily routine before the illness or disability.[14]

Given the uniqueness of home health care, modification of the environment to accommodate cognitive dysfunction is essential. Not only can function be enhanced, but safety issues can be addressed. Confusion and memory loss result in increased exposure to hazardous situations. The resulting risk of danger in the home may be the precipitating event for institutionalization. Substituting a microwave oven for a conventional stove or oven, and minimizing the risk of falls by concentrating the living areas on one floor, are examples of interventions to prolong independence in the client's own environment. Simplifying the home, eliminating clutter, and standardizing the location of necessary items such as keys will minimize the frustration and stress for a person in early stages of Alzheimer's disease. While environmental safety is a constant concern for the home health therapist, the presence of mental symptoms, especially memory impairment, requires that each session include assessment and reinforcement of safety factors (see Chapter 7).

Motivation

Motivation is always a factor in attempting to achieve therapeutic goals. In the home health setting it must be an integral part of therapy since the client is usually not seen daily and must depend on an inner sense to comply with the therapy program. According to Glickstein, motivation is defined as an "inner urge that moves or prompts a person to action" (ref. 15, p. 1). The actual Latin origin of the word "motive" is "to move." Taking movement as the critical factor, Kemp[16] developed a motive system based on the two bases of movement: direction and force. Applying these to behavior, he defines direction as choices, decisions, and selections, and force as the effort, persistence, or strenuousness. While there are many theories of motivation, the model presented by Kemp takes into consideration the cognitive, affective, perceptual, and environmental processes. Applicable to those in the home health environment, the model equation is:

$$\frac{\text{Wants} \times \text{Beliefs} \times \text{Rewards}}{\text{Motivation} = \text{Costs}}$$

As diagramed, motivation is the multiple result of a person's wants, beliefs, and rewards divided by the cost of the activity.

The term "wants" includes goals, desires, and wishes and refers to what the person wants to get, wants to do, and wants to express. In home health situations the most obvious application is the necessity to mesh the desires of the client with the goals of the therapist. "Assume," "conclude," or "think" are synonyms for the term "belief" in the model. The stumbling block is the therapist's assumption that the client's beliefs must be positive, rational, or reality oriented. Given this model, the therapist can understand motivational problems that occur when the person's beliefs are not in keeping with the reality of the situation. For example, a client who has sustained a hip fracture may believe that independent walking is now unattainable. Despite therapeutic intervention with independent ambulation as the goal, motivation will be a problem based on the client's beliefs. To be successful, the therapist must explore the origin of the misconception about walking, redirecting the client's beliefs, and enhancing motivation.

Given the common premise that behavior must be rewarded to continue, the therapist must provide positive reinforcement. If the client is elderly, the personal rewards that are important may differ from those of the young athlete who is motivated by the goal of playing sports again. For a person to be motivated, the combination of the above three factors — wants, beliefs, and rewards — must be greater than the costs involved in the process.

Costs can be physical, psychological, or social. As with beliefs, the costs may not be the reality of the situation, but what the person perceives they are or will be. If the person believes that the self-image of walking with a walker is strongly negative (psychological cost), the cost of this belief may outweigh the desire to walk independently, the belief that the task is attainable, and the reward of being independent. The therapist must explore the individual's personal wants, beliefs, rewards, and costs to determine the potential for motivation. In the above case it would be futile to keep rewarding the client for the efforts without addressing the feelings about the psychological perception of "looking old" associated with using a walker. Part of the client assessment is to determine the client's motivating factors. Information obtained during the interview will provide insight into the best method of approaching the client and of establishing achievable goals.

By viewing motivation as part of the treatment plan, the therapist can avoid the frustration of working with what is perceived as the unmotivated client. Actually, everyone is motivated. Unfortunately, when an individual's motivation is to not participate in the treatment plan, this is interpreted as a lack of motivation rather than a conflict of goals. Therapist may be unsuccessful if the therapist's goal is for the client to be able to live independently and the client's goal is to go and live with an adult child.

A common misconception is that people either are motivated or are not. When a person is labeled unmotivated, usually there is no understanding of the individual's behavior. Therapists must be aware that they can influence motivation after assessing a client's motivating factors using techniques or strategies to increase motivation. Strategies may include involving the client in goal setting, allowing the client to make choices about treatment modalities, and dividing activities into achievable tasks with appropriate positive reinforcement for success.

Compliance

Cooperation, or compliance, is a significant factor in all therapeutic situations. In the home, however, there is an even greater need to address the issue of compliance or cooperative behavior. The inpatient setting provides the structure to monitor follow-through. In the home, the focus is on client responsibility because the therapist rarely treats the client on a daily schedule. Therefore, the therapist must consider noncompliance a reality when structuring the program and planning the client's progress.

Three predictor variables—personality, social support, and instructional methods—are most often mentioned in the literature as causes for noncompliance.[17] Personality is an easy explanation for uncooperative behavior. The blame is put on the client with minimal expectation that change is possible. However, actual research data are not conclusive about the influence, if any, of personality on compliance. While the presence of a support system has been shown to influence compliant behavior, the interesting factor is that the influence may be positive or negative. Practicing in the home provides a greater opportunity for the therapist to observe the interaction between the client and family or caregivers. In some cases the support can be positive, encouraging and reinforcing the client to follow a treatment regime. On the other hand, the support system may sabotage the therapeutic program by questioning the method and not allowing the client to practice independent activities. Assessment of the support system and home environment will inform the therapist about potential cooperative behavior. For example, a marriage may be based on one partner's doing everything for the other partner. Attempts to make the client more independent may result in noncompliant behavior to prevent changing the dynamics of the marriage.

Home programs are an ongoing part of home health treatment. Client compliance to directions may vary depending on the instructional method. Research reviewed by Schunk[17] indicates that the combination of demonstration and an instructional booklet for teaching an exercise program will result in higher retention. Providing feedback to the client via a graph or log are also instructional methods that have demonstrated increased compliance.

Once compliance is viewed as a factor in successful outcome, the therapist must determine whether cooperation has been achieved. Without knowing if a client has followed the treatment regimen, the therapist may decide to change a treatment program because the client is not making progress. When compliance is investigated, the therapist may discover that the lack of progress is not due to inappropriate treatment modalities but to the client's failure to follow the original directions. In the home, self-report and observation is probably the most practical method of assessing compliant behavior. To minimize the client's tendency to report only positive compliant behavior, the question must be phrased in a nonjudgmental manner, in essence giving permission to be truthful and report noncompliance if appropriate. The method should not be accusatory: "Did you do your exercises?" but concerned: "Some people find it hard to do all the exercises; did you have any trouble completing the program?" If the client reports noncompliance, it is necessary to investigate the reasons behind the behavior.

A discussion with the client will often provide the therapist with information that can be used to facilitate cooperative behavior. Perhaps diagrams or a daily checklist can help if memory is a problem. As with motivation, the client must perceive that the benefit gained by following the program outweighs the cost. The relationship of the home program to the desired outcome is also a factor. If the therapist does not explain how a specific task is related to the desired outcome, the probability of follow-through is minimized. The important factor is the client's perception of the situation rather than the reality that decides the outcome.

When uncooperative behavior is an issue, health problems should also be considered. Some health disorders can create barriers to follow through with prescribed treatments.[18] Because therapy is based on educating the client, understanding and learning are essential elements. Communication and therefore learning may be hampered by sensory or language deficits that are often present in elderly people. Vision and hearing disorders may prevent a person from initially comprehending the program to be followed. An inability to read affects the design of instructions. If the lack of understanding is not exposed, the therapist operates on the assumption that the client understands the instructions when in fact the client may be too embarrassed to mention the sensory deficits interfering with cooperation. Cognitive dysfunction, discussed previously, affects an individual's ability to follow a prescribed regimen. Given the decline of memory evident with dementia and the indifference seen with a depressive state, the therapist should anticipate noncompliance and make appropriate adjustments to the treatment program when encountering these obstacles. Suggested adjustments are cues to enhance memory or increased involvement of a depressed client in establishing personal therapy goals.

SUMMARY

The goal of therapy, regardless of the setting, is to maximize the client's function to the highest level of independence. The influence of the psychological aspects of rehabilitation cannot be ignored if the therapist hopes to achieve treatment goals. In the home, the therapist has the unique opportunity to work with the individual in his or her own environment. Therefore, client and family problems with motivation, compliance, and cognitive dysfunction become more obvious. A therapist who is aware of the importance of these aspects of treatment and incorporates them into therapy will provide a total program for the client with a minimum of personal frustration.

REFERENCES

1. Odenheimer, GL: Acquired cognitive disorders of the elderly. Med Clin North Am 73:1383, 1989.
2. Hartke, RJ: The aging process: Cognition, personality and coping. In Hartke, RJ (ed): Psychological Aspects of Geriatric Rehabilitation. Aspen, Gaithersburg, 1991.
3. McCrae, RT: Age differences in the use of coping mechanisms. J Gerontol 37:454, 1982.
4. Lazarus, RS and Folkman, S: Stress appraisal and coping. Springer-Verlag, New York, 1984.
5. Manfredi, C and Pickett, M: Perceived stressful situations and coping strategies utilized by the elderly. Journal of Community Health Nursing 4:99, 1987.
6. Keefe, FJ and Williams, DA: A comparison of coping strategies in chronic pain patients in different age groups. J Gerontol 45:161, 1990.
7. Middaugh, SJ, et al.: Chronic pain: Its treatment in geriatric and younger patients. Arch Phys Med Rehabil 69:1021, 1988.
8. American Psychiatric Association: Diagnostic and Statistical Manual of Mental Disorders, ed 3 (revised). Author, 1987.
9. McKhann, GD, et al: Clinical diagnosis of Alzheimer's disease: Report of the NINCDS-ADRDA work group under the auspices of Department of Health and Human Services task force on Alzheimer's disease. Neurology 34:939, 1984.
10. Teri, L, et al: Behavioral disturbance, cognitive dysfunction and functional skill prevalence and relationship in Alzheimer's disease. J Am Geriatr Soc 37:109, 1989.
11. Haggerty, JR, et al: Differential diagnosis of pseudodementia in the elderly. Geriatrics 43:61, 1988.
12. Techendorf B: Cognitive impairment in the elderly: Delirium, depression, or dementia? Focus on Geriatric Care and Rehabilitation 3:1–8, 1987.
13. Mace, NL, Hardy, SR, and Rabins, PV: Alzheimer's disease and the confused patient. In Jackson, O (ed): Physical Therapy of the Geriatric Patient. J & A Churchill, London, 1989.

14. Hibbard, MR, et al: Cognitive therapy and the treatment of poststroke depression. Topics in Geriatric Rehabilitation 5:43–55, 1990.

15. Glickstein, JK: Motivation of older adults. Focus on Geriatric Care and Rehabilitation 3:8, 1990.

16. Kemp, BJ: Motivation, rehabilitation, and aging: A conceptual model. Topics in Geriatric Rehabilitation 3:41–51, 1988.

17. Schunk, CR: Prediction and assessment of compliant behavior. Topics in Geriatric Rehabilitation 3:15–20, 1988.

18. Stilwell, JE: Common health problems that threaten compliance in the elderly. Topics in Geriatric Rehabilitation 3:34–40, 1988.

19. Zillmer, EA, et al.: Comparison of two cognitive bedside screening instruments in nursing home residents: A factor analytic study. J Gerontol 45:69–74, 1990.

Chapter 12

Caregivers

BELLA J. MAY & JANCIS K. DENNIS

As home health therapists, we focus our attention on movement—movements associated with self-care and mobility in and around the home. Although the psychosocial aspects of disability are an integral part of our basic education, we are not educationally prepared to be social workers, sociologists, psychologists, or family therapists. Yet our therapeutic goals often carry implications for the social milieu in which our clients are situated. Attainment of the goals can depend more on caregiver and client follow-through than on the time we spend in the home. We cannot expect independent transfers to be achieved if the client is called on to transfer without physical assistance only when we are present. Nor can we project the blame for failure to achieve the independent transfers onto the client or the caregiver. Understanding the family relationships that can enhance or impede attainment of objectives is as much a part of our evaluation as the actual ability to transfer. Seeking ways to increase the caregiver's ability to structure practice time with an appropriate facilitator is as much a part of our care plan as is teaching the new skill in the first place. Family relationships are complex and dynamic. The caregiving function places some degree of burden on the family, however defined. In this chapter we examine some of the issues involved in the interaction between therapists and caregivers as they relate to the therapeutic interaction. In particular, we explore techniques of evaluation, consider some of the major stressors in caregiving, and suggest some approaches to handling family dynamics. Caregiving has been extensively researched in recent years, and the literature is replete with information and study results. The purpose of this chapter is not to provide an extensive review of related literature, but rather to consider research results as they might be used by home health therapists in their daily activities.

THE FAMILY UNIT

Definitions

The family is the primary source of caregivers. What aggregation of people constitutes a family? Traditionally, the family is considered to be the husband, wife, and children living together in a residential unit. However, there are many different types of family units. A generally accepted definition is "any significant group of intimates with a history and a future" (ref. 1, p. 1099). For our purposes, we will consider the family as the individual or individuals assuming responsibility for the care of the client either temporarily or permanently. The family can be a spouse, a single or married adult child with or without family, a significant other of the same or opposite sex, or friends and neighbors who may provide assistance to a disabled client living alone. Contrary to the popular myth that children do not take care of their parents in our society today, research indicates that most of the care given to frail or disabled individuals is given by the children with little assistance from formal provider organizations.[2,3] The aging of the population and the increased numbers of elderly individuals living well into their 80s and 90s is creating a large pool of caregivers, predominantly women in their 50s and 60s caring for parents or in-laws.[2]

Caregiving responsibilities vary with the needs of the client, the extent and scope of the disability, and the number of individuals available for caregiving. Caring for an ill or disabled family member is a generally accepted responsibility. However, few caregivers are prepared for the role, which usually occurs suddenly, and few are aware of the demands of caring for a chronically ill individual. Some caregiving may require personal sacrifice and some may be done out of guilt. Caregiving, whether temporary or permanent, requires flexibility and adaptation and places some degree of stress on the family unit.

Functional and Dysfunctional Families

Family systems are dynamic, not static. Families undergo constant change as children grow older and leave home, patients retire or change careers, and elderly members become ill and need assistance. Nontraditional families change similarly as individuals mature, partnerships are formed or disbanded, people change employment or move, or illness occurs. Individual family members face conflicting demands and changing roles. The illness of any family member may threaten the delicate balance within the family.

Functional families find ways to adapt to the new stresses placed on them by the addition of caregiving responsibilities. They balance individual and family needs without placing excessive expectations on one member. Functional families are characterized by this ability to adapt, by evidence of closeness and caring among the members, and by mutual respect for themselves and the care recipient. However, some families have difficulty adapting. Corgiat[4] identifies four basic dysfunctional family paradigms and discusses how each functions when faced with a problem situation.

The *closed family* works hard to maintain stability and constancy. Individuality in beliefs or opinion is not welcome and the family tends to shut out the outside world when problems arise. The family focuses on the ill member and uses that person's needs to keep everyone in line and to shut out other family problems. The therapist working with a closed family may find the caregiver unwilling to consider alternative approaches to client management and appearing to be threatened by the client's possible recovery.

Conversely, the *open family* has no leader. Each person is involved in problem solving and expected to participate in decision making. Family members may gather considerable information and will try to communicate all information to each other. However, the open family has difficulty using the information they gather. Different family members may seek information but there is little evidence of that information being shared or used by the group. The therapist may find it difficult to identify a primary caregiver and to obtain concensus on a plan of action.

The *random family* values independence and individuality and may feel threatened by a need to cooperate. In times of crisis family members may each institute an individual solution. The therapist may again have difficulty finding the major caregiver and the client may feel a lack of emotional support. The therapist may find that one family member may obtain one piece of adapted equipment only to have another family member introduce a different adaptation that does the same thing. In working with a random family the therapist may have to function as a coordinator.

The *synchronous family* works together and values cooperation rather than individuality. The primary caregiver usually expects other family members to "do the right thing" without being given specific instructions. Family members are expected to take the initiative, seek out what needs to be done, and do it. Problems may arise when a family member does not do what is expected. The caregiver may experience frustration, yet not be able to verbalize the cause of the feelings. Harmony will be apparent to the therapist at first because the synchronous family is difficult to identify.

Naturally, few families fit the extremes outlined above, but many present elements of one paradigm or the other. Most families can be considered functional; however, understanding the family situation can help the home health therapist select an effective approach to teaching home programs and generally working with the caregivers.

EVALUATING THE CAREGIVING SITUATION

General Concepts

You have a new client to see on your home health rounds today, Ms. V., who has recently been discharged from a nursing home by her family because they suspected mishandling. The client suffered her third stroke 6 months ago. The nurse, who initiated home care, stated that Ms. V. has just started to be responsive and communicate with family members.

On arrival, you find that the primary caregiver is the client's 52-year-old daughter, Diane Cartin, who is married and living with her husband. There are two young children living in the house, a 2-year-old and a baby about 3 months old. Ms. Cartin tells you that she looks after her eldest daughter's children while the daughter is at work. She will soon have another "charge" because another daughter will be returning to work after the recent birth of her first child.

You arrive at the house about 11:30 AM and start your evaluation. Soon you hear male voices asking, "What's for dinner?" You learn that Ms. Cartin's husband and two sons-in-law come home at noon each day for the main meal. When the men arrive, the client, who has a marked expressive dysphasia, gives you the impression that there is someone in the household group of whom she does not approve.

Evaluating the family situation is not easy and may not be completed during the initial visit. The therapist must identify key family members, learn how the family functions, and develop insights into important individual relationships within the group. However, asking probing questions could create the impression that the therapist is prying in areas unrelated to "exercises" and functional activities. Additionally, many therapists do not always feel comfortable asking "personal" questions. Some information can be collected as part of the routine data gathering:

1. Is this the client's usual domicile?
2. Who lives in the house at this time?
3. Is there an extended family in the area? How often do they visit?
4. What was the client's premorbid level of function? Is return to that level anticipated by the client? the family?
5. Who will be able to work with the client on home activities?
6. How does the client relate to that person?

These and similar questions can provide a wealth of information both by what is said and by what is left unsaid. Hasselkus[5] interviewed 15 caregiving families, starting each interview with the question: "Can you begin by telling me what your day is like?" (ref. 5, p. 61). Further questions evolved from the response to the first. Caregivers would identify major problems, raise concerns, and provide some indication of their emotional state in relation to the caregiving function.

Talking with Diane Cartin after finishing your evaluation, you mention home exercises. Ms. Cartin frowns a little and states that she would be the one to do whatever is needed for Ms. V. She indicates that she was concerned about the care Ms. V. was receiving in the nursing home and took her out as soon as she could. She wants to do everything she can to help her mother but is very busy during the day with the children. When you ask about other family members, Ms. Cartin responds rather curtly, saying, "They are not available."

It is helpful to spend some time talking with the client and caregiver independently. Compare the client's and caregiver's information. Is there congruence or disparity? Note the caregiver's perception of the family support system. Brummel-Smith[6] suggests documenting family relationships in a genogram. A genogram is a graphic outline of family members and relationships using standardized symbols. Figure 12–1 shows some of the major identification codes used with genograms. A genogram can be designed to focus on any aspect of the family such as the ancestors or the current members[7,8]. Working with the elderly, Brummel-Smith recommends focusing the genogram on the client's offspring. Figure 12–2 is a genogram of Ms. V. and her family. It is clear that the caregiver has minimal assistance and will need extra resources to prevent burnout. A genogram is easy to compile, and the information can be gathered as part of the regular initial interview.

Discussion with the client and caregivers can give the home health therapist some insights regarding family stress level and potential problem areas. Care must be taken in interpreting caregiver answers and comments. Without a professional psychological background, home health therapists may impute their own feelings and reactions to the caregivers. It is easy to categorize and judge families on the basis of our past experiences and our own biases. We bring our own values and beliefs about family behavior and evaluate the situation from that mindset. It is critically important to be cog-

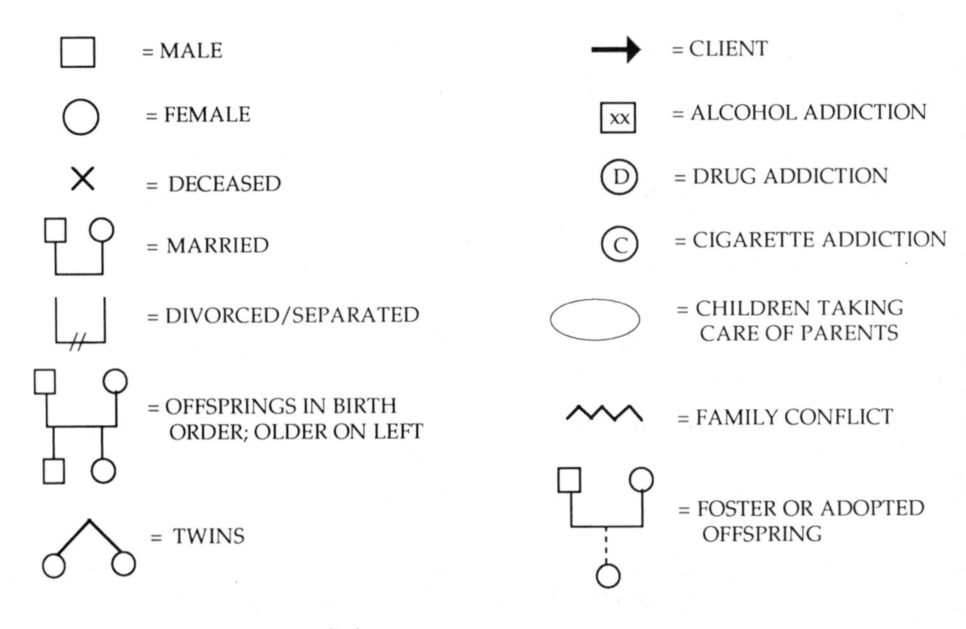

Figure 12–1. Genogram symbols.

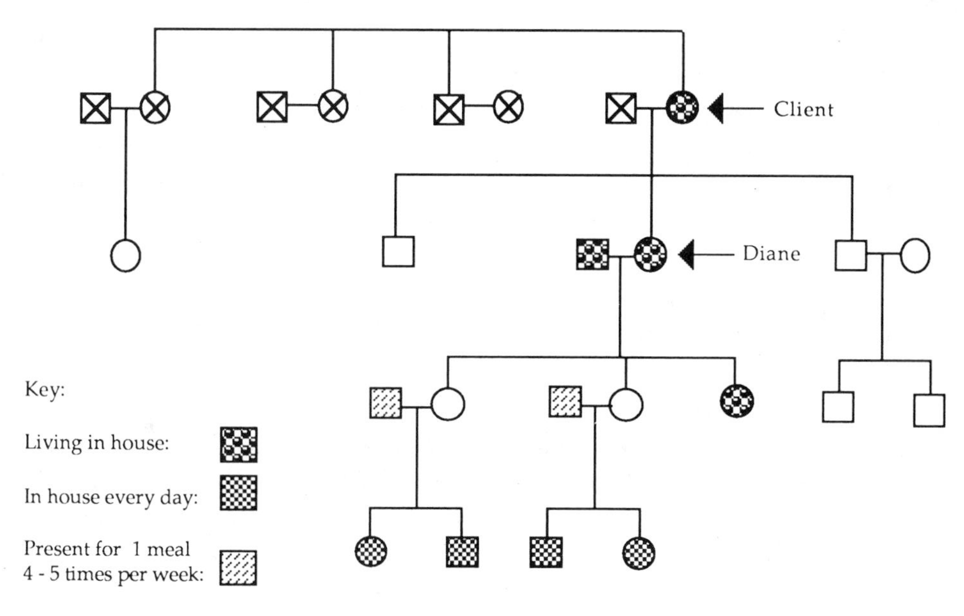

Figure 12–2. Genogram of the client, Ms. V, and her daughter/caregiver, Diane Cartin.

nizant of our own values and beliefs and of how they influence our perspective and the advice we give.

Because the home health therapist may be the first person to note caregiving problems, a careful evaluation of the family and caregiving situation is important. Potential caregiving problems may not be apparent to hospital personnel discharging the client because their contact with the family has been limited.

Identifying the Primary Caregiver

The home health therapist must identify the primary caregiver. Some caregivers, such as Ms. V's daughter, are easily identified. In other instances the primary caregiver may not be apparent.

Mr. R., 74 years old, has been living with his son Bob Davis, his daughter-in-law Jane Davis, and two teenaged granddaughters, Beth and Rose, since the death of his wife 2 years ago. The family lives in a small three-bedroom house in a housing project for low-income families. Mr. R. suffered a cerebral vascular accident resulting in a left hemiparesis about 6 weeks ago. He has just been discharged from the rehabilitation center and referred for home health care. During the day the home health therapist would probably find only Mr. R. and Mr. Davis in the home. Mr. Davis, unemployed because of a back injury, takes care of Mr. R. while Ms. Davis is at work and Beth and Rose are in school.

Without investigation, the therapist might assume that Mr. Davis is the primary caregiver and aim the interventions toward his involvement. However, exploring the family situation reveals that Mr. Davis takes care of Mr. R. only during the day. Rose is the one who spends the most time with Mr. R. She went to the rehabilitation center to learn the home program and now encourages her grandfather to be as independent as possible. Rose is also the one to whom Mr. R. relates the best.

The primary caregiver may, of course, not be the person to whom the client relates best. Clients and their caregivers bring old scripts into the relationship. "She'll do it for you, but she won't do it for me" is not an uncommon statement from caregivers. There are many reasons why clients and caregivers may have difficulty working together. Perhaps the client is reluctant to work in a dependent relationship with the caregiver; perhaps the caregiver is reticent because of a former dominant parent-child relationship, or one in which the now adult child felt that most efforts fell short of parental expectations. Clients and caregivers may not verbalize long-standing issues of trust but may find superficial reasons for their lack of cooperation. Sometimes the therapist can negotiate some sort of compromise focusing on the superficial conflict. The therapist may encourage each person to suggest a solution and help them find an approach both can support. On occasion someone outside the home, a friend or neighbor, can participate in the home activity and relieve the primary caregiver of some of the burden.

Evaluating Caregiver Needs

Caregiver needs fall into three general areas: (1) a need for information; (2) a need for specific recommendations or assistance for specific problems; and (3) an understanding of their fears and concerns.

Need for Information

Most individuals do not have a good understanding of the cause, treatment, and prognosis of different disabilities. Some clients believe that sustaining a fractured hip means a dependent life-style forever. Family members may be concerned that exertion will cause another stroke. In some instances the client or caregiver may know someone who recovered fully from the same disability without any therapy. Often the client is discharged from the hospital without anyone's taking the time to answer the family's questions. In some instances, information may not be heard or understood. Taking some time to talk quietly with the client and the caregiver can provide a desirable opportunity to voice issues and concerns. It is not necessary for the home health therapist to be able to answer all the questions. However, it is helpful for the therapist to be able to suggest resources. Many clients and family members simply do not know what to expect. Will grandmother be able to stop using the walker when the fracture is healed adequately? How long will that take? Can Mr. R. be taught to take care of his own needs? He loved to take long walks in the afternoon; is that now out of the question? What about all this medication? Care must be taken not to overwhelm the client or caregiver with information but rather to focus on the most imminent expressed needs. Providing a listening environment and allowing the caregiver or the client to raise issues and concerns is often most helpful and appreciated.

Need for Assistance

Suggestions or recommendations may be related to the physical environment, the specific care of the client, or emotional concerns. The therapist can provide specific assistance with certain types of problems. Helping to obtain equipment and supplies, making recommendations to improve the home environment, and making referrals to obtain external resources are all part of the therapist role. Obviously the therapist's role is limited and referral to the social worker may be required (see Chapter 13). The therapist also must avoid being placed in the middle of an uncomfortable situation.

Ms. V. has learned to transfer from bed to wheelchair and move her chair around the house, although she is a little unsteady and tends to run into things. Ms. Cartin states she wants Ms. V. to wait until she can be with her to get out of bed in the morning. Ms. V. indicates that her daughter is busy with the children and cannot always come to help her. They both look to you for an answer.

The therapist can function as a negotiator and help Ms. V. and her daughter find a mutually acceptable compromise. The therapist must guard against telling the client and family what to do and must encourage them to solve their own problems. Recognizing each person's point of view is important.

Fears and Concerns

Illness and disability create many fears and concerns among clients and caregivers. Parents of disabled children may feel guilt and worry about the future for the child. Caregivers of elderly parents fear a growing dependency and the change in life-style it might bring while often having some guilt at not being totally altruistic. Spouses fear the loss of companionship and an inability to care properly for the loved one. When the client first comes home, caregivers often express concerns about their ability to manage the care. Hasselkus[5] reports that caregivers first expressed fears about client safety, causing another stroke, and managing in general. Later, caregivers expressed concerns about long-term management and the continued general health of clients who were permanently disabled or chronically ill. The home health therapist often can help allay some of the management fears by watching and guiding the caregiver through such tasks as transfers, dressing, and toileting.

Often, understanding the stresses and issues faced by the caregiver and providing an empathic ear may be all that is needed or expected. The therapist often has a closer relationship with the family than does any other member of the health care team. The therapist frequently sees the client more often, although nursing personnel may work with a client and family over a longer period of time. As mentioned earlier, referral for social or psychological services may be necessary.

CAREGIVER STRESS

There have been numerous studies of caregiver stress and several review articles summarizing the findings. Barer and Johnson[9] indicate that researchers do not define caregivers in the same manner and rarely focus on the recipient's point of view. Gywther and George[10] comment that most studies use a questionnaire or the telephone rather than face-to-face interviews and focus on middle-class, nonminority respondents. Despite these limitations, the literature can provide insights into some of the issues that create the greatest stress among caregivers. The findings may, of course, vary with specific individuals as well as ethnic and cultural differences. The stresses, problems, and issues related to caregiving vary with the caregiver, the needs of the client, and the other participants in the interaction. A single adult daughter caring for a severely impaired parent in her home must cope with major restrictions on her work and social life, particularly if funds are not available to provide support and respite. A sick child affects not only the immediate family but the extended family as well. What if the disabled individual is the adult child, the member of the middle generation who is expected to provide care for the young and the old? Disability among the middle generation often creates havoc within a family.

Spouses and Other Elderly Caregivers

A large number of caregivers are spouses, elderly individuals who may have physical limitations themselves.[11,12] Although much of the research on caregiver stress has focused on the effects of care on the middle generation, there is evidence that spouse caregivers are also under stress.[12] On some occasions, the initial hospitalization of one spouse may seriously affect the coping ability of the remaining spouse. Someone who has been passive may have to become the family decision maker, taking responsibility for the care of the disabled partner as well as the personal affairs.[2] The caregiver may also have health problems. There is a direct relationship between the degree of caregiver stress and the amount of help needed by the client; the more dependent the client, the more the caregiver is stressed.

Mr. and Ms. J. have been married for more than 50 years and live together in a small apartment in a large city. Ms. J., 72 years old, has had rheumatoid arthritis for many years but has been able to care for her own needs, walk limitedly in the home and to the street, and help a bit with some household chores. For many years, Mr. J., 79 years old and a retired chemical engineer, has been doing most of the shopping, general housecleaning, and cooking. Mr. J. has high blood pressure and a history of a myocardial infarction, but he and his wife have been able to maintain themselves with very limited assistance from their daughter, who lives in the suburbs. They have paid help once a week for the major housecleaning and laundry. Recently Ms. J. fell while going to the bathroom at night and sustained a hip fracture, which was repaired with an open reduction and internal fixation. Following discharge from the hospital, nursing, physical and occupational therapy home health services were requested.

Over the first 2 weeks of treatment, the team members document finding Ms. J. in bed most of the time. On occasion the bed is wet and Ms. J indicates that she is afraid to try and get out of bed because "he's not strong enough to help me." The physical therapist reports that Ms. J. moves slowly and does not appear to be following her home program. The occupational therapist indicates that Ms. J. is not trying to dress herself or perform many self-care activities. All of the team members note that Mr. J. is not dressed as neatly or cleanly as he used to be and appears overwhelmed by the situation. The nurse who has been seeing Ms. J. reports checking Mr. J.'s blood pressure at his request and finding it high.

Elderly couples who have been able to maintain themselves in a particular pattern of function may encounter difficulties when illness or injury alters their routine. Assuming new roles may be difficult. Mr. J. may feel uncomfortable helping his wife with what are considered to be private functions of bathing and toileting. He may be afraid that Ms. J. will fall again if he helps her walk and he may be physically and emotionally unable to handle the extra responsibilities that have been thrust on him. Wives who have left decision making and financial deliberations to their husbands for all of their lives may encounter difficulty assuming these new roles if the husband has a stroke. A most difficult scenario occurs when the client requires 24-hour supervision projected to be permanent and the caregiver suffers major physical or cognitive limitations.

Similar problems exist when the family is composed of two elderly adults, related or not related. It is not uncommon to find two sisters or sisters-in-law, a brother and sister, or two unrelated elderly adults living together. If the caregiver is elderly, the problems of health, capabilities, and role changes remain.

Agnes B., 82 years old, and Joanna D., 80 years old, are widowed sisters living together in a small apartment in the inner city of a large metropolitan area. Ms. D. has severe rheumatoid arthritis and needs assistance for most self-care and mobility activities but can transfer and walk with a walker for short distances. Ms. B. has been taking care of her sister for the past 10 years but has osteoporosis and has suffered compression fractures of the thoracic spine. Ms. B. also has hypertension controlled by medication. Ms. D.'s greatest fear, which she verbalizes to the home health therapist who has come to help her regain some functional ability following hospitalization for ulcers, is that something will happen to her sister, forcing her to go into a nursing home.

Helping the family maintain the necessary balance between independence and care needs is an important role of the home health therapist. The therapist must be alert to evidence of a deteriorating home situation and, working with other members of the team, must make an appropriate social service referral early.

Children as Caregivers

Much has been written about the "sandwich" generation—adult children caring for elderly parents or in-laws, juggling work, marital, and family responsibilities and the needs of their own growing or grown children. Brody,[13] however, states: "The dependent elderly, who refill their aging children's 'empty nests' physically or in terms of psychological, emotional needs do not become children to their children, and the children do not become parent to their parent(s). Half a century or more of adulthood and of parent-child relationship cannot be erased or disregarded" (ref. 13, p. 274). Women are the predominant caregivers in our society, whether taking care of an ailing child, a disabled spouse, a parent, or an in-law.[14-18] Hooyman[19] makes the point that women are often the hidden victims of current health care patterns and policies. Traditionally in our society women are expected to assume uncompensated caregiving roles to dependents while continuing to perform regular homekeeping functions. The increasing number of elderly makes this a growing problem that has not been recognized as an issue in health care policies.

Hooyman[19] describes further some of the special burdens on women caregivers. Emotionally, a woman may feel very alone without anyone to share the burden. She suffers curtailed leisure and social time, may have difficulty meeting employment goals, may face financial limitations, and may experience an increasingly narrowed life-style. Stress is often manifested in physical illness that may become serious. Hooyman indicates that the single most frequently stated reason for seeking nursing home placement for an elderly family member is the death or serious illness of the caregiver. The burden is greatest on the single caregiver but has been manifested in families when other members do not assume part of the responsibility.[19] The problems faced by women as caregivers have increased in recent years with the greater number of women in the work force and the increased aging of our society.

Women, of course, are not the only children providing care for ailing parents. Male children do get involved, albeit at a much lower rate. Generally, male children provide assistance related to managing finances, repairs on the home, and transportation. If the parent is living in the son's household, the daughter-in-law is usually responsible for the day-to-day care. Unmarried male children may hire assistance from community agencies.

Problems that affect all caregivers, regardless of sex, are feelings of inadequacy, difficulty in planning for the long term and in responding to the client's physical and emotional needs, particularly if negative behaviors are encountered, and in obtaining assistance from siblings, other family members, or the community.[20] There is some evidence that cumulative stress can result from long-term caregiving situations even without changes in the client's health status. Townsend and associates[21] discuss the "wear and tear" hypothesis of caregiving, which suggests an increase in stress over time. They also support other findings indicating that caregiver stress is one of the major factors for institutionalizing the elderly.[22,23]

There is, however, another side to the negative aspects of caregiving. Townsend and associates[21] found that there is considerable adaptation to caregiving and that stressful events may be seen as opportunities for psychological growth and increased tolerance within the family. Some families and individual caregivers develop effective coping mechanisms, and caregiving often becomes a rewarding activity. In a study of 60 caregivers, Kinney and Stephens[23] report that client progress, affection, cooperation, and other positive responses are considered "uplifts" and reward the caregiving function. With good support systems, the caregiving function must not necessarily be visualized as negative.

Elder Abuse

> The therapist arrives at Mr. R.'s house around 1:00 PM. During the course of therapy Mr. R. states that he is hungry and that he does not get enough to eat. He complains that his son leaves him alone a lot during the day and does not always get him something to eat.

How does the therapist interpret statements such as this? Is the statement from Mr. R. accurate? If the therapist were to question Bob Davis, he might say that Mr. R. forgot that he ate earlier in the day. Elder abuse is difficult to assess, but a study of 2020 elderly individuals living with another person indicates that 32 out of 1000 suffer some form of abuse.[24] The same survey revealed that physical violence such as hitting, pushing, or throwing something at the victim is the most prevalent form of elder abuse and that neither age nor ethnic status is a factor. Finally, the survey indicates that spouses or adult children caregivers are equally likely to be the abusers.

Elder abuse is generally a hidden problem. Few victims report it, usually feeling shame because the abuser is frequently a member of the family, often a child. It happens in the home without witnesses and, even if it is suspected, it is often not reported. Elder abuse can be physical or psychological and includes such acts as withholding appropriate care and nourishment, misusing the elder's financial resources, verbal abuse, physical punishment, neglect, and mobility restriction. Filinson and Ingman[25] suggest that elder abuse is difficult for even professionals to detect and that all individuals working with the elderly should be alert to potential abuse. Elder abuse is more likely to occur if the caregiver

1. Has unrealistic expectations of the client;
2. Suffers from severe psychological problems and feelings of inadequacy or feelings of severe stress related to caregiving;
3. Has a history of substance abuse;
4. Feels forced into the caregiving role;
5. Has been abused as a child;
6. Is also impaired in some way.[25,26]

Kosberg,[26] while stating that any elderly person could be the victim of elder abuse, describes the high-risk elderly person as a woman who

1. Depends on the caregiver;
2. May abuse alcohol;
3. Tends to blame herself for her problems;
4. Is isolated;
5. Can be demanding.

Kosberg[26] identifies the high-risk family as one that does not get along well, has economic problems, lives in crowded conditions, accepts the caregiving role reluctantly, and may have marital conflict.

While the incidence of elder abuse may not seem high in comparison to statistics on child abuse or even other problems of the elderly, it is nevertheless a growing problem that still goes mostly unreported. In 1984, Congress passed the Family Violence Prevention and Treatment Act, which authorizes the development and implementation of state grant programs for prevention and treatment. Reauthorization of the Older American Act provides further funding for social services. Some states have developed fairly comprehensive programs of identification and treatment whereas others have little more than unfunded statutes. Many states have passed mandatory reporting legislation, which requires health professionals to report suspected incidents. Many communities have adult protection services agencies that provide some support for abuse victims. Interventions can include psychological services for the caregiver, support groups for the abused, and possibly a change in placement. Sometimes the knowledge that an outside agency is monitoring the situation can reduce the problem. The home health therapist must know appropriate reporting procedures and agencies and must be alert to potential incidents. The local adult protection services can provide information on reporting procedures.

The Client as the Caregiver

Many clients live alone, have no available family, and depend on neighbors and friends for caregiving. Some can afford the cost of paid caregivers until independence is regained; however, some are reluctant to spend their limited assets, while others do not have the necessary resources. Magaziner and Cadigan[27], investigating community resources for women living alone, report that people who live alone are at greater risk of institutionalization if they become ill but are generally healthier than elderly individuals living with someone other than a spouse. Magaziner and Cadigan[27] compared similar groups of elderly women to determine use of formal and informal support systems. Members of one group lived alone, whereas members of the other group lived with someone else. Women who lived alone appeared more knowledgeable about available systems and made greater use of both formal and informal support systems. The results of the study, although limited in scope, indicate the importance of community support to help maintain independent living. There are few reports of caregiving issues related to individuals who live alone.

THERAPIST INTERVENTIONS

Provide Information

Awareness of family needs and caregiver stresses can guide the home health therapist in family interactions. A therapist who understands that many caregivers are thrust into the role suddenly, sometimes unwillingly, and often with little information or understanding of the client's needs or disability can provide information, solicit and answer questions, and help the caregiver and family begin to plan for the future. It is important to provide information as it is needed and guide the caregiver to potentially useful publications.[28] Encourage the caregiver to voice concerns and doubts.

Ms. Cartin, Ms. V.'s daughter, is concerned that Ms. V. will fall and hurt herself if she transfers to her wheelchair alone. You have been working on wheelchair transfers; Ms. V. can perform this activity without assistance but occasionally forgets to lock the chair and sometimes gets dizzy when she first sits up. Ms. Cartin has been leaving the chair on the other side of the room when her mother goes to bed at night because Ms. V. usually wants to get up just when the children first arrive in the morning and Ms. Cartin is very busy. Ms. V. has taken to ringing her bell violently to get Ms. Cartin's attention when she wants to get up. You are aware of the frustration felt by both people about this issue and encourage them to express their concerns. Ms. V. has some communication problems secondary to expressive aphasia but lets it be known that she wants to get out of bed on her own because that is one of the few things she can do independently. Ms. Cartin is concerned that if Ms. V. falls or has another problem she will not be able to alert anyone. A compromise is worked out after you explain to Ms. Cartin that Ms. V. can transfer safely if the chair is in the proper position and locked. You remind Ms. V. to sit on the side of the bed for a few minutes after she first sits up. The chair will be left in the proper position at night when Ms. V. goes to bed. In the morning Ms. V. will ring the bell once when she is ready to get up and will wait until the older child comes in to watch her transfer.

The home health therapist must involve the family as well as the client in goal setting. Often the initial goals will be determined by activities that will ease the caregiving burden. "What does the client need to be able to do to make the caregiving easier?" is a valuable question.

Assist with Long-Term Planning

Difficulty with long-term planning has been identified by many researchers as one of the stressors of caregiving. Illness or disability happen suddenly. Often caregivers do not know what to expect and are unable or unwilling to make decisions regarding long-term management. Often it is difficult for the therapist to provide much information in the early stages of disability. In later stages the therapist can stimulate thoughts of long-term planning, particularly if the client will continue to need assistance. Both the client and the caregiver must be involved to the extent possible. Some clients with thoughts of independent living must eventually face their continued needs for assistance. On occasion, the client can return to independent living with support from nearby friends or relatives. The home health therapist can serve in a resource role and, although prognostication is difficult, can provide some idea of the long-term expectation for recovery.

Enhance Caregiver Confidence

Part of the home health therapist's role is to teach the caregiver proper methods of providing care. Teaching, in whatever capacity, must be at the learner's level. Learning a new skill, particularly for elderly caregivers, can be daunting. The home health therapist must provide the caregiver with support, positive feedback, and confidence-building skills. Creativity and flexibility are needed to find the most appropriate methods of carrying out required activities. It is important for the home health therapist to allow the caregiver to indicate which methods would be more comfortable and which would be more difficult. Given confidence in their abilities, caregivers can adapt techniques or find more efficient ways of helping clients: "The [therapist] always said to turn the wheelchair and put it back by the wall to get him up from the bed; but I just get him under the left arm and kind of whirl him right around into the wheelchair. It's a lot easier and a lot faster, and it seems like I can get him up a lot better this way" (ref. 6, p. 65). There are many reasons why the caregiver does not follow through with a home program. Perhaps the client and the caregiver share some old "scripts" that make it difficult for the caregiver to teach the client new skills; perhaps the client has never perceived the caregiver as a skilled or responsible person; perhaps the family has little time or patience for the goals set; perhaps the activity represents a threat—the caregiver is afraid that supervised independence will lead to premature attempts at unsupervised independence and result in a fall. It is important for the therapist to discern impediments and try to help the caregiver and client work through the difficulties. Sometimes, reassuring the client that the caregiver is capable of helping with the activity and having the caregiver perform during the therapy session will help build confidence.

Providing emotional support and anticipating problems is another role of the home health therapist. After a time, the caregiving role can wear thin because energy levels are down and frustrations are up. This is particularly true when the client requires considerable assistance, is incontinent, is up in the middle of the night, or is demanding. The home health therapist can listen and provide an opportunity for the caregiver to vent frustrations and angers. The caregiver may feel guilty at being angry and may need the opportunity to express those feelings without fear of judgment. Finances may also be a worry, and the therapist may be able to make an appropriate referral to social services or community agencies.

Suggest Other Resources

The "Care Partner" Concept

Grieco and Kowalksi[15] coined the term *care partner* instead of *caregiver* to suggest that the process must be a partnership of shared responsibilities. In a partnership both members are equal, both have responsibilities, and both are involved in problem solving. Grieco and Kowalksi make the point that it is important to understand the role of the family member prior to illness. Was the client the support for the rest of the family? Did the client live independently and see the care partner only occasionally? Was it a friendly relationship? Under this concept, the client shares responsibility for the interaction with the care partners. Most studies have focused on the caregiver's point of view and problems in the caring situation. There has been little consideration of the care recipient's perspective. The home health therapist is in a unique position to support the partnership concept by being open and listening to both points of views. Although mediating major conflicts is unlikely, enhancing cooperation in small activities may increase the likelihood of communication about major problems. This approach necessitates a client with a fairly intact cognitive and emotional system. If the client is not able to participate fully in the partnership, finding even small areas of mutual understanding can be beneficial. The partnership concept can be extended to the family as a whole.

Support Groups

Community support can be categorized as formal and informal. The formal system includes such services as Meals on Wheels, elderly transportation, home health care, homemaker services, and emergency communication systems, to name just a few. Informal systems include friends and neighbors, religious groups, and volunteers. Support groups such as church fellowships, neighborhood friends, or associations may provide respite to the primary caregiver and are usually responsive to needs when the client or caregiver has been an active group member. This is particularly important to the lone caregiver. The therapist must check the availability of such groups when the family genogram suggests that respite from caregiving will be limited within the family group. If paid caregiving is not a regular option, college students may be available to sit with the client for a few hours or a weekend, giving the primary caregiver some respite. Many communities also have adult day care centers. It is important for the home health therapist to be aware of community resources and offer the caregiver some alternatives for respite. The home health therapist must be aware of social services available within the home health agency and must work closely with the social service worker for optimum results. (See Chapter 13 for further details on the role of social services and on community resources.)

SUMMARY

Most caregivers are members of the client's family — a spouse, adult child, relative, or significant other. Most frequently the caregiver is a woman caring for a disabled parent or parent-in-law either alone or within the family. Caregiving is a demanding and often fatiguing activity that can upset family balance and create considerable stress. The home health therapist, working within the family milieu, is aware of family relationships and must find ways to enhance the attainment of therapeutic objectives while not increasing caregiver stress. Being open to the needs of the client and the caregiver, providing opportunities for both to express their feelings and frustrations, and moderating goals and activities in accordance with the needs of the care partners are all available tools for the home health therapist. The therapist must understand the dimensions of caregiver burden, be aware of family and community resources, and be willing to incorporate the caregiver's needs into the therapeutic interaction. The home health therapist also must be willing to make appropriate referrals when necessary.

REFERENCES

1. Ransom, DC and Vandervoort, HE: The development of family medicine: Problematic trends. JAMA 225:1098, 1973.
2. Brashler, R and Hartke, RJ: The caregiving family for the disabled older adult. In Hartke, RJ (ed): Psychological Aspects of Geriatric Rehabilitation. Aspen, Gaithersburg, 1991.
3. Biegel, DE and Blum, A: Aging and Caregiving: Theory, Research and Policy. Sage Publications, Newbury Park, 1990.
4. Corgiat, MD: Identifying dysfunctional families in geriatric rehabilitation. Topics in Geriatric Rehabilitation 4:16, 1988.
5. Hasselkus, BR: Rehabilitation: The family caregiver's view. Topics in Geriatric Rehabilitation 4:60, 1988.
6. Brummel-Smith, K: Family science and geriatric rehabilitation. Topics in Geriatric Rehabilitation 4:1, 1988.
7. McGoldrick, M and Gerson, R: Genograms in Family Assessment. WW Norton, New York, 1985.
8. Davis, CM: Patient Practioner Interaction. Slack, Thorofare, NJ, 1989.
9. Barer, BM and Johnson, CL: A critique of the caregiving literature. The Gerontologist 30:26, 1990.
10. Gywther, L and George, L: Introduction: Symposium on caregivers for dementia patients: Complex determinants of well-being and burdens. The Gerontologist 26:245, 1986.
11. Coward, RT, Cutler, SJ, and Schmidt, FE: Differences in the household composition of elders by age, gender, and area of residence. The Gerontologist 29:814, 1989.
12. Ory, M: The burden of care: A familial perspective. Generations 10:14, 1985.
13. Brody, E: Women in the middle and family help to older people. The Gerontologist 21:471, 1981.
14. Young, RF and Kahana, E: Specifying caregiver outcomes: Gender and relationship aspects of caregiving strain. The Gerontologist 29:660, 1989.
15. Grieco, AJ and Kowalski, W: The "care partner." In Bernstein, LH, Grieco, AJ, and Dete, MK (eds): Primary Care in the Home. JB Lippincott, Philadelphia, 1987.
16. Yaffe, MJ: Implications of caring for an aging parent. Canadian Medical Association Journal 138:231, 1988.
17. Brody, EM, et al: Women's changing roles and help to elderly parents: Attitudes of three generations of women. J Gerontol 38:597, 1983.
18. Brody, EM: Aging parents and aging children. In Ragan, PK (ed): Aging Parents. University of Southern California Press, Los Angeles, 1979, p 264.
19. Hooyman, NR: Women as caregivers of the elderly: Implications for social welfare policy and practice. In Biegel, DE and Blum, A (eds): Aging and Caregiving. Sage Publications, Newbury Park, 1990.
20. Smith, GC, Smith, MF, and Toseland RW: Problems identified by family caregivers in counseling. The Gerontologist 31:15, 1991.

21. Townsend, A, et al: Longitudinal impact of interhousehold caregiving on adult children's mental health. Psychol Aging 4:393, 1989.
22. Morycz, R: Caregiving strain and the desire to institutionalize family members with Alzheimer's disease. Research on Aging 7:329, 1985.
23. Kinney, JM and Stephens, MAP: Hassles and uplifts of giving care to a family member with dementia. Psychol Aging 4:402, 1989.
24. Pillemer, K and Finkelhor, D: The prevalence of elder abuse: A random sample survey. The Gerontological Society of America 28:51, 1988.
25. Filinson, R and Ingman, SR: Elder Abuse: Practice and Policy. Human Sciences Press, New York, 1989.
26. Kosberg, JI: Preventing elder abuse: Identification of high risk factors prior to placement decisions. The Gerontological Society of America 28:43, 1988.
27. Magaziner, J and Cadigan, DA: Community care of older women living alone. Women Health 14:121, 1988.
28. Rob, C: The Caregiver's Guide. Houghton Mifflin Co., Boston, 1991.

Chapter 13

Social Services and Community Resources

MARIANNE HART

Paul Raeborn, home health therapist, approaches the Conklin home with some concern. Mr. Conklin, 61, sustained a nerve injury about 10 years ago that left him with a flail right foot. He tripped over his toes last month and broke his hip. Mr. Conklin indicated to Paul that he used to have a brace but that the shoe is worn out and the brace does not fit anymore. Paul has obtained a prescription for a plastic ankle foot orthosis, but the Conklins have not purchased a new pair of shoes to take to the orthotist. Paul is concerned because Mr. Conklin is able to walk well with the walker but the drop foot is a safety hazard. The Conklins only income is Ms. Conklin's Social Security and a small income Mr. Conklin receives from personal investments. Finances are a problem because Mr. Conklin does not yet qualify for Medicare but the family's income is too high for Medicaid. Discussing the problem with the Conklins, Paul suggests a referral to the agency's social worker.

Social workers fill many roles in a home health agency. Most home health therapists are familiar with the resource director role but may not be aware that social workers also function as counselors, educators, advocates, and mediators or facilitators. Social workers interact with clients, families, and each member of the health care team. It is important for the home health therapist to remember that although social service is reimbursable under Medicare, Part A, it is not usually reimbursable under Medicaid. In most instances, social services must be requested by a primary team member such as the physician, the occupational, physical, or speech therapist, or the nurse. If team conferences are held regularly in the agency, social service referral can come from the discussion of client status. In this chapter, a brief outline of the major social worker roles is followed by a discussion of interventions. This chapter provides a better understanding of the role of the social worker as a guide to the home health therapist. The focus is on the medical social worker.

SOCIAL WORKER ROLES

Resource Director

The social worker informs clients and families of available resources and helps them make the necessary application. The social worker acts as a liaison between families and financial agencies. Social workers maintain current information on financial resources such as social security, social security supplemental income, Medicare, and Medicaid. They must know eligibility guidelines and application procedures. Social workers must also be aware of local community agencies and their services. In many communities, for example, The Easter Seal Society provides rental or loaner equipment; the Alzheimer's Association pays for respite care; the Multiple Sclerosis

Foundation has support groups around the country; and groups such as the Lupus Foundation, Muscular Dystrophy, the Multiple Sclerosis Foundation, and Chronic Fatigue and Immune Dysfunction Syndrome provide information packets and newsletters to let the client and family know more about the disease and available assistance. Appendix 13–1 lists national agencies with addresses and a brief description of activities.

Counselor

Personal or family counseling is frequently needed when illness or disability strikes suddenly. Normal coping mechanisms may not be adequate for the added and often complex pressures created by the disability.[1] Shapiro[2] outlines the goals of individual and family counseling as "a) to gain more insight into themselves; b) reach a more constructive level of action in dealing with each other; and c) learn to cope with the new or changing realities of their life situation" (ref. 2, p. 215). The social worker can reduce destructive environmental pressures and assist the client and the family in coping by suggesting alternative mechanisms and helping the family resolve conflicts that may have arisen around dependence and independence issues.[3]

Educator

As an educator, the social worker teaches the client and the family about their given medical situation. Romano[4] states that the social worker provides broad information about social, psychological, and environmental aspects of disability. The social worker can also teach the home health staff, helping them understand their feelings toward the client and family and providing insight into the etiology of the client and family interaction and crisis management. The social worker may also suggest which interventions might be most successful.

Advocate

The social worker may need to function as a client advocate. In the advocacy role, otherwise similar to the resource director role, the social worker may encourage the client to be more assertive or may intervene directly with the agency. This function may entail removing barriers, or developing new services in the client's and family's geographic area. Suppose the social worker has several clients who have had a cerebral vascular accident (CVA) and could benefit from a support group. The social worker can mobilize and develop a support group for clients in the area, or can encourage the clients and caregivers to organize a carpool to the closest existing support group for people with CVAs. Often the social worker must intervene with other agencies to obtain needed services. For example, an agency focusing on individuals with head injuries may have money for respite care. The social worker may have to advocate agency service for a client with acquired immunodeficiency syndrome (AIDS) that has primarily attacked the brain so that the family can obtain some respite care. If clients are denied services or if services are inappropriate or inferior, the social worker may intervene to ensure that the clients are treated properly and able to access all services for which they are eligible.

Mediator/Facilitator

Ms. Clarkson, a 58-year-old mother of three adult children, has been diagnosed with metastatic cancer of the lungs. She has already undergone one course of chemotherapy which has failed to reduce the tumor. She is receiving home health nursing services and spends most of her time in bed or sitting in a recliner for short periods. Physicians have recommended a second course of chemotherapy, but Ms. Clarkson has refused, stating that the treatment is too difficult and will not do any good. Her husband and children want her to try the chemotherapy. The nurse notices considerable tension between family members whenever she goes into the home and asks the social worker to visit the family.

The social worker may be able to mediate between the client and the family, or among family members. If Ms. Clarkson were a widow and did not have a terminal disease but were unable to continue living alone, the social worker could help the children determine which of them would be the primary caregiver, how they could take turns caring for the client, or if placement in a personal care home were a better option. Shapiro[2] states that mediation is to be used to

> a) alleviate fears; b) develop realistic expectation of an afflicted member; c) inform a specific agency of changed circumstances; and d) interpret the family's situation to relatives.

Mediation may also entail interpreting the client's and family's situation to other members of the home health care team. Social workers have considerable training in conflict resolution and role orientation. The home health care multidisciplinary team members must collaborate and use their particular training, knowledge, and skills to enhance comprehensive and high-quality care for the client. Working with Ms. Clarkson can be stressful and home health staff may have their own feelings about the efficacy of treating terminally ill patients. If their frustrations and other feelings are evident at team meetings, the social worker may suggest rotating some of the staff to avoid burnout and ensure high-quality services.

Social workers gather considerable psychosocial data in the course of their activities and can provide information of value to team members. For example, the social worker has access to information on the predictive value of psychosocial profiles following the onset of a myocardial infarction and can help the home health therapist interact more effectively with the client. Social workers are skilled in performing psychosocial evaluations. Information from these evaluations is shared with the multidisciplinary team to help them interact most effectively with the client and the support system. Social workers understand normal and abnormal cognitive and psychological processes and reactions to illness and disability. They are trained to provide evaluation, counseling, and referral services as well as interpretation and guidance for home health therapist.

Social workers occupy several roles, but none are their exclusive province. Romano summarizes the position social workers hold on the multidisciplinary team, stating:

> It may be that social work occupies a unique position in that it has its feet in health and mental health, its hands in the social sciences, its viscera in clinical intervention skills, and its head and heart in a commitment to the issues of the quality of life of disabled persons in society (ref. 4, p. 19).

Social workers can provide considerable assistance to home health therapists, but first the client must be referred for services.

REFERRAL REQUIREMENTS

Social service is not primarily reimbursed by most third-party payers. In many home health settings, therefore, the scope of social work function is limited by reimbursement practice. Most insurance plans make no provisions for social services. Health maintenance organizations offer little if any coverage. Medicare provides some reimbursement after careful documentation of social problems affecting the health and safety of the client.[5] Social workers, like other members of the health care team, must document appropriate goals, show a plan of care outlining interventions, and detail the course of activities. Any member of the health care team may make a referral to social services. Often it is the therapist or the nurse — someone who interacts frequently with the client and family — who is first aware of social, financial, or emotional problems requiring intervention.

SOURCES OF ASSISTANCE

Financial Resources

Many home health clients are senior citizens; a high percentage are women living alone. The client may have lost a spouse within the previous year and may be experiencing grief, the loss of social support, and fear of losing independence. The client may also face financial losses if the death of the spouse has changed family income. Additionally, financial stability may be lost through the illness and hospitalization of the spouse prior to death. One hospitalization can deplete a lifetime of savings and force the remaining spouse to seek community assistance. For many elderly people, the idea of seeking community assistance, even welfare and Medicaid, is difficult. Many senior citizens who have worked hard all their lives and tried to save enough money to care for themselves in their older years find it embarrassing to seek public assistance. This embarrassment becomes an emotional burden. Clients may go so far as to refuse further care or intervention, fearing the financial repercussions. The client may question the therapist about the cost of services and may need to be reassured that it is covered by available insurance. The social worker counsels the client about feelings and thoughts, as well as about available financial resources.

Social Security

Many individuals plan their retirement income around Social Security and are unaware that Social Security has always been meant as a supplement rather than the total retirement income. Many elderly persons today worked all their lives for minimum wages and for employers who did not provide any retirement or pension benefits. These individuals have no alternative than to rely on Social Security for their income. Others may have lost their savings through catastrophic illness. Financial fears are very stressful; some clients may believe that they will end up in poverty and be forced to live on the street. Many clients are not aware of available resources and need social service intervention to guide them through the maze of agencies and applications. Finding financial resources may be one of the more demanding activities of the social worker; however, there are alternatives for clients who meet qualifications. Several primary financial support programs are provided through the Social Security Administration.[6] These are Social Security, Social Security Supplemental Income, and Medicare. Most clients cannot evaluate whether they are entitled to any of the services. About 60 percent of all Social Security beneficiaries are receiving benefits because of retirement; however, the remaining 40 percent may be getting benefits because they are disabled, depend on someone who receives Social Security, or because they are a widow, widower, or child of someone who paid into Social Security before death.

Social Security Supplemental Income

Many clients may be eligible for Social Security Supplemental Income (SSI) depending on total income and the value of their belongings, including their homes. Income and asset guidelines vary significantly throughout the United States and the application process can be daunting. A client can become very anxious trying to fill out the multitude of forms involved in applying for Social Security or SSI. The data requested by the Social Security Administration is not difficult to provide and much of it is redundant, but the paperwork looks overwhelming to the client and family. The social worker can guide the client regarding the appropriate program, help complete application forms, and obtain the necessary supporting documents.

Social Security Disability

A client may be eligible for Social Security disability if less than retirement age and permanently disabled. Clients applying for Social Security due to disability must document correctly and completely the types of activities required in their previous employment and have proof that they are no longer employable. It may be difficult for the home health therapist to predict whether a client is permanently disabled, but a referral should be made if the possibility of qualification exists. If the application is rejected, the client is entitled to a review, and the social worker can help the client prepare for the hearings. Consider the following situation:

> Marie Drummond, a 54-year-old single woman living alone, was being seen by a home health therapist for a broken ankle and a broken humerus. She was in very poor health. A referral was made to the social worker, who determined that Ms. Drummond was narcoleptic and had just been denied Social Security and Medicare. The social worker filed for a review and sent the review board more specific information on narcolepsy and Ms. Drummond's specific symptom. Information was also provided by the Narcoleptic Association. On review, Ms. Drummond was awarded Social Security and Medicare.

Medicare

Medicare is a third financial program supported by the Social Security Administration. Medicare is a health insurance program for people more than 65 and other persons who are disabled and receiving Social Security or SSI. Medicare is administered through the Health Care Financing Administration. There are two parts to Medicare: hospital insurance (Part A) and medical insurance (Part B). Both parts of the program have annual deductible fees that must be met by the client.

Hospital insurance (Part A) pays for inpatient hospitalization, skilled nursing facility care (inpatient), home health care, and hospice care. Part A does not cover all costs because there is a deductible fee and payment is made on the basis of allowable charges. There is also a limit on the number of days a client can stay in the hospital. For home health care, Medicare pays 80 percent of the allowable charges. It is frustrating to health care providers that Medicare often does not cover durable medical equipment such as a bath bench or wheelchair adaption. Clients need supplemental insurance to pay for whatever portion Medicare part A will not pay. Supplemental insurance, however, can be quite expensive.

The second portion of the Medicare program, medical insurance (Part B), covers physician visits, outpatient roentgenograms, laboratory tests, ambulance transportation, blood transfusions, and outpatient physical and occupational therapy services. Part B also covers durable medical equipment such as wheelchairs, canes, and walkers as well as some supplies. Like Part A, Part B also covers home health care. (More detail on Medicare can be found in Chapter 14.) Clients often do not understand their benefits and worry about their coverage. The social worker can educate the client about coverage and rights of appeal.

Medicaid

Although not a specific program of the Social Security Administration, Medicaid is a source of financial assistance in health care for the indigent. Each state administers its own Medicaid program under broad federal government guidelines; therefore there are many variations in eligibility and benefits. Generally, to be eligible an individual must meet one of the following requirements: (1) receive Aid to Families with Dependent Children; (2) be more than 65 years of age and in financial need; or (3) be disabled and in financial need. For eligible clients, Medicaid pays the Medicare hospital insurance deductible. Medicaid also pays the 20 percent that Medicare does not cover on such expenses as physician visits, surgery, hospitalization, and laboratory work. For individuals receiving both benefits, Medicaid is the only program that covers most medical equipment, supplies, and certain medications.

Once again the social worker can help the client complete applications and determine for which program to apply. Medicaid can be a frustrating program for the home health therapist. Consider the following:

> Tim Jones, 22 years old, sustained a closed head injury in a motor vehicle accident. Because he was on welfare, Medicaid paid for his hospitalization, rehabilitation, and home health care. While in the rehabilitation center he was fitted with a wheelchair for which Medicaid paid. Now, he has improved to the point where he can ambulate with a quad cane, but Medicaid refuses to purchase the cane because it has already purchased the wheelchair. No notice is taken of Tim's improving condition.

There is no certainty with Medicaid. The social worker can contact Medicaid workers and try to obtain a more effective processing of the client's claim.

Even with the above programs a significant number of clients still "fall through the cracks" for one reason or another.

Trish Cellar, an 85-year-old widow, fell in her mobile home and broke her tibia and scapula. After hospitalization she moved into her daughter's house. Apart from this accident, Ms. Cellar has had no medical problem. She has received only Social Security and Medicare and has no supplemental insurance. Her hospitalization was very expensive. Although it appeared she would be eligible for SSI and Medicaid, she was denied benefits because she was not at present living in her mobile home. The family had to sell her home and put this money toward the hospital bills before she was considered eligible for SSI and Medicaid.

The social worker can counsel the family around the anger they have toward the system and direct this anger in a positive manner. The social worker can also intervene by procuring food from the local food bank and requesting funds from the local church organization so Ms. Cellar can pay her bills.

Community Resources

There is a vast network of community resources available to assist clients in a wide array of services. The problem with using these resources is that they are undersupported and overused. Those who are needy are growing in number every day. Organizations such as the Elks, Knights of Columbus, Junior League, and Veterans of Foreign Wars, among others, may have canned food, clothes, and medical equipment such as bedside commodes, wheelchairs, canes, and bath benches available for clients. International service organizations such as Kiwanis, Lions, Rotary, Pilot, and Soroptomist require their members to volunteer time for community service. Members of these service clubs may visit individuals who are alone or transport a client to the physician's office.

Most communities have some support groups, with the most extensive networks in larger urban settings; there are also telephone networks for clients who live in more rural settings. Appendix 13–1 lists the national offices of many community service organizations and support groups, but it is not meant to be all inclusive. Clients are often unaware of social service programs for which they may be eligible. The medical social worker can make the client aware and prevent a feeling of being overwhelmed by needs. Among the lesser-known community programs are: Lifeline (a home alert program for senior citizens and the disabled); Homemaker Services (a home health aid paid for by the county); and National Odd Shoe Exchange (an exchange for shoes and gloves). Social workers are knowledgeable about resources in the local and surrounding communities and make necessary referrals.

CLIENT INTERVENTIONS

> Jessie Camden, 69, is a retired realtor, married with grown children. She is an elder in her church and often gives the sermon at Sunday services. She suffered a CVA that left her paralyzed on the right side with a loss of speech. She has now lost her role as a leader in the church, as well as her role of homemaker for her husband. She used to be the caregiver; instead, she needs to be taken care of.

The home health therapist is frequently faced with situations where the illness has changed family roles, creating stress, conflict, and frustration. Consider a 42-year-old man, married and head of a household, who develops end-stage renal disease needing home dialysis; or a 32-year-old single working woman who sustains multiple fractures in an accident and is without family or caregiving support. (The caregiver role is explored in greater detail in Chapter 12.) All of these individuals have lost their status in society, have lost income, and are faced with a crisis situation. The social workers can counsel Jessie Camden, help the wife of the client with renal disease to develop head-of-household skills, and find support for the woman temporarily disabled.

Working with the Client

The client in the home often has difficulty accepting the physical limitations and loss of independence imposed by chronic disease, illness, or accident. The first issue many clients face is coping and adapting to multiple losses, such as loss of status, possible loss of a loved one, forced retirement from work, loss of eyesight or hearing, and peripheral sensorineural losses. Effective crisis intervention requires the social worker to understand the client's and family's coping mechanisms, recognize the effects of the problem on emotions and life-style, and find interventions that address primary problems relevantly without creating additional difficulties.[5]

Working with the family is an integral part of the team approach to home health care. (In this section the terms "family" and "caregiver" are used interchangeably.) The term "family" is used in a generic sense because in today's society families may be spread out or separated. Many people build their own family or support system apart from their blood relatives. This may be the support system with which the health care team must connect. However defined, the family is an important resource. Family members are usually involved in the care given by home health therapists. They can be a catalyst in working with the client, or they can become a major roadblock. If they do become a roadblock, the social worker can facilitate a working relationship between the caregiver and the home health therapist.

Fears

Clients can have many fears. They may fear abandonment, being a burden to their family, becoming more dependent or having to change living arrangements, or dying in pain or alone. They may also fear changing sexual capacities or loss of cognitive abilities. Counseling from the social worker can help alleviate many of these stressful feelings and can aid the client in gaining insight.

A primary role of the social worker is collaboration with the home health care team regarding significant losses or fears the client may have, which may directly influence the outcome of the client's rehabilitation. Consider the following situation:

Tom Crane is 45 years old and has diabetes mellitus, visual disturbances, and diabetic neuropathy involving lower extremities and balance. He has been referred for home health care. The home health (physical and occupational) therapists report that Mr. Crane does not seem motivated and does not follow through with his home exercises and activities. They further report that Ms. Crane left him recently. The therapists request a social worker evaluation. While gathering data, the social worker learns that the Crane's 15-year marriage had been shaky for some time. Mr. Crane has had two affairs during the marriage.

The social worker can counsel Mr. Crane and try to guide him to find a more constructive method of coping with issues surrounding his wife and their marriage. It is important for the social worker to collaborate with the physical and occupational therapists regarding Mr. Crane's situation, how he is coping, and what intervention strategies are being used. Consultation among these professionals will ensure that all provide consistent care specific to the client's needs and life situation.

During illness, clients experience a wide range of emotions. They may be distressed that they need home health care and may feel uncomfortable with strangers coming into their homes. The nurse may be educating the client and family on how to use a glucose monitor while the physical therapist teaches the client to use a walker after an amputation, the occupational therapist works on activities of daily living such as maintaining balance while dressing, a home health aide comes to bathe the client, and the social worker assists a healthy adaptation to the amputation. Such a scenario may cause confusion and distress for the client and family. The social worker can help the client and family express such feelings to empower the client to find ways of maintaining control in daily life while benefiting from the services. Empowerment means that the client and family feel in control of their daily lives rather than overwhelmed by the disability and the attendant demands and activities of home health care. Empowerment is enhanced when each home health team member gives the client the respect expected from guests coming into the home.

Fear of death and dying is another issue some clients may face. Issues surrounding death and dying may be especially difficult for the health care providers to approach. Health care providers are in the business of assisting their clients toward improved lives, not watching their lives be taken away. In terminal situations, the home health care agency may be working in conjunction with a hospice organization (see Chapter 16). Social workers are trained in the area of death and dying and can provide counseling services and assist the client in the grief process. The social worker, with the client's consent, may make a referral to a member of the clergy. The client's grief can directly affect perception and involvement in therapy. Some clients may not access the services from the physical and occupational therapist. The social worker will work with the client if services are being refused.

Depression

Depression is another condition that affects many clients. Depression can present as pessimism, loss of interest in life, fatigue, loss of sexual desires, withdrawal, or changes in sleeping and eating habits. It is very difficult to treat the client with any of the above symptoms. Lack of motivation may be encountered in the client with, or without, depression. See chapter 11 for a greater discussion of emotional issues. The social worker needs to counsel the client toward positive adjustment to present circumstances. The social worker also attempts to find out what will engage a client to be motivated, what kind of control the client needs to exert and what goals the client wants to achieve.

Working with the Family

Families have many of the same issues as the client, and some unique ones, because they are in the caregiving role. As Bishop[7] states:

> Considerable skill is required as family functioning in the face of significant disability is a complex system to understand. Care must be taken to not gloss over areas or make assumptions with little or no data on which to base them. This requires a clear conceptual model of family functioning, assessment, and treatment (ref. 7, p. 59).

Being a caregiver requires learning to manage and treat the client when members of the home health care team are not in the home. To some caregivers this is an overwhelming task. Most of them are not health care workers and may feel unqualified to perform certain duties such as suctioning, caring for a decubitus ulcer, or giving insulin injections. The social worker enables the caregivers to believe in their ability to care properly for the client, and facilitates coping mechanisms that enhance their ability to provide the necessary care. The caregiver may be under financial stress. Often families take care of other family members by helping pay for medication or having them move in to their homes. This may occur because the family is unaware of available financial assistance programs.

Some clients appear to have no family or support system. Often the social worker can find available support that may be appropriate and safe enough to keep the client out of a skilled nursing care facility. Social workers may also help find respite care for overworked caregivers; this subject needs to be approached gently because caregivers may feel that their ability to care properly for the client is in question.

SUMMARY

Social workers have much to contribute to the multidisciplinary team. This chapter has provided information on the diagnostic and management abilities the social worker has to offer, and on the mechanisms social workers use to integrate many complex systems at one time and to exhibit the profession's evaluative abilities.

REFERENCES

1. Lane, HJ: Working with problems of assault to self-image and life-style. Soc Work Health Care 1:191, 1975–1976.
2. Shapiro, E: Family and long-term treatment or care at home: Implications for social work. In Browne, JA, Kirlin BA, and Watt, S (eds): Rehabilitation Services and the Social Work Role. Williams & Wilkins, Baltimore, 1981.
3. Aldrich, SJ: The role of social work in long-term health care. Arch Phys Med Rehabil 54:572, 1973.
4. Romano, MD: Social worker's role in rehabilitation: A review of the literature. In Browne, JA, Kirlin, BA, and Watt, S (eds): Rehabilitation Services and the Social Worker Role. Williams & WIlkins, Baltimore, 1981.
5. Powell, WE: The Social Worker's Perspective. In Meisenheimer, CG.: Quality Assurance for Home Health Care. Aspen, Rockville, 1989, p 163.
6. Social Security Administration: Understanding Social Security. SSA publication No. 05-10024, US Department of Health and Human Services, Washington, DC, January 1991.
7. Bishop, D: Social work in rehabilitation: Identity dilemma, strength, and cautions. In Browne, JA, Kirlin, BA, and Watt, S (eds). Rehabilitation Services and the Social Work Role. Williams & Wilkins, Baltimore, 1981.

Appendix 13–1

Community Resources*

1. **Alzheimer's Association**
   70 E. Lake St., Suite 600
   Chicago, IL 60601
   1-800-621-0379; in Illinois 1-800-572-6037
   Combats Alzheimer's disease and related disorders. Promotes research to find the cause, treatment, and cure for the disease; provides educational programs for the public, the media, and health care and medical professionals; represents the continuing care needs of the affected population before government and social service agencies.

2. **Alzheimer's Disease Research**
   Alzheimer's Family Relief Program and Information
   15825 Shady Grove Road, Suite 140
   Rockville, MD 20850-4022
   1-800-227-7998
   Provides free public information booklets on various aspects of Alzheimer's Disease. Booklets include Alzheimer's Diseases: A Family Survival Guide, and Caring for the Alzheimer's Patient at Home: Tips for Coping.

3. **American Amputee Foundation**
   P.O. Box 55218, Hillcrest Station
   Little Rock, AR 72225
   (501) 666-2523
   Provides free peer counseling to new amputees and their families to aid their adjustment to amputation. Other services include legal assistance, information and referral, rehabilitation, resource database, and technical and scientific information concerning prosthetics. Provides financial assistance for the purchase of prosthetic equipment, wheelchairs, crutches, braces, and modifications to the home.

4. **American Cancer Society**
   1599 Clifton Rd., N.E.
   Atlanta, GA 30329
   (404) 320-3333
   Sponsors Reach to Recovery (for women who have had a mastectomy), Can-Surmont, and I Can Cope support groups for client and family.

5. **American Diabetes Association**
   National Service Center
   P.O. Box 25757
   1660 Duke St.
   Alexandria, VA 22314
   (703) 549-1500

*From Burek, D: Encyclopedia of Associations, ed 25. Gale Research, New York, 1991.

Promotes the free exchange of information about diabetes mellitus by educating the public in early recognition of the disease, the importance of medical supervision in its treatment, and the development of educational methods designed for people with diabetes.

6. **American Heart Association**
   7820 Greenville Ave.
   Dallas, TX 75231
   (214) 373-6300
   Mission statement is "The prevention of premature death and disability due to cardiovascular disease and stroke." Each state is an independent affiliate with local chapters in counties or other geographic localities.

7. **American Juvenile Arthritis Organization**
   1314 Spring St., N. W.
   Atlanta, GA 30309
   (404) 872-7100
   Advocates the needs of those affected by juvenile arthritis.

8. **American Kidney Fund**
   6110 Executive Blvd., Suite 1010
   Rockville, MD 20852
   (301) 881-3052
   Goals are: to alleviate the financial burdens caused by renal disease; to improve the quality of life for renal disease patients; to promote renal health care nationwide.

9. **American Lung Association**
   1740 Broadway
   New York, NY 10019
   (212) 315-8700
   Makes policy recommendations regarding medical care of respiratory disease, occupational health, hazards of smoking, and air conservation.

10. **American Lupus Society (The)**
    East 2617 Columbia Ave.
    Spokane, WA 99207
    Assists lupus patients and their families in coping with the daily problems associated with lupus. Collects and distributes funds for research.

11. **American Narcolepsy Association**
    P.O. Box 1187
    San Carlos, CA 94070
    (415) 591-7979

12. **American Paralysis Association**
    500 Morris Ave.
    Springfield, NJ 07081
    (201) 379-2690
    Encourages and supports research aimed at finding a cure for paralysis caused by spinal cord injury, head injury, or stroke. Gives grants to research laboratories and to individuals for post-graduate study.

13. **American Red Cross**
    17th and D Sts., N.W.
    Washington, D.C. 20006
    (202) 737-8300

Serves members of the armed forces, veterans, and their families, aids disaster victims, and assists other Red Cross societies in times of emergency. Other activities include blood services; training volunteers for chapters, hospitals, and other community agencies; community services; international activities; service opportunities for youth.

14. American Spinal Injury Association
250 E. Superior, Rm. 619
Chicago, IL 60611
(312) 908-3425
Comprises physicians trained in the care of patients with spinal paralysis, and who are either actively engaged in the field and acknowledged to be competent by their peers or who have contributed significantly to the advancement of the basic sciences or a clinical field of practice applicable to the treatment of the spine.

15. Arthritis Foundation
1314 Spring St., N.W.
Atlanta, GA 30309
(404) 872-7100
Seeks to discover the cause of and improve treatment methods for arthritis and other rheumatic diseases; increase and improve treatment facilities; increase the number of scientists investigating rheumatic diseases; provide training in rheumatic diseases for more physicians; and extend knowledge of arthritis and other rheumatic diseases to the public, emphasizing the socioeconomic as well as medical aspects of these diseases.

16. Associated Services for the Blind
919 Walnut St.
Philadelphia, PA 19107
Helps blind and visually impaired people live independently. Maintains a counseling service for blind and visually impaired people and their families, and a radio reading service that reads newspapers and magazines over closed-circuit radio. Offers referral and job placement services.

17. Cancer Information Services
N.I.H. Bldg., Rm. 10A24
Bethesda, MD 20892
(301) 496-5583
Provides information about cancer causes, prevention, detection, diagnosis, rehabilitation, and research.

18. Candlelighters Childhood Cancer Foundation
1312 18th St., N.W.
Washington, D.C. 20036
(202) 659-5136
Serves as clearinghouse and liaison between parents, groups, and medical and psychosocial professionals. Offers 24-hour crisis line and babysitting and transportation services; sponsors blood and wig banks and immune programs; and establishes Ronald McDonald houses for families of children requiring extended care away from home.

19. Chronic Fatigue and Immune Dysfunction Syndrome
P.O. Box 220398
Charlotte, NC 28222-0398
(704) 362-CFID
Advocates continued research into the cause and cure of the syndrome. Awards research grants.

20. City of Hope
1500 E. Duarte Re.
Duarte, CA 91010
(818) 359-8111
Sponsors treatment, research, and medical education in catastrophic diseases including cancer; leukemia; blood, heart and lung diseases; certain hereditary disorders; and metabolic disorders such as diabetes. Patient care is available on a national and nonsectarian basis.

21. Compassionate Friends (The)
P.O. Box 3696
Oak Brook, IL 60522-3696
(708) 990-0010
This nondenominational, informal, self-help organization assists parents who have experienced the death of a child. Promotes the positive resolution of parents' grief; fosters the physical and emotional health of bereaved parents and siblings.

22. Corporate Angel Network
Bldg. One
Westchester County Airport
White Plains, NY 10104
(914) 328-1313
US corporations that own aircraft volunteer empty seats to cancer patients in need of transportation to or from recognized treatment centers.

23. Cystic Fibrosis Foundation
6931 Arlington Rd., #200
Bethesda, MD 20814
(301) 951-4422
Supports medical research, professional education, and care centers to benefit people with cystic fibrosis.

24. Disabled American Veterans
P.O. Box 14301
Cincinnati, OH 45250-0301
(606) 441-7300
Helps veterans with service-connected disabilities. Provides services in areas including emergency relief, disaster relief, employment, legislation, advocacy, and transportation.

25. Easter Seal Research Foundation
70 E. Lake St.
Chicago, IL 60601
(312) 726-6200
Administers grants-in-aid for applied research investigations concerned with the management and treatment of physical and associated disabilities.

26. Emphysema Anonymous, Inc.
P.O. Box 3224
Seminole, FL 34642
(813) 391-9977
Helps people with emphysema through education, encouragement, and mutual assistance. National office provides nonmedical counseling for clients and their families.

27. Epilepsy Foundation of America
4351 Garden City Dr.
Landover, MD 20785
(301) 459-3700
Goals: to prevent and control epilepsy and improve the lives of those who have it. Provides federal government liaison. Supports medical, social, rehabilitational, legal, employment and information, education, and advocacy programs.

28. Hear Now
4001 S. Magnolia Way, Suite 100
Denver, CO 80237
Provides financial resources to people who are hearing impaired. Purchases hearing-assistance devices such as hearing aids and cochlear implants.

29. Hospice Association of America
519 C St., N.E.
Washington, DC 20002
(202) 546-4759
Hospices, home health agencies, community cancer centers, and interested health care professionals. Promotes concept of hospice.

30. Leukemia Society of America
733 Third Ave.
New York, NY 10017
(212) 573-8484
Raises funds to combat leukemia through research, patient service, and public and professional education.

31. Lupus Foundation of America
1717 Massachusetts Ave., N.W., Suite 203
Washington, D.C. 20036
Provides patient education, services, and human support to members; educates the medical community and the public about lupus to obtain earlier diagnoses and better treatment; encourages research into the cause and cure of lupus.

32. Make Today Count
101 1/2 S. Union St.
Alexandria, VA 22314
(703) 548-9674
Brings people with life-threatening illnesses, their families, and other members of the community together to discuss openly the false implications and the realities of the disease. Takes a positive approach to the problems of serious illness to lessen the emotional trauma for all concerned.

33. Muscular Dystrophy Association
810 Seventh Ave.
New York, NY 10019
(212) 586-0808
Supports international programs of more than 500 research awards, major university-based neuromuscular disease research and clinical centers, and 230 outpatient clinics in hospitals. Local chapters provide services including diagnostic examinations, follow-up medical evaluations, orthopedic appliances, physical therapy, flu shots, and summer camps.

34. Myasthenia Gravis Foundation
53 W. Jackson Blvd., Suite 1352
Chicago, IL 60604
(312) 427-6252
Funds research and professional and public education programs. Sponsors low-cost prescription service.

35. National AIDS Network
2033 M St., N.W., Suite 800
Washington, D.C. 20036
(202) 293-2437
Serves as a resource center and networking agency for members; provides information on AIDS service organizations. Makes financial aid available to organizations that provide AIDS education or services.

36. National Amputation Foundation
12-45 150th St.
Whitestone, NY 11357
(718) 767-0596
Fosters and helps all amputees in employment, social, and mental rehabilitation. Provides services including legal counsel, vocational guidance and placement, social activities, liaison with other groups, and psychological aid.

37. National Association For Down Syndrome
P.O. Box 4542
Oak Brook, IL 60522-4542
(707) 325-9112
Comprises parents of children with Down Syndrome and persons interested in their treatment and welfare. Encourages medical and educational research on Down Syndrome; helps organize community parent groups.

38. National Association of the Physically Handicapped
76 Elm St.
London, OH 43140
Seeks to advance the social, economic, and physical welfare of the physically handicapped.

39. National Braille Association
1290 University Ave.
Rochester, NY 14607
(716) 473-0900
Helps obtain Braille equipment and materials for blind individuals.

40. National Burn Victim Foundation
308 Main St.
Orange, NJ 07050
(201) 731-3112
Maintains a 24-hour emergency referral and crisis intervention team of professionals that counsels burn victims and their families, addressing psychological problems and physical disabilities remaining after treatment. Provides free blood services to burn victims. Sponsors Burn Recovered, a self-help group.

41. National Easter Seal Society
70 E. Lake St.
Chicago, IL 60601
(312) 726-6200
Offers a broad range of services and support for handicapped individuals;

funds education programs, research, publications. Works through local affiliates.

42. National Hemophilia Foundation
110 Green St., Rm. 406
New York, NY 10012
(212) 219-8180
Supports research through postgraduate fellowship program; disseminates literature for the public.

43. National Hospice Organization
1901 N. Moore St., Suite 901
Arlington, VA 22209
(703) 243-5900
Promotes standards of care in program planning and hospice care.

44. National Kidney Foundation
30 E. 33rd St.
New York, NY 10016
(212) 889-2210
Supports research, patient services, professional and public education, organ donor program, and community service.

45. National Multiple Sclerosis Society
205 E. 42nd St.
New York, NY 10017
(212) 986-3240
Stimulates, supports, and coordinates research into the cause, treatment, and cure of multiple sclerosis (MS); provides services and aid for persons with MS and related diseases and their families; aids in establishing MS clinics and therapy centers.

46. National Neurofibromatosis Foundation
141 Fifth Ave., Suite 7S
New York, NY 10010
(212) 460-8980
Provides patients and their families with information about the disorder and assists them in finding medical, social, and genetic counseling.

47. National Odd Shoe Exchange
P.O. Box 56745
Phoenix, AZ 85079
(602) 246-8725
Brings together persons with mutual shoe problems (foot amputees and persons having feet that differ physically due to disease, injury, or accident). Also operates an odd glove exchange program.

48. National Rehabilitation Information Center
8455 Colesville Rd., Suite 935
Silver Spring, MD 20910-3319
(301) 588-9284
Maintains library of research reports; conference proceedings; books; microfiche; audiovisual material; material on individuals who are blind, hearing impaired, developmentally disabled, spinal cord injured, and emotionally disturbed.

49. National Reye's Syndrome Foundation
426 N. Lewis
P.O. Box 829
Bryan, OH 43506
(419) 636-2679
Comprises families of children who have had Reye's syndrome. Goals: to disseminate information to the public and the medical community; to raise and provide funds for research into the cause, treatment, cure, and prevention of Reye's syndrome through research grants to individual scientists and the support of a research laboratory.

50. National Spinal Cord Injury Association
600 W. Cummings Park, Suite 2000
Woburn, MA 01801
(617) 935-2722
Supports research toward curing paralysis from spinal cord injury; provides public and professional education programs and services; helps individuals to reach their personal goals.

51. National Wheelchair Athletic Association
1604 E. Pikes Peak Ave.
Colorado Springs, CO 80909
(719) 635-9300
Supports male and female athletes with significant permanent neuromuscular-skeletal disability (spinal cord disorder, poliomyletis, or amputation) compete in various amateur sports events in wheelchairs.

52. North American Society for Dialysis and Transplantation
c/o Robert Mendez, MD
1893 Wilshire Blvd.
Los Angeles, CA 90057
(213) 483-6830
Promotes education and research and disseminates current knowledge and technology in the field of renal dialysis and transplantation.

53. Paralyzed Veterans of America
801 18th St. N. W.
Washington, D.C. 20006
(202) 872-1300
Comprises veterans who have incurred an injury or disease affecting the spinal cord and causing paralysis. Sponsors wheelchair sporting events in table tennis, basketball, swimming, bowling, archery, and track and field. Promotes projects that publicize employment of handicapped individuals. Sponsors research, rehabilitation, and educational programs.

54. Parents of Down Syndrome Children
c/o Montgomery County Association for Retarded Citizens
11600 Nebel St.
Rockville, MD 20852
(301) 984-5792
Provides parent-to-parent counseling; contacts new parents of children with Down Syndrome to offer support and information on community resources.

55. RP Foundation Fighting Blindness
1401 Mt. Royal Ave., 4th Floor
Baltimore, MD 21217
(301) 225-9400

Conducts fund-raising to support research on retinal degenerative diseases including retinitis pigmentosa, macular degeneration, and Usher's syndrome.

56. Siblings of Disabled Children
535 Race St., Suite 220
San Jose, CA 95126
(408) 288-5010
Provides support and information about brothers' or sisters' illness or disability and gives an opportunity to express and understand feelings of resentment, embarrassment, jealously, anger, or guilt in a therapeutic environment.

57. Spina Bifida Association of America
1700 Rockville Pike, Suite 540
Rockville, MD 20852
(301) 770-SBAA
Goals: to develop an information service of materials relating to spina bifida; to conduct research into the causes of the birth defect; to improve vocational training of individuals with spina bifida; to monitor development of legislation applying to the handicapped.

58. Tuberous Sclerosis Association of America
1305 Middleborough Row
Middleborough, MA 02346
(508) 947-8893
Goals: to promote patient service, public education, and physician awareness; finds cases of tuberous sclerosis (TS) and identify the disease as early as possible; to expand tuberous sclerosis movements at local, state, and national levels; to stimulate development and support local, state, and national representation of human service to make the delivery system more responsive to the needs of TS patients and their families.

59. United Parkinson Foundation
360 W. Superior St.
Chicago, IL 60610
(312) 644-2344
Supports scientific research on the disease; assists clients and their families through medical referrals, education, and other means.

60. Very Special Arts
John F. Kennedy Center for the Performing Arts Education Office
Washington, D.C. 20566
(202) 662-8899
Goals: To ensure that disabled individuals have year-round opportunities to participate in educational programs demonstrating the value of the arts; to provide experiences to help them become active participants in mainstream society. Sponsors programs and festivals. Provides training and technical assistance for teachers, artists, and administrators in schools, museums, libraries, and recreation and art centers.

Chapter 14

Reimbursement and Documentation

DONALD E. JACKSON & MAUREEN K. KAVALAR

Reimbursement and documentation are intimately interrelated. The entire reimbursement system for home health care depends on the documentation provided by the home health agency. This chapter is heavily weighted with information related to Medicare; however, the reimbursement and documentation issues addressed here carry over into all aspects of home health care.

REIMBURSEMENT

Reimbursement for home health services is driven by the federal Medicare program. Home health rehabilitation services (physical therapy, occupational therapy, and speech-language pathology) are reimbursed individually. Medicare reimburses each of the three services in a distinctly different way. Physical therapy is affected most significantly by federal salary equivalence regulations. Occupational therapy is not an allowable service unless another skilled service is being provided. All three services are effected by cost caps that limit reimbursement to the home health agency.

Home Health Agency Reimbursement by Medicare

Home health agencies (HHAs) that receive payment from Medicare are required to be similarly organized. They must successfully meet and maintain certain standards as delineated in the Medicare Conditions of Participation for Home Health Agencies. An HHA is required to provide skilled nursing services (RN) and may offer physical therapy (PT), occupational therapy (OT), speech-language pathology (SP), medical social work (MSW), and home health aide services. HHA clients must receive at least one skilled service, RN, PT, or SP. OT, MSW, and home health aide services may be provided only if the client is receiving RN, PT, or SP services. The client may continue to receive OT if all other skilled services have been discontinued, but OT cannot be the only skilled service initially provided to the client.

HHAs are reimbursed by Medicare on a cost-based system. However, several demonstration projects are being organized by Medicare to test a prospective payment reimbursement system. The cost-based system allows the HHA to bill Medicare its actual costs for providing care, but the costs must fall within specific cost caps established by Medicare. Hospital-based HHAs receive an additional "add-on" amount because, according to Medicare, hospital-based HHAs have higher general and administrative costs than do free-standing HHAs and therefore deserve a higher cost cap.

Each HHA service has a separate cost cap determined by the Health Care Financing Administration (HCFA) for each standard metropolitan statistical area (SMSA). (HCFA is the agency within the Department of Health and Human services that administers the Medicare program). Rural areas outside each SMSA have their own cost caps. The cost caps are published periodically by HCFA and are used by Medicare auditors to determine annually the maximum allowable costs for the HHA.

Each HHA must submit an annual cost report to its Medicare fiscal intermediary within 90 days of the close of the HHA's fiscal year. (Fiscal intermediaries are private insurance companies that contract with Medicare to pay HHA claims.) Medicare uses the cost caps as a component of the cost report to determine the allowable costs for each service. If the HHA exceeds its allowable cost for any service, it is not reimbursed for the excess. In addition, Medicare reviews all the HHA's costs to determine whether they are reasonable or allowable. If specific costs are determined not to be reasonable or are not allowable, they are not reimbursed.

Medicare often reviews the salaries of key administrative staff to determine whether or not they are reasonable. The same is true of business travel and automobile leases. Nonbusiness travel and club memberships are not allowable expenses. Medicare pays the HHA monthly on the basis of the claims submitted and of Medicare's estimate of the HHA's cost for each service. A reconciliation occurs after Medicare audits the HHA's cost report. As a result, some HHAs may not be fully reimbursed for their costs until several months after the close of their fiscal year.

The payment the HHA receives each month is based on the claims the fiscal intermediary (FI) has approved. The FI is required to pay each "clean claim" within 30 days of the date it is received. "Clean claims" have no technical deficiencies and the appropriateness of the service provided is not challenged by the FI. The FI may determine that further review is necessary and therefore not pay within 30 days. If the FI denies a claim, either the client or the HHA may appeal the denial to the FI. If the claim is still denied, either the client or the HHA may appeal the claim to an administrative law judge, with further review through the Social Security Appeals Council and federal courts.

Reimbursement to Independent Contractors Who Provide Rehabilitation Services

Reimbursement to independent contractors who provide PT services to the HHA is limited by federal salary equivalence regulations passed in 1975.[1] These regulations do not affect OT or SP. The cost caps are the primary limitations on fees paid to independent contractors providing OT or SP services. The salary equivalence regulations also affect all Medicare-reimbursed health care organizations that are paid on a cost-based system (e.g., skilled nursing facilities, rehabilitation agencies, rehabilitation hospitals, and certified outpatient rehabilitation facilities). Services provided by acute care hospitals (unless billed as outpatient PT) are not affected by the salary equivalence regulations because acute care hospitals are reimbursed by Medicare through a prospective payment system.

The salary equivalence regulations have been written to be specific when applied to HHAs. The basic regulations are fairly simple. However, many exceptions make interpretation much more complicated. The regulations are used to determine whether fees paid to a PT independent contractor are allowable. (Hereafter, references to "PT" include both individuals and organizations that provide PT services to the HHA under a written arrangement with the HHA). They limit the amount the HHA can pay the PT and are applicable independently of whether the HHA's costs for physical therapy are within the cost cap limitations. Medicare allows the HHA to pay for the PT's professional time with each client, including treatment, travel, charting, and conferencing time. Medicare also allows the PT to be paid for travel mileage or expense. The PT may be paid a flat fee-for-service for each visit as long as the PT's total compensation for each visit does not exceed the standard HCFA allowances for that geographic region. If daily time or travel records are not kept, the HHA is not allowed to pay the PT any amount that exceeds the standard allowances. The standard allowances include 1 hour for treatment, charting, and conferencing; ½ hour for travel; and 10 travel miles for each client.

The HHA may require the PT to keep actual time or travel records. It is allowable for the HHA to pay the PT on the basis of actual records if the hourly and mileage rates do not exceed the published salary equivalence rates. The HHA may choose to pay the PT according to time records for professional time but use the standard allowance for travel expense. Conversely, the HHA may pay the standard amounts for professional time but pay actual mileage for travel expense. (HCFA refers to the hourly rate for professional time as the "Adjusted Hourly Salary Equivalence Amount"; see Table 14–1) The methodology for paying the PT must be consistent for each cost reporting period.

Most HHAs pay the PT on a flat fee-for-service basis. The HHA generally bases its payment on the standard allowance for professional and travel time as well as the standard allowance for travel expense. Therefore, the PT may not realize that the fee offered by the HHA is based on the allowable sal-

TABLE 14–1
The Home Health Agency's Options for Paying the Physical Therapist

	Standard Time Allowances	Actual Time Records	Standard Travel Expense	Actual Travel Expense
Method 1	X		X	
Method 2	X			X
Method 3		X	X	
Method 4		X		X

ary equivalence rates. Generally, the PT can negotiate a much more favorable rate by learning the maximum allowable salary equivalence rates for the area. For example, if the adjusted hourly salary equivalence amount for a specific geographic area is $33.00 per hour, the standard allowance is calculated by adding $33.00 plus $16.50 (half the adjusted hourly salary equivalence amount for travel allowance) plus $3.00 (Government Services Administration [GSA] travel rate for 10 miles). The total allowable rate would then be $52.50, whereas the HHA may be paying only $40.00 per visit (Table 14–2).

In this situation the PT obviously has room to negotiate. Salary equivalence applies to the HHA, not to the PT. The PT may charge the HHA any negotiable fee. The HHA must aggregate all of its costs incurred by contracting for PT services. The HHA is not disallowed a cost solely because a single PT is over the salary equivalence limit. Therefore, the HHA may contract with various PT providers at various rates and in some instances may pay above the salary equivalence rate. As long as the HHA does not exceed the salary equivalence allowance for all of its PT service provided under arrangement, it is not disallowed the cost. Therefore, in some situations, the PT provider may be able to charge successfully in excess of the salary equivalence rate. This is particularly likely if the HHA contracts with several independent practitioners at a rate well below the allowable salary equivalence rate.

Determining the adjusted hourly salary equivalence amount for a specific area can also be confusing. The amounts were last published in the Federal Register on September 30, 1983 with an effective date of October 1, 1982 (Table 14–3). The amounts for each HHA are based on the first day of its fiscal year. HCFA allows an upward adjustment of .006 for each month from October 1, 1982 until the first day of the HHA's cost reporting period. The adjusted hourly amount is calculated by multiplying .006 times the number of months from October 1, 1982 until the beginning of the HHA's current fiscal year. For example, if the HHA's fiscal year began on January 1, 1993, the salary equivalence amount would be .006 × 123, which is the

TABLE 14–2
Sample Calculation of Standard Home Health Salary Equivalence Rate

Standard treatment, conference, and charting time rate (1 h: adjusted hourly salary equivalence amount)	$33.00
Standard travel time rate (½ h at $33.00/h)	16.50
Standard travel expense rate (10 miles at $.30 per mile)	3.00
Standard home health salary equivalence rate	$52.50

TABLE 14-3
Adjusted Hourly Salary Equivalence Amounts
Effective October 1, 1982

STATE	ADJUSTED HOURLY SALARY EQUIVALENCE AMOUNT	STANDARD TRAVEL ALLOWANCE	STATE	ADJUSTED HOURLY SALARY EQUIVALENCE AMOUNT	STANDARD TRAVEL ALLOWANCE
Alabama	$17.14	$ 8.57	Missouri	$16.97	$ 8.49
Alaska	26.39	13.20	Montana	18.24	9.12
Arizona	21.11	10.56	Nebraska	16.97	8.49
Arkansas	16.79	8.40	Nevada	21.11	10.56
California	21.11	10.56	New Hampshire	16.71	8.36
Colorado	18.24	9.12	New Jersey	18.79	9.40
Connecticut	16.71	8.36	New Mexico	16.79	8.40
Delaware	18.79	9.40	New York	19.58	9.79
District of Columbia	17.83	8.92	North Carolina	17.83	8.92
Florida	18.42	9.21	North Dakota	18.24	9.12
Georgia	16.55	8.26	Ohio	18.65	9.33
Hawaii	25.33	12.67	Oklahoma	16.79	8.40
Idaho	19.52	9.76	Oregon	19.65	9.83
Illinois	18.96	9.48	Pennsylvania	17.24	8.62
Indiana	19.13	8.57	Rhode Island	16.71	8.36
Iowa	16.97	8.49	South Carolina	17.14	8.57
Kansas	16.97	8.49	South Dakota	18.24	9.12
Kentucky	17.83	8.92	Tennessee	17.63	8.92
Louisiana	16.79	8.40	Texas	16.79	8.40
Maine	16.71	8.36	Utah	18.24	9.12
Maryland	17.82	8.91	Vermont	16.71	8.36
Massachusetts	16.71	8.36	Virginia	17.83	8.92
Michigan	20.19	10.10	Washington	19.45	9.73
Minnesota	16.97	8.49	West Virginia	17.83	8.92
Mississippi	17.14	8.57	Wisconsin	17.92	8.96
			Wyoming	18.24	9.12

Source: Federal Register, Part VIII. Department of Health and Human Services Publication 48:191:44922, Medicare and Medicaid Programs: Schedules of Guidelines for Physical Therapy and Respiratory Therapy Services, September 30, 1983.

number of months between October 1, 1982 and January 1, 1993. The next step is to multiply that amount (.738) by the original adjusted hourly salary equivalence amount for the area. Using Illinois as an example, the October 1, 1992 adjusted hourly salary equivalence amount was $18.96 ($18.96 × .738 = $13.99). The product ($13.99) represents the increase in the base salary equivalence amount for the area.

The next step is to add $13.99 and $18.96, which equals $32.95. This is the adjusted hourly salary equivalence amount for HHAs in Illinois for cost reporting periods beginning January 1, 1993 (Table 14-4).

To carry this discussion one step further, the standard allowable sal-

TABLE 14-4

Calculation of Adjusted Hourly Salary Equivalence Amount in Illinois for Home Health Agency Cost Reporting Periods Beginning January 1, 1993

Step 1

Count the number of months between October 1, 1982 and January 1, 1993. This number is 123.

Step 2

Multiply 123 by .006 (monthly adjustment factor):

$$123 \times .006 = .738$$

Step 3

Multiply .738 by $18.96 (October 1, 1982 adjusted hourly salary equivalence amount):

.738 × $18.96 = 13.99 (increase in adjusted hourly salary equivalence amount)

Step 4

Add $13.99 + $18.96 = $32.95.

$32.95 = Adjusted hourly salary equivalence amount for HHA Cost Reporting Periods Beginning January 1, 1993.

HHA = home health agency.

ary equivalence amount for HHAs as described above is then determined as follows: $32.95 + $16.48 (½ hour standard travel allowance) + $3.00 (assuming the GSA rate at that time is .30 per mile). The standard allowable amount would then be $52.43 per visit (Table 14–5).

The HHA may contract with the PT to provide supervisory or administrative functions for its organization. There are special allowances for each of these situations. PTs are considered to be in supervisory roles if they supervise one or more PTs or other professional staff in addition to carrying their own caseloads. PT assistances, OT assistants, and aides are not considered professional for the purposes of this allowance. Medicare considers supervision of assistants or aides to be part of the responsibility of any PT, OT, or SP, and therefore not supervisory in nature. A PT who is supervising a staff of OTs or SPs as well as PTs could include all professional staff in the equation. Medicare regulations are vague on this point except that the supervisor must spend at least 20 percent of the time supervising other therapists. The

TABLE 14-5

Calculation of Standard Home Health Salary Equivalence Rate in Illinois for HHA Cost Reporting Periods Beginning January 1, 1993

Standard treatment, conference and charting time rate (adjusted hourly salary equivalence)	$32.95
Standard travel time rate (½ adjusted hourly salary equivalence)	16.48
Standard Travel Expense Rate* (10 miles at $.30 per mile)	3.00
Standard home health salary rate in Illinois for HHA cost reporting periods beginning January 1, 1993	$52.43

*The GSA Travel Rate is assumed at $.30 per mile. The actual rate may be different.

purpose of the supervisory allowance is to adjust the salary equivalence guidelines to reflect the supervisor's additional responsibilities. The FI bases the amount of the allowance on the differential between PT and PT supervisor salaries in home health settings in the same area. The regulations also require that the differential reflect the extent of the therapist's supervisory responsibilities, the number of individuals supervised, and the amount of time performing supervisory functions versus the amount of time providing direct client care. The supervisory rate applies to all the work the supervisor performs for the HHA, regardless of whether it represents time spent supervising other individuals or time spent providing direct client care.

The HHA administrator may not be familiar with the allowance for supervisory services. The contracting therapist may have to provide the appropriate reference.[2] The method used to determine the additional allowance must be reasonable. The optimal method would be to use actual salary data for the same geographic area. However, comprehensive data of this nature are generally not available.

These authors have found that one method accepted by an FI is to increase the salary equivalence amount by three percent for each full-time equivalent professional staff person supervised, with a maximum increase in the allowance of 15 percent. An industry-accepted definition of a full-time equivalent is an individual who treats between 25 and 30 clients during a regular 5-day work week. See Table 14–6 for a step-by-step approach to implementing this methodology.

A PT providing administrative services to the HHA is not governed by salary equivalence. The HHA can pay the PT any amount as long as the FI considers it to be reasonable. The difference between this provision and the supervisory allowance provision is that the PT providing administrative services cannot treat any clients for the HHA. If the PT were to provide direct care for the HHA, the FI could determine the PT to be a supervisor instead of providing administrative services. Administrative services may include assignment of referrals, review of documentation, preparation of appeals, supervision of clinical staff, and recruiting activities.

Another quirk in the salary equivalence regulations is that the HHA is allowed to pay the PT for only one visit per day to the HHA's office. Therefore, most HHAs are reluctant to reimburse the PT for either travel time to the office or professional time in the office. This is particularly true if the PT is being paid a standard fee for service. In these circumstances, the HHA is not able to allow for travel or professional time related to meetings in the HHA's office. In spite of this fact, some HHAs still pay the PT a fee for time in the office, but only if the HHA's overall cost for PT is well within its salary equivalence constraints. Some HHAs refuse to pay the PT an amount equal to the allowable salary equivalence rate because of their concern with the cost cap limits for the agency. HHA administrators frequently use this reason to keep payment to the PT at a lower rate.

TABLE 14–6

Example Methodology for Calculating Additional Supervisory Allowance

Assumptions

1. Three percent additional allowance is given each FTE supervised.
2. Adjusted hourly salary equivalence amount is $32.95 (see Table 14–4).
3. The average number of visits provided each month by all professional staff supervised is 485.
4. A month has 21 working days.
5. Five visits per working day is a full-time case load.

Methodology

Step 1. Determine the number of home health visits per month by one FTE by multiplying 21 working days per month times 5 visits per day:

21 days × 5 visits/day = 105 visits/month/FTE

Step 2. Determine the number of FTEs supervised by dividing the total number of visits for the month (485) by 105 (visit/FTE):

485 ÷ 105 = 4.6 FTEs supervised

Step 3. Determine the percentage of increase of the additional supervisory allowance by multiplying 4.6 FTEs by .03 (the amount of increase per FTE):

4.6 × .03 = .138, or a 13.8% increase

Step 4. Determine the amount of increase by multiplying the adjusted hourly salary equivalence amount ($32.95) by .138 (the increase factor):

$32.95 × .138 = $4.55 (amount of increase)

Step 5. Determine the adjusted hourly supervisory amount by adding $4.55 (amount of increase) and $32.95 (adjusted hourly salary equivalence amount):

$4.55 + 32.95 = $37.50 (adjusted hourly supervisory amount)

FTE = full-time equivalent.

The HHA has more flexibility in controlling its cost caps than may be readily apparent to the PT. First, administrative and general costs are added to the cost caps to determine the final cost per visit for each service the agency provides. Therefore, an agency that is burdened with heavy administrative and general expenses may be more concerned with cost cap limits than an agency with lower administrative and general costs. In addition, as mentioned earlier, a hospital-based HHA will have higher cost cap limits than a free-standing HHA. Second, as discussed previously, all PTs contracting with the HHA are not necessarily paid at the same rate. The HHA's average cost per visit for PT service (exclusive of administrative and general costs) is very likely lower than the allowable salary equivalence rate. It is not uncommon for a PT to contract with a therapy business (usually providing PT, OT, and SP services) that has contracts with one or more HHAs. In this circumstance, it is the HHA's payment to the PT business that is governed by the salary equivalence regulations. PTs, OTs, and SPs who contract with PT businesses instead of directly with the HHA are paid less money for their work. However, the therapy business may provide many benefits that are not available directly from the HHA, such as obtaining referrals from several

HHAs in the same geographic area, negotiating contracts with the HHA, and providing more peer contact for the therapist.

Home Health Reimbursement by Non-Medicare Payers

Third-party payers other than Medicare can be generally classified as traditional insurance companies, health maintenance organizations (HMOs), or state public aid programs. Most traditional insurance companies reimburse the HHA according to the reasonableness of its cost for service. Traditional insurance companies generally have a ceiling on the amount they are willing to pay per visit for any specific service. These ceilings are generally, but not always, at least as high as the Medicare allowable rates. Very few HHAs have the majority of their referrals paid through traditional insurance reimbursement. However, for the purpose of the Medicare discussion, Medicare cost caps and salary equivalence allowances apply only to those HHA clients for which the HHA is paid by Medicare. Therefore, when traditional insurance is the primary payer for an HHA, the PT may be able to negotiate a higher fee for service.

HMOs have the opposite impact on HHA reimbursement. They generally reimburse the agency at a rate lower than the Medicare rate and therefore make it difficult for the HHA to pay the therapist at a rate approximating the allowable salary equivalence rate. Some HMOs pay the HHA on a fee-for-service basis. Most prefer to pay at a capitated rate; that is, a predetermined amount of money for each client serviced by the HMO in a specific geographic region. The HHA agrees to accept all clients within this region and to provide whatever care is necessary for the client. The fee is generally paid to the HHA monthly and has no bearing on the number of referrals provided to the agency. Many HHAs (and other health care provider organizations as well) have found capitated reimbursement by HMOs to be a financial disaster. PTs who are working in these environments find the agency placing significant pressure on the PT to keep the number of visits down.

Public aid (often referred to as Medicaid) reimbursement for home health services varies widely from one state to another. There is no consistency and no pattern. The program, if one exists, is generally housed in either the state's Department of Public Aid or its Department of Public Health (or their equivalents).

In summary, HHA reimbursement, whether paid to the agency or to the therapist, is driven by the Medicare program. Because HHAs are ideally suited for serving geriatric populations, the vast majority of HHAs receive most of their funding from Medicare. PTs and other rehabilitation professionals who contract with the HHA need a keen understanding of Medicare to negotiate adequately with the HHA for a reasonable fee for service.

DOCUMENTATION

Documentation in medical practice is the key to successful reimbursement, especially in closely regulated Medicare health facilities such as home health agencies. As funding becomes increasingly limited, rehabilitation professionals can expect to see more requirements for specific documentation and more denials.

Diagnosis and the client's condition are the first elements scrutinized to determine the required level of competency and the sophistication of the skilled clinician. The documentation must show that the treatment provided could only have been delivered effectively and safely by a qualified therapist. The program design should be restorative, with the expectation that the client's functional status can be upgraded.

Medicare and Medicaid

A good working knowledge of Medicare and Medicaid rules and regulations is essential. The key elements for coverage of services for a home health client are (1) the client is considered homebound, (2) skilled services are needed, and (3) services are ordered by a physician. To meet the homebound criterion the client must be generally confined to the home and must either require an assistive device or obtain medical advice against leaving the home without assistance to obtain treatment due to the considerable and taxing effort necessary. Absences from the home should be infrequent and of relatively short duration (e.g., for physician visits). Homebound eligibility is not affected by frequent absences from the home when the reason is to receive medical care, such as dialysis.

Skilled service must relate directly and specifically to an active written treatment program established by the physician after any needed consultation with the therapist. The service must be reasonable and necessary to the treatment of the client's illness or injury. Services must be considered specific and effective treatment for the client's condition and must be so complex and sophisticated, or the condition of the client must be such, that the services required can be safely and effectively performed only by a qualified therapist or under his or her supervision. The therapist's notes must reflect this skilled level of activity and must correlate the treatment with the patient's condition. In the past, the restorative potential of the client was a deciding factor in determining whether skilled services were needed. This is not the case currently, and denials may be overturned if the client requires skilled services to prevent further deterioration or preserve current capabilities. Maintenance programs are generally not considered skilled services. However, establishing a maintenance program and teaching family caregivers associated with the program are considered skilled services.

Medicaid regulations vary from state to state depending on allocated funding for home services. Some states do not fund home care services, but some are more liberal than the Medicare regulations and allow for ongoing continuous maintenance care requiring the skills of a therapist.

The Initial Assessment

At the time of the initial visit, the client's history is obtained to determine the extent of prior therapy, the onset date of the current condition, the prior level of function, and the physical environment in which the client must function. Objective tests and measurements of range of motion (ROM), strength, and function are used for baseline information. (The initial assessment is detailed in Chapter 4.) At the conclusion of the assessment process the therapist should identify and list the significant clinical findings, the goals (short-term and long-term if appropriate) and the plan of treatment. The significant clinical findings identify those areas that affect function and require intervention. They include motor deficits, deviations from the norm, and degree of functional impairment. The goals are stated in functional terms, are measurable, and should be time specific. The plan of treatment must relate to the stated goals. The following is an example of the significant clinical findings, goals, and plan of treatment for a cerebrovascular accident (CVA) client with prior rehabilitation:

Significant Clinical Findings

1. Left lower extremity (LLE) indicates abnormal flexor tone synergy.
2. Transfers require moderate assist of one: sit to stand and bed to chair.
3. Gait requires maximum assist of one with quad cane and ankle-foot orthosis (AFO) due to poor dynamic balance and poor LLE step-stride length, swing phase, and heelstrike.

Goals

1. Inhibit abnormal tone to facilitate functional movement of LLE in 4 weeks.
2. Achieve independent sit to stand and bed to chair transfers in 2 weeks.
3. Achieve independent gait with quad cane and AFO on level surfaces in 4 weeks, supervised on stairs.
4. Become independent in home exercise program in 1 week.

Plan of Treatment

1. Inhibition and facilitation techniques to LLE.
2. Transfer training: sit to stand and bed to chair.

3. Therapeutic exercises.
4. Gait training with appropriate assistive device.
5. Instruction in home exercise program.

Duration: Twice a week for 4 weeks.

The Progress Note

The daily progress note should reflect skilled treatment provided, functional progress, remaining goals, problems, and plan of treatment. Progress should be stated in measurable terms: for example, "Client now comes to standing with supervision; minimal assist to complete pivot transfer."

Using the SOAP format for visit notes is one way to relay the above information in a concise, organized method. The subjective (*S*) part of the note refers to what clients or their families tell you and often indicates how clients feel about their condition, therapy, and so on. While the client's or family's comments may not be detailed or accurate, they allow for further discussion and can assist the therapist in identifying the problem areas. The objective (*O*) portion of the note identifies what was done during the treatment session (i.e., the skilled care performed) and the client's response to the treatment. The assessment (*A*) analyzes progress made since the last session or in the last week, identifies new problems, and allows for new or upgraded goals. The plan (*P*) indicates upcoming plans for treatment and revisions of the original plan.

Example of a Physical Therapy SOAP Note: *Four weeks ago the client had a right total knee replacement and has a history of arthritis, hypertension, and postoperative respiratory problems.*

S: *Client notes pain in right knee but that it is feeling "looser."*

O: *ROM—Right knee extension-flexion actively 7 to 94 degrees supine at start of treatment session. After active assistive exercise 5 to 100 degrees supine and 8 to 96 degrees sitting.*

Strength: *Tolerating 5 lb with straight leg raise, hip adduction, hip abduction, terminal knee extension, and prone knee flexion; 10 to 15 repetitions each.*

Gait: *Right knee moves within normal limits (WNL) during gait cycle, but weight does not shift fully onto right lower extremity due to knee pain. Client requires use of quad cane for ambulation. No longer using walker. Practiced stair climbing with quad cane and one minimal assist because four steps have no railing.*

A: *Client tolerates increased number of repetitions with 5 lb weight and increased ROM following exercise. Gait improving as client no longer relies on walker.*

P: *Continue therapy two times per week with anticipated discharge in 2 weeks. Progress client to independent stair climbing with quad cane.*

In addition to the specific client related data, documentation of communication and conferences with other members of the health team is critical. It indicates the coordination of services between the various members of the team and ensures progress to accomplish stated goals. Communication also prevents duplication of services by the different therapy disciplines. While treatment protocols may appear to be similar, outcomes and specific goals are usually different. For example, the PT may be working on static and dynamic standing balance to facilitate improved gait, whereas the OT may be doing the same to facilitate independence in dressing. Documentation of the activities is related in terms of the specific outcomes. In general, the PT focuses on restoring the client's ability to ambulate (or wheelchair mobility) and transfer. Documentation of client problems should include motor deficits and degree of functional impairment. Established goals must be related to functional skills. Transfer skills, gait, and bed mobility should be addressed. The OT concentrates on Activities of Daily Living (ADL) training, homemaking skills, compensatory techniques, perceptual training, ordering and teaching use of adaptive equipment, fabrication and fitting of upper extremity orthoses, fine motor upper extremity coordination, energy conservation, and work simplification. OT documentation of client problems and goals must be functionally stated and task oriented.

Communication disabilities and swallowing difficulties are the areas that the SP attends to. Specific activities include esophageal speech, graphic skills, word retrieval exercises, electrolaryngeal therapy, speech intelligibility exercises, swallowing, expressive exercises, oral motor exercises, dysphagia therapy, and language-based exercises. When identifying problems, the SP must indicate functional impairment using terminology indicative of such impairments, for example, "aphasia," "dysphasia," "dysarthria," "dyslexia," "agnosia," and "dysphagia."

Example: *Wheelchair positioning for a client with a history of multiple CVAs whose significant clinical findings include: (1) increased extensor tone lower trunk and both lower extremities, (2) increased flexor tone of left upper extremity with 90 degree elbow flexion contracture, (3) normal strength and ROM of right upper extremity, (4) right laterally flexed head and neck, and (5) dysphagia and dysphasia.*

Physical Therapy: *Improve wheelchair position to promote independent wheelchair mobility within apartment and 50 ft in hallway.*

Occupational Therapy: *Improve wheelchair position to promote oral hygiene, and face and upper trunk bathing.*

Speech-Language Pathology: *Improve wheelchair position to improve head positioning to facilitate swallowing.*

The Discharge Summary

The discharge summary is a review of the client's course of therapy. The length of service, the treatment received, and a comparison of the client's functional level at discharge to that at the initiation of therapy are detailed. The client's current level of function is described. Progress towards a goal, or lack of progress, is identified and reasons are given for goals not met. Follow-up activity by the client or caregivers may be indicated and is noted. The summary also gives a reason for the discharge.

Denials

Denial of reimbursement is almost always a function of documentation. The most common reasons for denial are (1) The services provided are not reasonable and necessary for the diagnosis, that is, the amount, type, frequency, and duration of services are not effective and specific for the client's condition; (2) the services provided did not require the skills of a therapist; (3) the client did not make significant functional progress in a reasonable time; and (4) the client is not homebound. To ensure reimbursement of services, referrals should be screened by appropriate agency personnel (rehabilitation coordinator or therapy director) to determine that the client meets the criteria for homebound status and need for skilled service. On complete review of the case in question, the denial can be appealed. Most denials should be appealed because the services provided are intended to reach an optimal level of functioning.

Documentation Tips

The following documentation tips will serve as an additional guide.

DO's

- **DO** document what was found (problem list) and what was done (intervention) in objective, measurable terms:
  - **ROM**—degrees lost, gained, passive or active
  - **Strength**—Muscle grades, percentages, number of repetitions, resistance used, progressive resistive exercise, techniques used
  - **Endurance**—Distance and time
  - **Muscle tone**—Status (hypertonic, hypotonic, or appropriate), relation to function (ROM, pain, motor control)
  - **Pain**—Severity (on a scale of 1–10, amount if limits function), irritability (ease of provocation, level and duration of incapacitation)
  - **Balance, Transfers, Gait**—Amount of assistance needed for accomplishment or safety, necessary assistive device, weight-

bearing status (non–weight bearing, partial weight bearing to tolerance, toe touch), quality of and deviation from norm of activity
   - **ADL**—Document specific level of function, highlight remaining deficits (avoid using this term unless specific activities are noted and do not conflict with OT).
- **DO** document home program instruction, which family members can be taught program and which cannot (e.g., client lives with disabled child; spouse is elderly and has severe congestive obstructive lung disease).
- **DO** describe intervention in therapeutic terms.
- **DO** document safety hazards and precautions—carpeting, stairs, lack of railings, pets, clutter, inaccessible rooms or furnishings (toilet, refrigerator).
- **DO** document all conferences with all health team members (physician, RN, HHA, other therapists, MSW, etc.).
- **DO** document the reason the client is homebound.
- **DO** be as brief and concise as possible, leave superfluous or unimportant items out of note.
- **DO** document plan for discharge from the first visit (i.e., frequency twice per week for 2 weeks, decrease to once per week for 2 weeks, then discharge).

DON'TS

- **DON'T** say client has stabilized if discharge is not pending soon.
- **DON'T** repeat "same," on each visit note.
- **DON'T** say "reviewed exercise program" unless you state how client's comprehension is limited and what repeated instruction is needed.
- **DON'T** say family is unwilling to give care.
- **DON'T** say ROM or strength is WNL and continue to treat the client for those deficiencies.
- **DON'T** use arrows to indicate increase or decrease without specific measurements (e.g., increase from 20 degrees flexion to 45 degrees flexion).
- **DON'T** say client is "doing well," "improving"—state what client is doing to overcome limitation on basis of previous assessed level.
- **DON'T** mention your agency's staffing problems (e.g., client not seen because therapist not available").
- **DON'T** mention personnel problems with other disciplines.
- **DON'T** mention "maintain."

REFERENCES

1. Federal Register, Part VIII: Department of Health and Human Services Publication 48:191:44922, Medicare and Medicaid Programs: Schedules of Guidelines for Physical Therapy and Respiratory Therapy Services, September 30, 1983.
2. Health Care Financing Administration: Health Insurance Manual 15: Provider Reimbursement Manual, Baltimore.

BIBLIOGRAPHY

Community Health Section bulletin, Vol 22, No 3, Fall, 1987, p 8.

Dale, EM: An Advocate's Guide to Medicare and Medicare Appeals. Legal Assistance to Medicare Patients, Willimantic, 1988.

Federal Register, Part VIII. Department of Health and Human Services Publication 51:104:19734, May 30, 1986.

Health Care Financing Administration: Health Insurance Manual 11: Home Health Agency Manual, Baltimore.

Hill, JR: The Problem-Oriented Approach to Physical Therapy Care. American Physical Therapy Association, Washington, DC, 1977.

Home Health Coverage Provider Training Manual, Health Care Financing Administration, Baltimore.

Jackson, DE: Medicare Documentation Guidelines for the Home Health Therapist: Unpublished material. American Physical Therapy Association, Combined Sections Meeting, Washington, DC, 1988.

Jackson, DE and Wilhoite, MJ: Home Health Physical Therapy: Considerations for the Provision of Care. Clinical Management 3:10, 1985.

Jackson, DE: Physical Therapy Cost Caps for Home Health Care. Progress Report. American Physical Therapy Association, Washington, DC, November 1985.

NovaCare, Inc: Home Care Orientation: Unpublished material, 1990.

Code of Federal Regulations: Title 42, Parts 400–429. US Government Printing Office, Washington, DC.

Chapter 15

The Child in the Home

MARGARET E. STROLLE GOSSENS

Children with a chronic illness or a disabling condition and their families are a client population that can be well served through home health care. Although a child can usually be transported to another setting to receive therapy, there are many advantages to providing therapy in the child's home. Several trends within the provision of services to children with disabilities support the benefits of home care. The evolution of interventions for clients with neurologic impairments emphasizes regaining function by learning to master functional tasks in an environment that makes sense to the client.[1] The concept of broadening the therapeutic focus from the child to include the child's family and community is addressed on a national level in Public Law 99-457 of 1986. A child is molded by the family and the community in which he or she lives. Thus, working in the home is a logical way to gain this family based, community centered environment for the provision of care.

ADULTS AND CHILDREN AS HOME HEALTH CLIENTS

Home health care for adults and children shares many similarities but also differs significantly. Both adult and pediatric caseloads can vary by age, diagnoses, or complexity of problems.

Similarities

Adult and pediatric clients receive therapy in the comfort of familiar surroundings, using their own furniture or household structures for functional tasks, with easy access to other family members. The therapist is able to observe the home environment, the layout of rooms and stairs, and obstacles that may be present either inside or outdoors. The therapist, as a guest in the home, may become aware of social or cultural differences that may influence the therapeutic approach. The child or adult client is one part of a family structure in which there are many competing priorities. The family may be more comfortable interacting with health care providers in its own home and may assume more responsibility for determining treatment goals and priorities.

Differences

There are some important differences between the adult and the child as a home health care client. Most adult clients are essentially homebound, either temporarily or long term, leaving home only for medical treatment. Receiving home health care may be the only option for therapy. Some adult clients may live alone and be able to complete the therapy programs independently; others may depend on family members or hired help for many aspects of their care. The adult client may have preferred times for a visit but is generally available at any time. On the other hand, pediatric clients are generally not homebound, as they leave home with their parents or to attend school. Thus therapy in the home is a choice, not a necessity. Pediatric clients usually depend completely on their parents or caregivers. Scheduling is a particular concern because nap times, fatigue at the end of the afternoon, and school schedules for the client or siblings must be considered. There are also administrative differences, related to reimbursement, between providing services to children and to adults. Options for payment usually include Medicaid, private insurance companies, private pay, or funding from programs available in some states. There is great variability among companies regarding what will or will not be reimbursed.

HOME-BASED PROGRAMS

Home health services for children are generally optional; only a small percentage of children receiving such services can be considered actually homebound because of the type or degree of disability. The therapeutic techniques are generally similar whether the service is provided at home or at a center. Therapeutic techniques are portable and probably vary more among therapists than from one setting to another. Providing therapy in a treatment center may be more efficient than home health care: (1) Each therapist can treat a larger number of clients through tight scheduling; (2) a variety of equipment can be assembled in one location; (3) several different service providers are close at hand and available for consultation or provision of service; and (4) the therapist can more easily try out different functional equipment such as standing boards, adapted high chairs, or chairs. However, equipment may be more effectively selected at home. In the center, the therapist can see only what fits the child and what he or she can use. In the home, the therapist, besides fitting the child to the equipment, can evaluate the space available for its use, determine whether it will be convenient or possible to use in the home, and decide whether there is an accessible place to store the equipment when not in use. Finally, the therapist can get a better sense from the family of whether the equipment will actually be used. In the practice of home health care, be it with adults or children, all sorts of expensive equipment remains in closets, under the bed, and in attics. Equipment that clearly appeared to be a good idea in the clinic may be impractical in the home.

There are other advantages to home health care for children from both the family's and the therapist's point of view. Children are in their own setting, with their own toys and are usually much more comfortable than in the less familiar setting of the clinic. The home program is taught and practiced in the same setting in which it will be given. The family will not have the disruption of the travel time and, if siblings have different nap schedules, parents do not have to awaken children to get to an appointment on time. When going to a center, parents must either bring the siblings or make arrangements for their care. When at home, the siblings have the opportunity to be in their own play area. While siblings often demand the parent's attention in any setting, it may be more distracting in the clinic, where there are other patients and activities.

THERAPEUTIC CONSIDERATIONS

Assessment

Many assessment scales and standardized tests are available for therapists to use as part of the information collected for an initial database or for ongoing assessments. The therapist's choice of assessment tool will vary according to the age and impairment of the child but also according to the requirements set by other individuals or agencies that may be collaborating in developing a comprehensive program for the child. Educators often need specific scores from standardized tests to determine eligibility for their program. Since many tests are standardized in centers, the question might arise as to whether tests done in the home might or might not be accurate. A study done in Hamilton, Ontario by Rosenbaum and associates[2] partially addresses this question. Fifty children referred to a rehabilitation center for initial assessment were divided into two groups. One group received their initial assessment at home and one at the center. One hypothesis posed in the study was that the home assessment would show more typical behaviors. However, no statistically significant differences were found in the rates of typical behavior in either setting. If the therapist must adapt a standardized test because it has been administered in the home, this can be appropriately noted. The assessment is primarily a good tool to use in planning treatment programs, setting goals, or judging progress. In addition, when the parent is involved with the assessment process, a standardized test may be helpful for education or provision of information. The parent may not, for example, be familiar with the normal acquisition of motor skills. Discussion of the assessment results during or after the test assists the parent in recognizing the child's abilities and also helps the parent identify the areas to be addressed in the home program. Over time, the reassessments can also be educational for families. Some families enjoy reviewing old data to see how far their children have progressed. For the very slowly developing child, a retest may show discouraged parents that progress has actually occurred.

Three examples of assessment tools for infants and children that can easily be used in the home are the Bayley Scales of Infant Development,[3] the Peabody Developmental Motor Scales,[4] or the Early LAP or LAP.[5] For the gross motor portion, very few modifications are needed. Stairs may vary in height or steepness but, for retesting, the child will be using the same set of stairs. If the family's home does not have stairs, the therapist might accept by report how the child negotiates stairs at a grandparent's house or at another home that the family visits. A balance beam is harder to come by, but many families can find a two-by-four in the basement or may have a raised threshold that could substitute. Outside, there may be a platform edge around a sandbox or a low wall around a garden. A 10-ft line can be a stripe in the carpet or a strip of masking tape placed on the kitchen floor. The therapist may need to assemble more items and bring them to the home for the fine motor portion of the tests. For consistency, these items—for example, specific puzzles, a doll without a head, or blocks—must be standard; it would take excessive time to assemble them from the toy chest in a child's home. In addition to using standardized assessments or tests, it is very helpful for the therapist to develop an individual database. This database may include the variety of components necessary for developing motor skills that may not be specifically addressed in an assessment form. Included could be such items as muscle strength, joint range of motion, trunk rotation, midline crossing, posture, respiratory patterns, assessment of balance in greater detail, and a continuing list of items developed by each individual therapist. The database can also include medical history, medication, surgical procedures, and any other information that might influence the planning of the therapy program. For the older child, this database may give the therapist a more complete assessment necessary to develop a treatment program.

Dunst and associates[6] discuss several assessment tools that provide a format for family members to identify needs not usually included in client assessments. Instruments such as the Family Needs Scale, the Family Support Scale, the Support Functions Scale, or the Family Resource Scale have been developed to help the family articulate needs in the areas of housing, finances, emotional support, time management, gaining additional information, and so forth. At times, any one or any combination of these needs may overwhelm a family and make it difficult for them to even consider doing a therapy program with their child. The therapist, if aware of these areas of need, can provide information or become an advocate for the family in gaining other community resources and services.

Therapeutic Interventions

A treatment plan is a part of the logical progression from assessment to attainment of goals. From the assessment, the therapist can outline the sequence of short-term and long-term goals and the therapeutic techniques that can be used to reach these goals. Many therapeutic techniques can easily be adapted for use with children in their own home. The key to success is negotiation and innovation with inclusion of the parent in all parts of the planning. The wide variety of home environments provides an interesting challenge for the home therapist. The therapist may not have a mat or therapy ball but can find a rug, a blanket, or maybe a hassock or large beach ball. As a treatment goal, the therapist may want to establish a routine in which a baby can play on its stomach on the floor. However, if the therapist finds four dogs, a chicken, and three active children playing on the same dirty floor, the options for achieving the above goal may be limited. If the therapist and the parent decide that a logical goal is having the baby prone for play, together and on the spot the two can figure out how and where this might be accomplished. In such a case, the therapist has worked with the reality of the home and has joined with the family in setting priorities for the therapeutic goals and working out routines to meet these goals that make sense to the family.

As another example, when children start to cruise or walk they are in a natural environment. There are sofas, chairs around tables, and other objects to hold on to, walk around, or bridge between. There are also the natural obstacles to ambulation such as throw rugs, thresholds, and moving children or animals. The stairs may or may not have carpeting or railings, but it is on these stairs that a child must be safe. In good weather therapy can be moved outside, for instance to try ambulation on rough terrain, or the client or family can discover how well the wheelchair can be pushed in the yard with grass, stones, and mud. A family's swimming pool can be used to do an exercise routine. The variety within each home environment provides multiple sites where a therapeutic program can take place. Functional skills can be practiced in context in various areas, possibly facilitating a transfer of learning. For example, if standing is a goal for a child with cerebral palsy, the therapist, parent, and child can discuss the various places where the child could practice standing and then try them out (Fig. 15–1). This is the advantage of

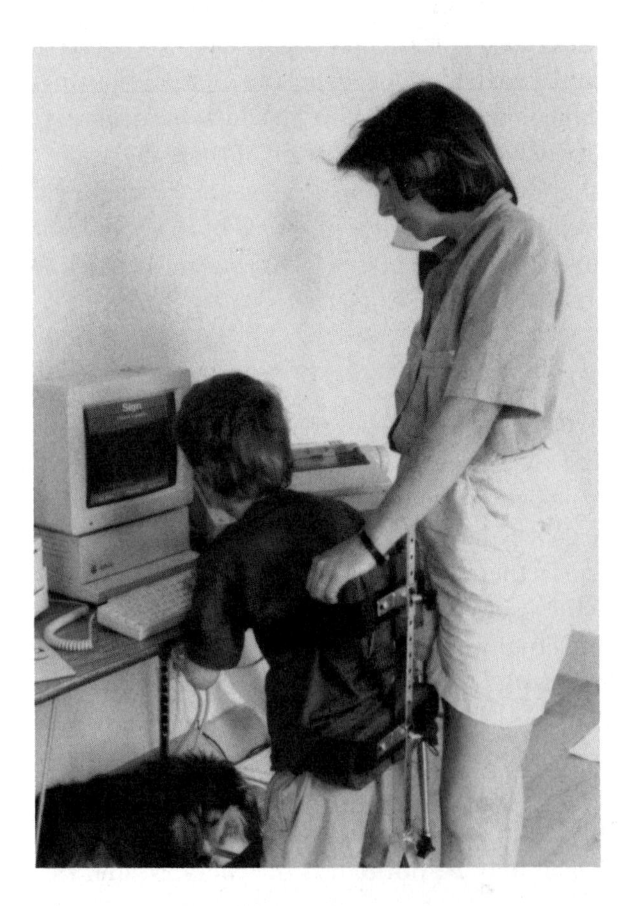

Figure 15–1. Child client, with his mother watching, uses a standing aid at the computer.

working with a child and the family at home with a functionally oriented therapeutic program.

"Problem solving in context" can refer to the child, parent, or therapist. The child learns to do things independently while doing normal activities throughout the day, whether maintaining balance while dressing, creeping downstairs, or learning to get up into a chair. The parent learns how to adapt a normal home routine by incorporating therapeutic goals into the regular daily routine. By being in the home with the family, the therapist can match therapeutic skills to the available resources, as well as to the family's abilities and their routine. The therapist and the family can then organize a therapeutic program that the family can do on a regular basis. This process can increase the parents' level of comfort and enhance their sense of competence in their ability to provide the therapy needed to reach the established goals. They see that the exercises can be done in various settings in their home. They are also using the child's own toys or household items such as bowls, spoons, and other natural toys. They are involved in observing results and setting goals in the context of their own home and with whatever is available to them.

Equipment

Much of the equipment the therapist might choose for a child is large. In many homes, space is limited, furniture is in the way, and architectural barriers such as stairs separate one area of the house from another. Bathrooms often are not designed to be handicapped accessible, or the house and its rooms are small or crowded. Additionally, the amount of time needed either to move the equipment to a useful spot or to get the child into or out of the equipment may not fit into the family's schedule. In the home, the limitations of many pieces of equipment become readily apparent. Often the family chooses not to use special equipment even though from the therapist's point of view it would be useful. The challenge is to determine, with the family, which activities are important and which cannot be done without special equipment. The activities and equipment most frequently identified are (1) seating for eating, playing, toileting, and bathing; (2) car seats or safety equipment for use in cars; (3) easily portable wheeled equipment for use in the yard or on trips to stores or malls; and (4) adapted play equipment, such as swings or tricycles, that allows the child to participate with siblings or friends in recreational activities.

Seating for the young child often starts with the high chair. Simple inserts can be built to fit the chair but often a homemade Norwegian hitch and blanket padding (Fig. 15–2) works just as well. Any long tie can be used for a Norwegian hitch. The tie is attached at the center back of the high chair, comes forward between the child's legs, then up over the thighs, and finally ties behind the chair. It is one of the most effective ways to seat securely a large child with poor sitting balance in a high chair. As the child grows, the

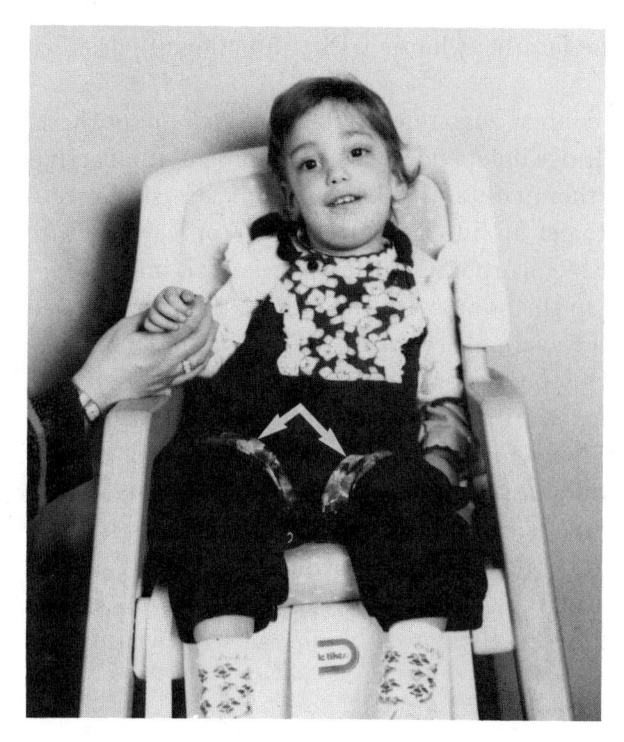

Figure 15–2. Child secured in high chair with Norwegian hitch.

family often prefers an accommodation that allows the child to join the family at the kitchen or dining room table. A sassy seat that hooks onto the table (Fig. 15–3) or a Trip Trapp chair (Fig. 15–4) that is easily adjustable to a variety of table heights is frequently used. Corner seats and trays (Fig. 15–5) are useful for play, but often families prefer to use a bean bag chair or the corner of a sofa or large chair. Trays can be made from cardboard boxes.

Bathing aids such as small tubs, sponges, or bath rings work well for small children. Webbed bath chairs often are too high above the water level to allow play in the tub, but some families have found that they work well in the yard or at a beach or pool. Wheelchairs are often necessary for a child's mobility, but many families find them cumbersome for family walks or for quick trips to the store, Umbrella strollers do not provide the support some children need but are easily portable and allow families to include a nonmobile child in regular family activities. In rural areas a baby jogger is often a cheaper alternative and easier to push for a family that likes to spend time outside. In all cases the piece of equipment must fit in with the family's priorities, finances, and level of tolerance for that extra step needed to use a piece of equipment and to deal with it when it malfunctions.

The purchase of a wheelchair is a big step for a family. It is expensive and, because it must last for several years, the fit and provision for growth must be carefully considered. The appearance of the chair is often important to the child. Along with the cost and appearance, a more difficult problem for many families is the acceptance of the fact that their child is not and may

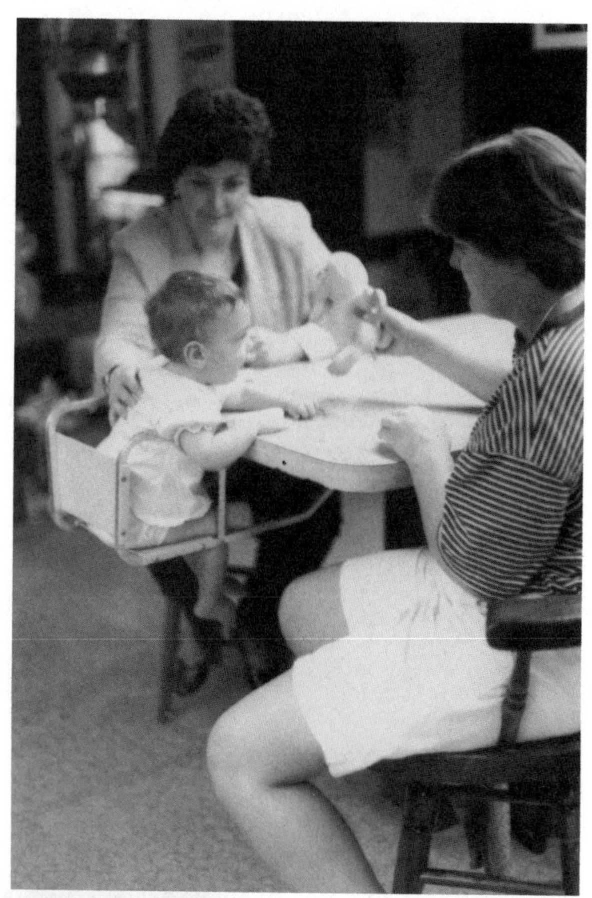

Figure 15–3. The Sassy Seat allows the child to eat and play at the table.

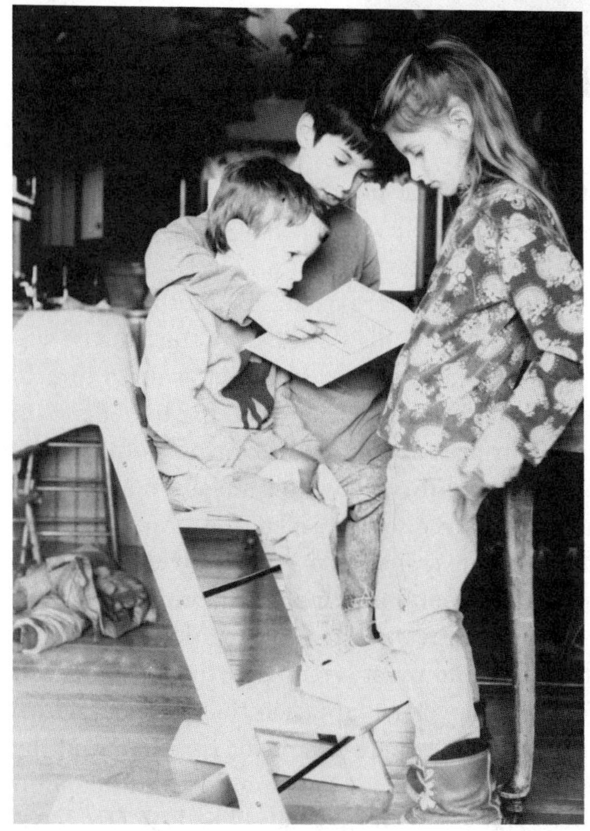

Figure 15–4. The Trip Trapp chair allows the child to maintain an erect posture and play with his siblings.

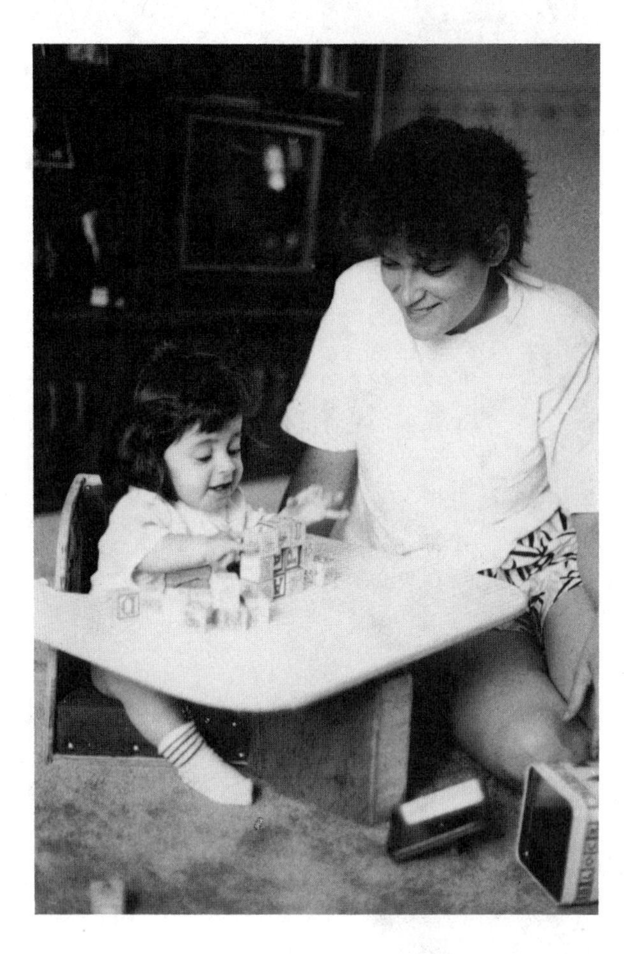

Figure 15–5. A corner seat provides support for the child in play.

never be a functional walker. The therapist must introduce the idea that a wheelchair may be needed as soon as possible. Michael has severe arthrogryposis; when he was 2 years old it was suggested that an electric wheelchair should be purchased before he entered kindergarten. His mother Roxanne burst into tears because her heart was set on his walking. By the time he was 5, however, the push for an electric chair was her idea. She wanted him to have the freedom to keep up with his friends without having to depend on her. Michael does walk on level surfaces at home but continues to use the electric wheelchair for independent mobility. How to transport a child with special needs by car or school bus is a frequently asked question. There are several points to keep in mind when transporting an individual with a wheelchair. Because wheelchairs are not built for crash protection, it is always safer for the child (or adult) to be transferred to a regular car seat and be safely secured in that seat. If the child must be transported in the wheelchair, the chair should face forward, have an adaptation that provides whiplash protection, and feature separate restraint systems for the chair and the occupant. In a bus or van, tie-downs for a wheelchair should be a four-point system with attachments above each wheel of the chair. The E-Z-ON-Vest[7] is one restraint system that can be used to secure children in wheelchairs, car seats, or school bus or van seats. The child wears the vest, which then is attached to the appropriate mounting strap in the vehicle or on the wheelchair. Thus a child with one vest can be transported in any vehicle that has been fitted with a mounting strap system. Richards[8] provides a comprehensive review of crash standards, product testing, specific adaptive devices, and resources for gaining more information on transportation.

The greater dilemma is choosing the functional equipment for the child with multiple handicaps, especially for the child with poor head control. Normal pieces of furniture are harder to adapt and the therapist must be careful to assist the family in determining their priorities. Loaner equipment can provide great advantages, particularly when the family is evaluating expensive equipment. Loaner equipment allows the family to try out the equipment and increases the odds that it will be useful to and used by the family. Standers are typical of the kind of equipment that is more effectively loaned than purchased (Figs. 15–6 and 15–7).

Finding the safe car seat or restraint system for the larger child who does not have good postural control is another problem. The few safety-approved seats are expensive. Multipurpose car seats are often difficult to move in and out of the car, especially with the child in the seat. The family may

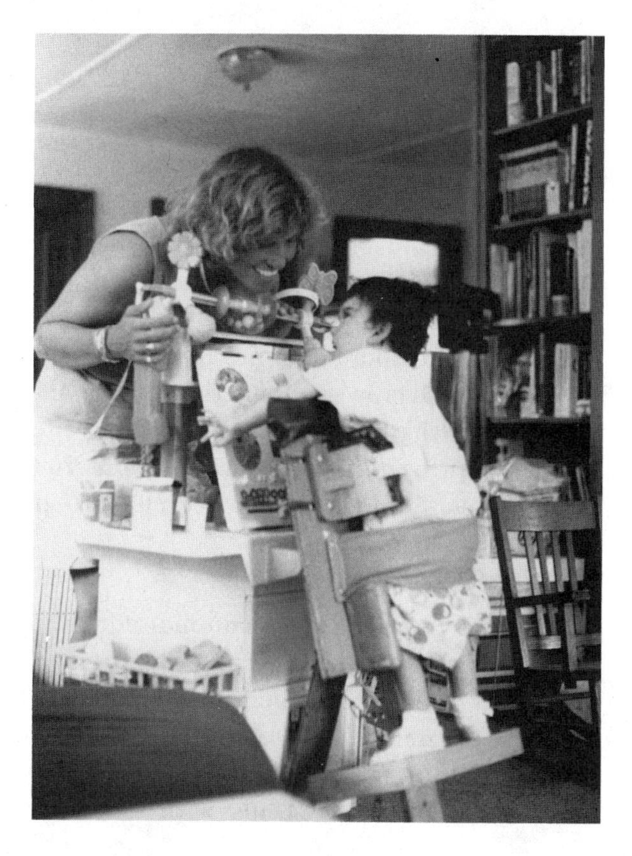

Figure 15–6. Loaner equipment such as the stander combines therapy and play.

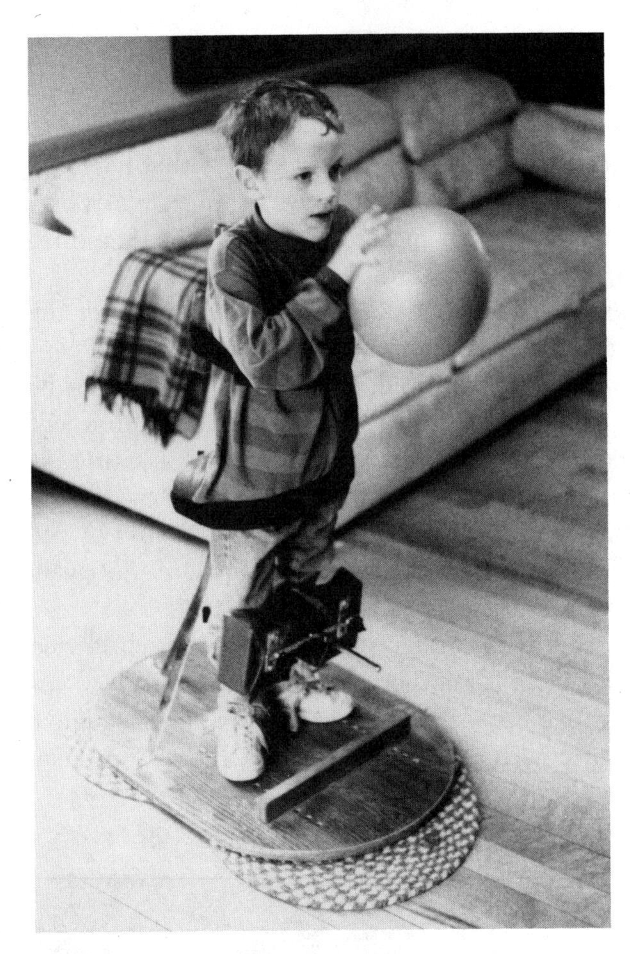

Figure 15–7. A stander allows a child to play catch with his sister.

also prefer a chair other than the car seat for mobility outside of the car; if so, this chair then must be transported. A wheelchair van as an alternative is also expensive. There are no good answers to this difficult question and, without safe transportation, a family's ability to participate with the child in activities outside the home becomes limited. The need for new equipment continues as a child grows and functional needs change. Recycling of equipment is a problem shared by therapists in all settings. Often the home therapist may be more aware than the family of outgrown equipment that has ended up in the closet and can then recycle it to another family.

Special Considerations

It is becoming more common for children who depend on oxygen, ventilators, feeding tubes, or other high-technology equipment to be cared for in their own homes rather than to remain in the hospital. When planning a therapy program for these children, the therapist must be familiar with the support machinery and the medical parameters for gauging the exercise capabilities of the child. Along with motor goals, which include working toward gaining maximum functional capabilities, an additional challenge is trying to facilitate the child's growth in all other areas, such as cognitive and language ability. The child may be too weak to manipulate toys or objects and may not be able to hold the toys where they can be seen. The child may not be able to tolerate certain positions that would commonly be used for play and learning. The therapist, in partnership with the family and other service providers, must adapt the child's environment.

Use of positioning or adaptive equipment such as supported seating allows the child to gain a variety of positions so that normal learning can occur in spite of the child's less-than-normal ability to move. These children often require very critical choices of goals and often many individuals must make decisions on each phase of the program. In our area, Addison County, Vermont, care conferences are held in the child's home. In each conference the family, physician, and all other service providers carefully discuss and plan the goals and program for the next week or month. These conferences are expensive in the short run, but at least three of my clients have been able to remain at home for long periods when otherwise they would have required repeated hospitalizations.

Some children have an illness or a genetic condition that will limit life span severely. Any planning done by the family and therapist is tempered by the reality that the child will not live past 2 or 5 or perhaps 12 years. Some families or providers might consider all program planning or services useless. However, there are frequently many services that therapists can provide. Every child needs access to food, play, rest, and interaction with family members or with others in the community. Parents want their child to be as comfortable as possible and to do as many age-appropriate activities as possible within their life span. Families also want to live from day to day as normally as possible despite the reality and fears of impending death. Assessments, goal setting, and planning for therapeutic interventions or adaptations must proceed. Emotional support, which is important in all cases, must be an integral part of the plan. Capricia's death at 3 years of age, though anticipated, was very difficult. Her abilities had been limited throughout her life, but the family could remember with pleasure the adaptations they devised so that she could sit with her brothers and sisters for songs and games.

THE FAMILY

Parents

Provision of therapy for children in their homes fits in nicely with the current trend of early intervention, being family centered and community based. However, a therapeutic program for a child can be just as isolated and non–family centered, whether at home or at a treatment center, if the parent is not an active participant in the treatment planning, provision of therapy, and setting of goals. Besides the encouragement of parent involvement, several other considerations are more obvious in a home setting. The therapist as the service provider is a guest in the home. There is a greater opportunity to observe interactions of family members, thus giving the therapist an understanding of possibly competing views on child care or priorities for activities. Issues that are important because of religious or cultural values may be more easily expressed or understood. In addition to or because of these factors, the family may have very clear goals for their child. Although the therapist may disagree with these goals and have competing priorities, the therapist must respect the family's choices. This should influence the approach with the family and the interaction with the child. The family can and should control all aspects of the visit and therapy session. Family members should feel more comfortable in their own home and it is the therapist's job to facilitate this. The family routine is important. A busy parent may see the therapist's visit as a convenient time to do chores while the therapist works with the child. There may be days when this is the easiest thing to do, but this does not facilitate the family-centered process. If the therapist's goal is to use skills of evaluation and treatment planning in partnership with the parent, the therapist must plan with the parent a time when the child is alert and the parent can participate in the session. The therapist also has the option of seeing the child with other caregivers who are interested in understanding and augmenting the child's program. When the child has a full-time babysitter, the therapist may need the flexibility to occasionally meet with the parents after their work time. Often other family members, such as grandparents or other relatives, may be available to help. If the parent is interested, a visit could be made at a time when that family member can be present. For some families the therapist may help the parent by talking with other family members during a visit, thus providing additional information or reinforcing the parent's position.

Siblings

Siblings often add an interesting dimension to a treatment session. They can help provide a normal model for a skill or actually assist with a therapeutic procedure (Fig. 15–8).[9] At various times, they can provide a distraction that may be disruptive. A parent may feel embarrassed by what they perceive as the misbehavior of the sibling and may feel compelled to send the child away to play. The siblings themselves may often be jealous of the attention their sister or brother with a disability is receiving and by the fact that most of the people coming to the home are not coming to play with them. There are several ways to cope with these situations. The therapist or the parent can plan a parallel activity for the sibling or spend some time with the sibling before or after the session. The therapist can also figure out a way to include the sibling in the treatment session. Often, if the therapist is com-

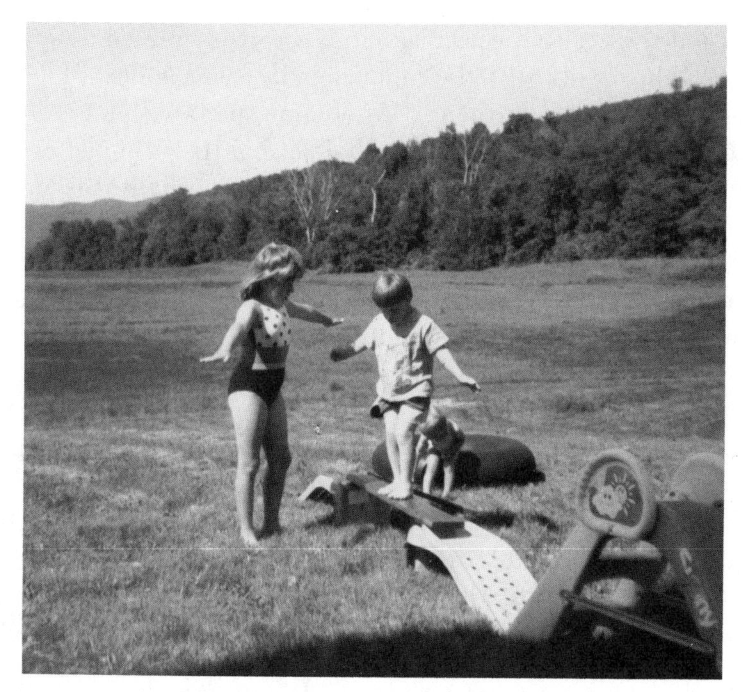

Figure 15–8. Megan designed this obstacle course for her brother.

fortable having the sibling be a part of the session, the therapist must assure the parent that if the parent approves, the sibling's help is welcome. Siblings' feelings are often an important issue for a parent and are a good topic for parents to discuss between themselves, in a support group, or through informal contacts. Several parents in our area have been organizing a sibling group in which the siblings will write and produce a newsletter for other siblings like themselves. The sibling group was the idea of two mothers, each of whom was concerned that there was too much focus in their family on the child with the chronic condition. Even though siblings Sarah and Megan were included in all therapy programs and sessions, everyone coming to the home was there primarily to work with the involved child. The mothers' goal was to provide a separate activity specifically for Sarah and Megan, but they also wanted to use the activity as a mechanism for the girls and other siblings to explore their feelings about their brother or sister.

Scheduling

The geographic location of the families seen by the traveling therapist has a major impact on the scheduling of visits. However, when working with children, the therapist must balance the logical progression of the day with the reality that children have specific times when they perform well. Also, if parent participation is wanted, the therapist must be aware of the parent's schedule as well. These accommodations may burden the therapist's schedule, but the positive aspect is that, if the visit is timed well, the therapist will be able to work with the child when he or she is awake and alert and not exhausted by a trip in the car. After time spent with a family in their home, their familiar routine is more obvious and the therapist can identify good times to visit. Because the pediatric client is usually not homebound and young families normally are frequently out of the house running errands or visiting friends, the therapist must take this into consideration when setting up a schedule. Many families have regular schedules and can plan ahead. For them it is often helpful to schedule the next visit before the therapist leaves; if the family has a calendar they can record the date and time of the next visit. For the families less likely to remember a scheduled visit, a call the day before or on the day of the visit may be necessary to prevent visiting an empty house. For some clients, coming on the same day at the same time is helpful. Frequency of visits will vary with individual therapists. However, when working with a family in their home, the therapist can get a better sense of how busy or hectic the family's schedule is; this may influence the evaluation of what visiting frequency is best for that family and may also allow therapeutic goals to be met.

Coordination of Services

It is astounding to see how many different services and providers are involved with any one child and family. Besides coping with different people coming into their home each week, the family also must cope with the variety of suggestions, programs, and goals proposed by these individuals. In addition, time must be found for visits to physicians or clinics. A home-based program provides a number of options, one of which is to make joint visits. This works well if the parent and the home visitors work together to combine goals and routines. One hazard to avoid is the tendency of two professionals to talk to each other in their own technical language and at times exclude or confuse the parent. Another option is for each professional to decrease frequency and to alternate visits. This works well if goals are clear, if each individual has a clear family-set role, and if the therapists communicate often. Another option is to have one therapist be the primary home visitor, with others providing evaluation and consultation. In choosing any of these options, the family must be at the center of the decision making process. If at any time additional services are needed, the therapist can, with the family's permission, act as an advocate and make the appropriate referrals to other services and service providers. Alternatively, the therapist can provide the information and have the family make the contacts themselves.

Community

Every community has a variety of recreational and educational programs available to children. What is available depends on the weather, the terrain, and local resources but, more important, on the enthusiasm and abilities of local individuals who develop and sustain each program. The children's participation may depend on skill, money, support of parents, or the vision of those running the program. Frequently the family with a child who has a disabling condition finds limited opportunities to involve their child in these community activities. The family may be isolated from community involvement by the demands of the daily routine connected with their child's care in addition to other responsibilities, or by the arrangements required to bring the child and possibly equipment from home to the activity. The family may also hesitate to participate because of the fear that their child may not be accepted or that the child may fail to do the activity at a perceived acceptable level. The therapist may help to bridge this gap by providing information about local programs that are already in place. If the family is interested, the therapist can be an advocate and resource in making programs accessible to their child. Ideally, with a little imagination, existing programs can be adapted to include a child with a disability. Other options include parallel activities such as Special Olympics or therapeutic horseback-riding programs (Fig. 15–9). Consideration of participation in these programs must be part of the planning process when the therapist and family are developing the home program. Goals for some children can be met through community activities. If participation in the community activity requires additional equipment, added costs, or possibly a non–family mem-

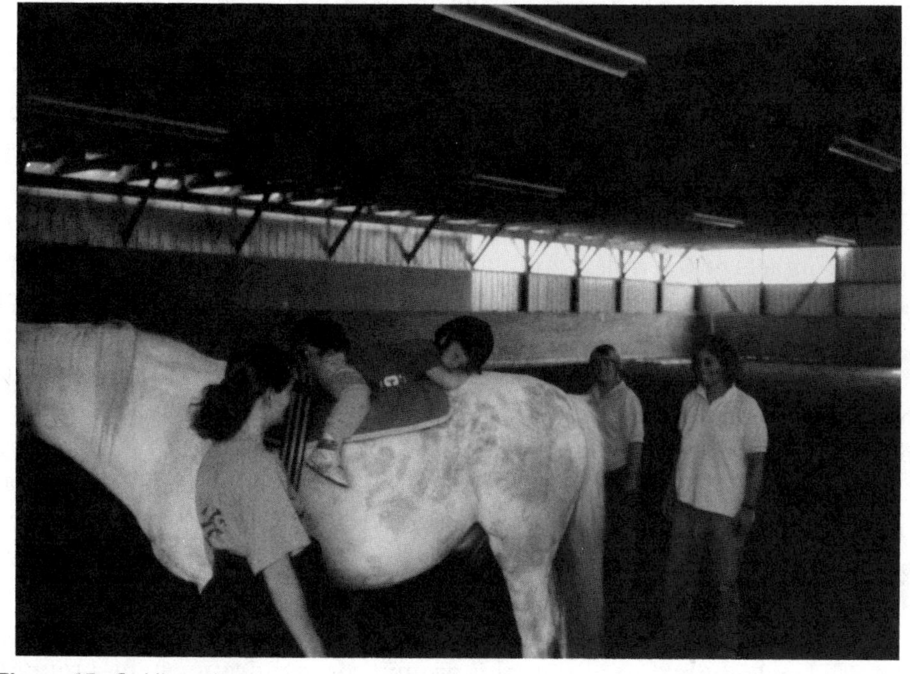

Figure 15–9. Hippotherapy.

ber assistant, these items must be addressed when a community program is being planned for a child. Parent support groups can play an important role in expanding community resources available to a family whose child has a disability. Families can share successful methods of gaining access to normal community activities. Frustrations held in common, or shared dreams, may be a positive spur for individuals to change community attitudes or lower barriers to their children's participation in sports or other programs.

Developing a Caseload

The development of a home-based program to provide therapy services to children may be initiated for various reasons. There may be no services available in an area, or a therapist may have a strong bias regarding where the provision of service might be most effective. In some rural areas, there may be limited access to center-based or hospital-based therapy departments within a reasonable traveling distance. Many local hospitals with therapy departments may not provide specialized services to children. Therapists interested in working with children and their families in rural areas therefore must be creative. It may be possible to develop a pediatric therapy program in a center or hospital with appropriate support. One option is to develop a community-based pediatric program that includes home care. In urban areas, where center-based programs are more readily available, an interested therapist might by choice develop a pediatric caseload through a home health agency or as a home-based private practitioner. This would provide an alternate service for families when they are developing the care plan for their child. The therapist who chooses to provide pediatric therapy through home health care may find a job that has an intact caseload. However, in most cases, it will be the therapist's responsibility to increase or develop a pediatric caseload. The children and families who would benefit from home therapy are there. Contact with the local pediatricians and family practitioners is essential because they treat most of the children in an area and often are the first to hear parental concerns. Another important source of initial contacts or referrals is from other community resources, such as parent-child centers or programs and infant-toddler programs, or possibly from clinics that screen graduates from neonatal intensive care departments. An active public health program that provides nursing services to families could be a basis for referrals. As more infants requiring high-technology equipment are surviving and arrangements are being made for them to go home, they provide an essentially homebound group of clients with a logical home health care base. If the initial contact with the client originates from a source other than the client's physician, the therapist should contact this physician as soon as possible and include him or her in the planning process. This contact helps to ensure comprehensive, coordinated, community-based care for the child and family. In addition, this prompt communication helps promote collaboration between the therapist and physician. The physician will be more likely to think of therapy options in later cases and begin to make earlier referrals. With a good physician-therapist colleague relationship, the therapist will find clients referred at younger and younger ages.

RESEARCH

The bias toward the advantages of providing therapy to children in their homes presented in this chapter is a result of my experience working with families through home health care. Exploration of this preference through research is limited. Several studies have been completed that investigated several aspects of provision of home care to chronically ill children. A common finding is that families prefer home care. In the Pediatric Ambulatory Care Treatment Study at the Albert Einstein College of Medicine, Bronx Municipal Hospital Center, Stein and Jessop[10] found that, although changes in functional status were equal in home care and standard care groups, the mother's satisfaction with the child's medical care and psychological adjustments were significantly better in the home care group. In the Early Intervention Collaborative Study completed in Massachusetts and New Hampshire, Shonhoff and associates[11] report that, in parent appraisals of their early intervention experience, home visits were described as the most helpful of all services received. Good therapeutic results for children and families can be achieved in a variety of settings. Whether client comfort and satisfaction can influence functional outcomes over time remains an interesting question. However, when you first contact a parent and indicate that you will treat the child in the home, do not be surprised to hear a sign of relief at the other end of the telephone.

REFERENCES

1. Gordon, J, et al: Movement science: Foundations for physical therapy. In Gordon, J, et al: Rehabilitation. Aspen, Rockville, 1987, p 1.
2. Rosenbaum, P, et al: Home or children's treatment centre: Where should initial assessments of children with disabilities be done? Dev Med Child Neurol 32:888, 1990.
3. Bayley Scales of Infant Development (0–2.5). Psychological Corporation, 757 Third Avenue, New York, NY 10017.
4. Peabody Developmental Motor Scales (0–83 months). DLM Teaching Resources, One DLM Park, Allen, TX 75002.
5. Early LAP (0–36 months) and LAP (36–72 months). Kaplan Press, PO Box 5128, Winston-Salem, NC 27113-5128.
6. Dunst, CJ, et al: Family needs scale. In Dunst, CJ, Trivette, CM, and Deal, AG (eds): Enabling and Empowering Families: Principles and Guidelines for Practice. Brookline Books, Cambridge, MA, 1988, p 149.
7. E-Z-ON Products, Inc. of Florida. 500 Commerce Way West, Jupiter, FL 33458.

8. Richards, DD: The challenge of transporting children with special needs. American Academy of Pediatrics, Safe Ride News, Spring, 1988 (Special insert).
9. Craft, MJ, et al: Siblings as change agents for promoting the functional status of children with cerebral palsy. Dev Med Child Neurol 32:1049, 1990.
10. Stein, REK and Jessop, DJ: Does pediatric home care make a difference for children with chronic illness? Findings from the Pediatric Ambulatory Care Treatment study. Pediatrics 73:845, 1984.
11. Shonkoff, JP, et al: Early intervention collaborative study. Brief report of Phase One. Unpublished material, 1990.

Chapter 16

Hospice Care*

Rick Reuss

*This chapter is written in the first person as I look back on my experiences as a hospice therapist. The use of first names for clients and health professionals reflects the closeness and personal nature of interactions among team members and with clients. The opinions presented in this chapter are mine alone and do not necessarily reflect the opinions of the editor or publishers of this book.

As I approached the client's house, I wondered what I would find. The home health referral read: "Dx: Terminal CA. PT to see patient." Being aware of the many difficult circumstances surrounding the care of terminally ill clients, I wished again that my small community had a hospice program. I had worked with a hospice program in another town and knew its many benefits. As was my habit before making the first home health visit, I had read the client's inpatient chart.

Crystal Donner was a 60-year-old woman who had had a right radical mastectomy 4 years before for breast carcinoma. Several months later, a total hysterectomy was performed to decrease hormone production. She had no further problems until 2 years later, when a liver scan showed metastasis. Ms. Donner underwent a successful course of chemotherapy and remained relatively well for about 1 year. She then developed middle back pain from further metastasis and underwent more chemotherapy and 10 radiotherapy treatments. Next, central nervous system signs were detected and brain metastasis was discovered. This time she received 10 radiation treatments to the involved brain area as well as to the coccyx where she had developed recurrent pain.

The Donners lived in a midsized, well-kept two-story house in a residential part of town. I was greeted at the door by the client's husband, Clarence Donner, a self-employed paint contractor. He took me on a brief tour and I made mental notes of the environmental details. There were two steps from the outside to the front door. A stairway went up from the right side of the foyer and the family room opened from the left side. The family room was carpeted and had a sofa, chairs, and a table around the fireplace. There was also a television set and bookshelves. Mr. Donner's office and a bathroom opened off the family room. The kitchen and dining room were in the rear. The four bedrooms were all upstairs. A full bathroom and shower were adjacent to the master bedroom, which was furnished with a full-sized bed, vanity, and dresser. Mr. and Ms. Donner had lived in this neighborhood for 3 years and in this town for the last 17 years.

Crystal Donner was asleep in the master bedroom but awoke as we approached. She was lying in a fetal position and appeared in extreme pain. Clarence stated that her pain had continued to increase to such a degree that she slept only sporadically and was in bed most of the day. She had not walked for the past 3 or 4 weeks due to pain and weakness. Crystal said she had two narcotic pain medications that she used only when the pain became so bad she could not "stand it any longer." It was obvious from the conversation that the pain medication was not taken on a regular schedule. Her primary pain was in her lower abdomen. She related that her "ovaries, which aren't there, feel like they're pulling apart!" Careful palpation of her lumbar spine, elicited moderate secondary pain, which she said she continued to have despite radiotherapy. I said that I had a device known as a transcutaneous electric nerve stimulator (TENS) which I had used with other clients for the type of pain she was having. Both Crystal and Clarence said they would try anything to help lessen her pain. I excused myself to go to get the TENS from my car. (Through years of home care experience, I had equipped my car to convey the modalities I would routinely use, as well as acquiring standing orders to use them).

DIMENSIONS OF HOSPICE CARE

As I walked to the car, I thought of the paradox of Crystal's situation. For the last 30 years there has been information available to the medical community on the subject of death and dying. Elisabeth Kubler-Ross[1] introduced the five stages of dying (denial and isolation, anger, bargaining, depression, and acceptance) and made the dying process an open topic for discussion, exploration, and research. She and other writers have provided the public and medical community with insight into the nuances of one's own mortality and ways of responding to this challenging life event. Cicely Saunders is generally credited with introducing the modern hospice movement in 1967, although acknowledging that other institutions offered special services for the terminally ill prior to that time.[2–5] Saunders founded the St. Christopher Hospice in England and developed the modern theories of hospice care, which advocate pain and symptom control, consideration of the psychological and social needs of the client and the family and continuous care by an interdisciplinary team of health professionals.[3,5] Richard Lamerton, also involved in early hospice activities, responded in 1975 to a question in which he was asked what he would do if he walked into a hospital room and saw a "vegetable" in the hospital bed. Lamerton replied: "I would eat it. What kind of vegetable are you talking about? A radish? A broccoli? If you are talking about a human being, I would take care of him!"[6]

The term "hospice" originally referred to places of shelter for travelers; hospices in medieval times were usually run by religious orders as stopping places for pilgrims. Gradually, hospices became places were people in need went for shelter, care, and comfort. There is evidence that the Irish Sisters of Charity of Dublin opened a place for the terminally ill in the mid-1800s and called it a hospice.[4,23] The Hospice of Connecticut is credited with being the first American hospice; it started providing care to a single patient in March 1974. Most hospice programs in the United States are home based rather than facility based. Many were started by nonmedical personnel, usually clergy, consumers, or social workers. In 1978 the National Hospice Association was created; in 1982 hospice services became reimbursable under Medicare. In 1984, through the efforts of the Joint Commission on Accreditation of Hospitals and the National Hospice Organization, a voluntary accreditation program went into effect with nationally accepted standards of hospice care.[3-5] Briefly, the standards for accreditation include:

- The client and family are the unit of care.
- Interdisciplinary team services available to the patient/family must include at least physician, nursing, psychological/social work, spiritual, volunteer, and bereavement services.
- Intervention focuses on the management of physical and psychological symptoms.
- Hospice services must be available 24 hours a day, seven days a week.
- Inpatient services must be available as well as home care, and continuity of care across both settings must be assured. (ref. 3, p. 4)

In 1985 it was estimated that there were approximately 1694 active hospice programs in many different settings in the United States.[7] Unfortunately they do not exist in all communities and the concepts of pain management not always used. Hospice care would surely help Crystal with pain control and other important aspects of her home care. The hospice concept of care serves as the appropriate medical model for all disciplines working with the terminally ill.

I surveyed the "tools" I always carried in my car since my hospice experience: (1) a TENS unit with postoperative electrodes and batteries, (2) a folding adjustable walker, (3) a fracture pan, and (4) a legal pad for written instructions. In this instance, I wished I had a portable durable medical supply store on wheels. The usual supplies ordered for delivery the next day for most hospice clients are (1) an electric hospital bed with a trapeze, (2) a bedside commode, (3) a fracture pan, and (4) an adult wheelchair with removable desk arms and elevating legrests. A hydraulic patient lift was not usually necessary on the first visit but was readily available.

As I prepared the TENS for application, I thought of the National Hospice Organization's definition of "hospice":

> Hospice is a centrally controlled program of palliative and supportive services. It provides physical, psychological, social, and spiritual care for dying patients and their families. A medically supervised interdisciplinary team of professionals and volunteers provides hospice services. Hospice services are available in both a home and inpatient settings. The hospice team provides home care on a part time, intermittent, regularly scheduled, around-the-clock, on-call basis. Bereavement services are also available to the family. Admission to a hospice program is on the basis of patient and family need (ref. 8, p. 8).

As I walked back to the house, many thoughts occurred to me. It appeared that facets of Crystal's care were not being addressed—errors of omission rather than commission. The problems she encountered in this small town were similar to problems faced by terminally ill clients in any location without benefit of hospice: a busy, caring physician (oncologist) in another city treating the primary disease; a busy, caring hometown physician responsible for all other aspects of care; and a busy group of caring home health personnel used to directing care toward the curative nature of medicine—helping clients become well. The goal of hospice intervention is to affirm and promote the quality of life until death, not to prolong life through extraordinary means. A primary aim is to keep the client pain free but alert. In this way, the client and family can achieve a level of satisfactory mental and spiritual preparation for death. Hospice intervention is designed to help the client successfully remain at home as long as possible, ideally until death. Inpatient facility care serves as a choice should the client no longer be able to remain at home. Later, hospice bereavement services provide direction in preparation for the client's death. Hospice care provides follow-up support for the family after the death for as long as the support is needed. The primary unit of care is the client and the immediate family.

While applying the electrodes on Crystal's back and lower quadrants, I gave the Donners a brief explanation of how and why the TENS would probably work for her pain. I told them I would call their hometown physician and suggest an increase in medication adequate to control her pain when taken on an around-the-clock basis; I would also confer with her primary home health nurse regarding the importance of the around-the-clock administration of the pain medication. The electrodes were placed to cross over and concentrate the paths of stimulation on both the primary and secondary sites of pain. The stimulator's pulse width was set at 120 μsec. The intensity and pulse rate were adjusted to her level of comfort and sensation of stimulation. All nuances of electrode placement and changes were discussed and written instructions (in large type) were provided. I gave Clarence my pager and home telephone numbers in case questions or problems regarding the TENS occurred. Both Clarence and Crystal were pleased with the visit, but I knew that this pleasure would be short-lived if her pain were not indeed reduced in the next few days. I assured them that I would be back the next day to check on her. If they needed me sooner, I would even break away from my softball game that night! They both smiled warmly.

ROLES OF HEALTH CARE PRACTITIONERS ON THE HOSPICE TEAM

Driving away from their house, I reflected on the importance of pain control in the dying process. Wistfully I though of how the Donners' circumstance could be improved with the hospice team I had worked with several years before. An effective hospice team works in concert for the alleviation of physical and mental pain. The multidisciplinary approach to client care is intrinsic to the hospice philosophy. Most home health practitioners are well acquainted with this approach. While only a small percentage of health care practitioners practice in formal hospice settings, the principles of hospice care transcend any practice setting. An intermingling of roles is inherent in the hospice concept of care. The team members not only know their specific roles but also draw on resources from other team members. There is a great need for coordination and communication, and team meetings are an integral part of hospice care.

The basic interdisciplinary hospice team consists of physician, nurse, social services, volunteers, and chaplains. Additionally, Medicare requires that a hospice must provide, either directly or under contractual arrangement, the following services when needed: physical therapy, occupational therapy, speech-language pathology, home health aide and homemaker services, medical supplies (including drugs and biologic agents for palliation), and short-term inpatient care.[9] In contrast, skilled care under a Medicare-certified home health program routinely provides skilled nursing services. In addition, a home health program must provide, either directly or under contractual arrangement, one of the following services: physical, speech, or occupational therapy; medical social services; or home health aide services. (See Chapter 2 for further information on the function of the home health care team.)

The most important member of the team, of course, is the client. The client and family watch and guide the success of all plans of intervention. As with restorative care, the client and the caregiver must be actively involved in the care process. As I drove on to my next home health client, I reminisced about my former hospice "teammates."

Medical Staff

Ralph Datzman retired from medicine in his early 50s when he saw so many of his peers dying from the stress and rigor of this profession. Financially secure, he pursued his interests in Civil War history, genealogy, and archeology. It was not until he learned of the hospice concept of care that he entertained the notion of coming out of retirement. "Datz" made a tremendous impact. The frequent sight of this physician carrying a golf seat around so he could stay at eye level with the client became famous in the area. On one of his visits to a 74-year-old man dying of disseminated carcinoma of the prostate, he wore a 200-year-old military uniform because the client had volunteered as a guard at a historic old fort. Datz was the primary team consultant and coordinated all physical care efforts while protecting the autonomy of all team disciplines. His responsibilities as hospice physician included client visits and assessments to determine appropriate pain and symptom intervention, clarification of the dying progress to the client and family, referral of client care needs to appropriate team members, assumption of the responsibility for regulation of appropriate medicines, provision of comprehensive physical and psychological care for the client and family, and collaboration with attending physicians. Hospice physicians may have any background but must share an interest in people as well as patience and compassion. A strong knowledge of pharmacology is also important.[5]

Datz wrote notes to himself on index cards and encouraged all team members to keep similar index cards. "Datzman's Observations,"[10] a set of informal guidelines, was the result of his index card collection from many different client visits. The Appendix lists some of the informal rules and procedures. Obviously, the list is not a "how to" set of instructions and has no official organizational permission.

Not all hospice organizations have a primary physician; often the client's personal physician serves in the capacity of a hospice physician and coordinates the care. Clients may be under the care of several physicians and the coordinating role may fall to the hospice nurse.

Nursing Services

Hazel Ryan was an experienced hospice nurse who exhibited clinical competence and a caring nature. One of the integral parts of the hospice concept is staffing by nurses skilled in pain management and symptom control. Hazel Ryan and the other nurses helped keep team members apprised of each client's physical and psychological condition, notifying us of changes by telephone or at the team meetings. Hazel was skilled in patient care delivery and gifted in supervising the total nursing program.

The nursing role is directed toward helping the client participate as fully as possible in day-to-day living.[1] Direct nursing services include routine nursing visits, client assessment to determine health care needs, identification of alterations in health status, initiation of a plan of individual nursing care, and participation in an on-call schedule to meet the emergency needs. Good nursing care basically consists of ensuring that (1) the pain medication is being taken by the client or given to the client in the appropriate timely manner; (2) the side effects of medications are watched for and taken into account; (3) the medication is doing what it is supposed to do; (4) good skin care is maintained; and (5) the client is not constipated.[3,5]

In the last several years there seems to have been movement away from the model of a formal hospice team with specific training in this specialized concept of care. In many instances hospice services are being incorporated within neighborhood visiting nurse or home health organizations. Nurses consult with other health care practitioners case by case rather than as part of an interdisciplinary team. In some instances, neither the consulting nurses nor the consulted health care practitioners have had formal training in the hospice concept of care. Further, there is confusion in some nursing communities regarding what actually is the hospice concept. A popular premise I have heard advanced by some home health nursing administrators is that if one takes care of terminally ill clients, one is providing hospice services! Providers in these situations lack the specific training and often do not understand the differences between the hospice care focus and that of curative care. Practitioners must understand the difference between care given through formal hospice programs and that given through the quasihospice parts of home care agencies. Many hospice agencies require clinical experience and advanced degrees for hospice nurses.[3,5] Recently, specialized formal education in hospice care has been advocated.[11]

In addition to direct patient care, nurses are also responsible for supervising nursing aides, who are critical to helping the client and the family cope with daily activities such as bathing, homemaking, and personal care.

Physical Therapy

I look back on my own experience with hospice care as the most rewarding period in my professional life.[12] It was not depressing, as some people not associated with hospice care suggest. It was, conversely, a joy-filled time replete with memories that most people could not imagine.[13,14]

As a hospice physical therapist I was responsible for helping clients in all areas of mobility, exercise, pain control, and bed positioning. No effort was wasted on the client's or family's part to attain reasonable short-term goals in the face of diminished pain. I also arranged for delivery of equipment that would reduce the effort of daily activities. One of my favorite interventions was an adjunctive role in pain control. One of the primary reasons clients entered the hospice program was the palliation of physical pain. The primary method of pain control was the conscientious administration of narcotic medication.

For some clients, the window between overmedication and undermedication was slight, with the client being either asleep or in pain. TENS bridged this gap well for most clients, regardless of the location of their pain.[15] Three hospitalized hospice clients who suffered severe acute pain and shortness of breath as a result of rib fractures from further metastasis come to mind. Their chronic pain had been controlled by medication and TENS. The onset of pain resulting from the rib fracture was controlled within 15 minutes by rearranging the electrodes without the need for more medication. The use of TENS has become standard protocol for the clients of some physicians for the treatment of traumatic rib fractures not related to metastasis.

The hospice experience served me well later in my professional career. I knew that, when Crystal's pain was reduced to a satisfactory level or eliminated, it would be rather easy to evaluate her from a functional and neurologic perspective. It would probably be appropriate to progress her from rolling in bed to sitting on the side of the bed. Depending on the course of her disease, Crystal might be able to stand with a walker and take a few steps around the bed. As with all home health clients, these activities would be performed as a nonrushed, confident process to maximize safety and minimize fatigue. Clarence would be encouraged to help his wife with sitting and walking and instructed in helping her progress to other tasks as she conceivably became stronger. If Crystal developed enough walking endurance to leave the bedroom, I would establish "way stations." Chairs would be positioned at comfortable intervals between the bed and other rooms of the second floor. (Many years ago, calling them "way stations" appealed to my sense of irony; the original meaning of the word "hospice" was a medieval shelter for tired travelers.) At some point it would be appropriate to suggest to Crystal and Clarence that a hospital bed be placed in the living room so that she could again be part of daily activities in their house. Chairs could then be placed so that she would have comfortable access to the kitchen, dining room, bathroom, and her husband's office. From her bed she could also look outside to see children playing in a park and to watch neighbors walking along the street.

As the dying process progressed, necessitating more time in bed, I would instruct the Donners in the most effective method of transfer and lifting. These techniques were no different from those used in any home health setting. Most important was the fact that Crystal did not have to be needlessly fatigued by being the subject of transfer training. If Crystal was too weak, Clarence and neighbors could practice on me or each other.

I remembered a similar situation 10 years before with June Bauer, a pleasant 56-year-old woman who had oat cell carcinoma of the lung with metastasis to the lower spine. Using a large bath towel as an abdominal binder to splint against the pain of spinal metastasis, she was able to sit up with the help of her husband and walk with a walker from the bedroom to her favorite reclining lounger in the living room. She used this binder even when she became weaker. Her husband became quite adept at helping her roll from side to side to replace the binder, position a draw sheet for transfers, and exchange bed linen at the same time. Fatigue was reduced by an adjustable bed, trapeze, bedrails, and bedside commode. The practical advantages of good body mechanics, gentleness, and patience could not be overemphasized in view of June's disease-weakened bones.

Occupational Therapy

The occupational therapist knows that a balance exists among work, rest, and play. This balance influences a client's mental state and physical capabilities and has a significant affect on quality of life. Clients must be allowed to experience natural order in daily living. Being denied the opportunity to engage in occupational roles or fulfill basic self-care tasks deprives clients of the opportunity to be members of society and of their families. This sets into place the pain of isolation and abandonment and a lowering of self-esteem.[16] Until recently, occupational therapists were only rarely involved in hospice care. Medicare requirement and an increase in available practitioners has increased their participation. Although my hospice program did not have an occupational therapist, my thought went to Sandy, an occupational therapist at my last clinical internship. Sandy and I worked together in the care of a 12-year-old boy named Al.

Al was a baseball fan who had enjoyed participating in sports until he underwent a craniotomy for a medulloblastoma, a highly malignant brain tumor. Within the understanding of his 12 years, Al provided Sandy with insight into his feelings. He spoke of knowing that he was getting stronger, but not ultimately well, despite surgery, chemotherapy, and radiotherapy. He had concerns about how members of his family were going to cope with his illness. Sandy completed an occupational therapy assessment and found that Al had decreased strength, mild incoordination, and a mild sensory loss in the left upper extremity. His balance was fair in sitting and poor in stance. He required minimal help with upper body bathing and dressing and moderate assistance for his lower extremities. He was independent in self-feeding.

A treatment plan was developed to foster Al's independence in self-care and to relieve his family from the task of caring for him 24 hours a day. Sandy instructed Al in hemiplegic dressing techniques, initially working in supported sitting and supination. She gradually withdrew the amount of help provided as he grew stronger. Al used primarily his right upper extremity, with his left upper extremity as a stabilizer assist. Sandy had explored the use of self-help devices, but Al did not have much patience with "gadgets" other than a reacher he used initially to obtain objects outside his grasp. Sandy also worked closely with Al's parents, teaching them ways to help Al while supporting his need for independence. She also listened well as Al's mother voiced her fears and concerns. When Al and his family became involved in the adaptation process, the quality of Al's life was enhanced and the transition home was made smoother.

Sandy asked Al if there was a specific activity he would like to do. Al chose to attend a professional baseball game in his hometown. Sandy arranged for a light-weight wheelchair for Al to use in traveling from the car to his seat in the stadium. This conserved his strength to watch the game. He discussed players and plays and thoroughly enjoyed his night out.

Al went home to his family 6 weeks after the initial craniotomy. He had progressed from being hemiparetic with a walker to being ambulatory with the occasional use of a cane. He could take care of all his personal needs, including getting in and out of the shower. Right before discharge, Al was even able to throw a baseball and swing a bat, albeit with a widened stance. Al retained some independence in the presence of advancing functional loss until his death 6 months later.

Occupational therapy for the hospice client does not differ in kind from that given to any client. Assessment and treatment are individualized and communication skills are paramount. The occupational therapist can help each client perform meaningful activities that enhance the quality of life.[17,18]

Chaplaincy

The Reverend Dale Jerome brought good humor, competence, and compassion to the hospice team. Dale was the coordinator of several chaplains of different religious faiths who worked with hospice clients. He met regularly with the team and provided support to clients and families. Dale never pushed theologic dogma on either clients or staff members. He was well aware that his basic responsibility to the clients and team was to be available for spiritual, religious, and philosophic guidance.

Dale coordinated community pastoral care services in addition to his other duties. He would contact a client's personal minister, priest, or rabbi or find appropriate religious support if none were locally available. If the client held no formal religious beliefs, this too was honored by Dale within the hospice concept. This liaison provided many volunteers to aid in the care of clients. I remembered Dale's value at the weekly hospice team meetings when all clients were discussed. He afforded us insight into the client's and family's religious background. He also served as an ethical consultant to the interdisciplinary team and counselor for the spiritual concerns of the staff members on request. In the nature of a hospice team member, Dale was available on a 24-hour-basis, providing spiritual support for clients and their families. He respected the privacy and maturity level of the client's belief's or lack of belief. He knew that persons who had a strong religious belief system or those who strongly held no religious convictions had an easier time accepting their own dying. For those who wanted to pray, Dale was very careful to listen to their concerns, thoughts, and fears. He would then craft prayer rephrasing the client's, family member's, or staff member's own words. Priority was given to the client's opportunity to voice particular beliefs.

I remembered Dale's genuine gift of nonverbal communication. Late one night in the fall, Arnold Jacobson, a 71-year-old man with histolytic lymphoma, was dying without pain in his favorite reclining chair in his living room. He was in a relaxed semicomatose posture and his wife, Thelma, knew that his death was imminent. She had become upset with this knowledge and called the hospice nurse who, in turn, called Dale and me. When I arrived to check on Arnold's TENS, Dale was in the kitchen with Thelma helping her prepare coffee and baking rolls. There was really nothing else to be done for Arnold. Thelma was reassured that the hospice team would be there in whatever situation would comfort her in the last hours of her husband's life. She had felt so secure with the situation that when Arnold died at

4 the next morning, she did not call the hospice team until 3 hours later so "everyone could get a good night's sleep." Dale officiated at Arnold's funeral, as their regular clergyman was out of town.

Pharmacology

My thoughts kept returning to how relatively easily pain can be reduced in terminally ill patients if there is enough medication and if it is given regularly. How many changes have occurred since the oral Brompton's mixture was used extensively in the 1970s?[5] In the 1990s there are intravenous morphine pumps at the bedside of selected postoperative clients who control their own doses. These pumps were originally developed for the pain of terminally ill clients, but now even clients with total hip replacements are using them. Even these pumps are becoming obsolete with the development time-delayed morphine tables of varying strengths. Also available are 72-hour analgesic narcotic medication patches by which the medication is given transdermally, thereby reducing nausea. (See Chapter 9 for more detail on medications.)

The hospice pharmacist is an important member of the team. I remembered how skillful Steve Schneider, the hospice pharmacist, was in making sure that pain control was successful by helping the team understand the basic concepts of clinical pharmacology and the nuances of pain control. There indeed is an art and science involved in hospice pharmacology. Steve was responsible for consultation with the client and family to ensure an adequate daily drug supply to lessen the pain and possible concomitant symptoms of constipation, depression, nausea, and vomiting. He was creative in making the oral pain medication more palatable by offering cola, cherry, wild cherry, or peppermint flavors. In concert with the team, Steve maintained the drug profile, monitoring individual dose titration for analgesics and displaying mastery in the use of equianalgesic charts.

Weekly team meetings and frequent telephone calls provided daily information about clients to all the staff including Steve. Hospice team members are sensitive to each other as well as to client and family needs. Shared social functions and long discussions helped bridge stress lines. I remembered fondly how Steve, at a team St. Patrick's Day party, was adept in mixing beverages and in formulating the green coloring for the beer.

Social Services

Jody Mallory worked the complexities of medicine, finance, and community resources into a simplified form to spare clients and their families needless trial and error and wasted time and energies. Before her involvement in the hospice program, she had enabled a most effective network of medical professionals, medical equipment companies, and volunteer agencies to work with hospital clients. Jody exhibited the expertise and maturity necessary for constructive individual, marital, and family counseling. Clients, families, and staff benefited from problem solving experiences including social crisis intervention, improvement in the method and mode of communication, helping the family to work as a unit in facing the process of terminal illness and bereavement, and facilitating appropriate team dynamics. Jody demonstrated that, even with the process of dying, there are still reasons for hope. Individual, marital, and family problems confront everyone. Terminal illness does not change or eliminate these challenges. Relationships can be restored. A client or family member can start growing or continue growing emotionally even when days are numbered. Memories can be recorded for succeeding generations. (See Chapter 13 for more detail on social services.)

Volunteer Services

Hospice volunteers are a unique group of people. I reflected happily about one of the most outstanding individuals I had been privileged to meet. In established hospices, a committee of hospice team members select volunteers through formal recruitment procedures. Elly Sampson was chosen to join the original team because of her interest and enthusiasm, without benefit (and at times encumbrance) of established procedures. The joy this special woman brought to all her clients, their families, and each staff member served as a standard against which I have measured each subsequent volunteer.

In established programs a volunteer coordinator trains the volunteers in the hospice concept of care. Elly had no teacher or model to learn from in gaining her tools of caring and compassion. Volunteer services run the gamut from direct client to family care. Volunteers provide nontechnical bedside care (bathing, lifting, feeding, dressing, shopping, etc.), run errands, and offer personal support and companionship. They are also available at the time of death if a family member cannot be present. Volunteers provide an atmosphere of warmth and understanding for the family and help in bereavement follow-up after the client's death.[3,5]

Elly was not satisfied to read the many articles the team had available for reference. She journeyed to England to spend time at St. Christopher's Hospice with Cicely Saunders.[2] On her return she related that there are no set ways to provide peace and comfort to dying clients and their families. The willingness to be honest and to take risks in caring for people is primary.

Only those who have cared for dying people understand that closeness to dying clients and their families is not something to be avoided. The loss is indeed sad and grief occurs. This grief becomes supplanted by an even greater sense of love and the ability to care. Platitudes are useless because they are not honest to the dying or their survivors. Who can seriously deal with loss if one has not experienced loss? Loss has many faces. The tasks are many in both the anticipatory and actual grief processes. Only through the knowledge of one's own mortality can a volunteer or other team member effectively assist clients working through their imminent death.

PAIN CONTROL

Despite the many advances in pain control that have occurred in the last 20 years, a survey involving over 1000 oncologists revealed that most physicians (85%) still do not give enough medication to ease the physical pain of cancer clients. These findings were presented at the 1991 meeting of the American Society of Clinical Oncology.[19] Nearly two thirds of the physicians indicated that they do an inadequate job of even learning whether their patients are in pain. The primary reason physicians do not treat pain aggressively is the belief that they will not be able to deal with the side effects of the medication. About one third of the physicians indicated they do not currently prescribe the highest levels of pain medicine unless they believe the client has less than 6 months to live.

When I returned to the hospital I called Crystal's general practitioner. I had worked with this physician before in the treatment of terminally ill clients. Indeed, he had been unaware of the level of Crystal's pain and was amenable to suggestions for pain control prescribing the appropriate pain medication for Crystal's situation.

As has been stated, one of the main reasons for referring a client for hospice care is to alleviate physical pain. In most instances, the around-the-clock administration of narcotics accomplishes pain control. The client, a family member, a caregiver, or an external medication device can control the amount of medication. The main point is that the client should receive enough medication to lessen the pain. Generally, the client and family must be aware that on the first day the client generally feels better. On the second and third days, the client may feel quite drowsy and sleep a lot. On the fourth day the client is usually alert again, but without pain. It is important that the client stay on the prescribed schedule and not skip a dose, even when not feeling pain. The client must be maintained on a plateau of comfort rather than be allowed to suffer through episodic periods of agony. Addiction to the prescribed, around-the-clock pain medication is not an issue in the face of successful pain reduction. In fact, studies have shown that individuals who go into remission or whose pain is alleviated through other forms of treatment can be withdrawn from narcotics quite easily.[5] Practitioners must be aware that symptoms of constipation (abdominal distention, cramping, diarrhea) often follow administration of narcotic pain medication. These symptoms may affect the client's ability to do activities comfortably.

SYMPTOMS OF DYING

Once Crystal's physical pain was controlled, Crystal and Clarence would be able to deal with the mental and emotional aspects of her terminal disease. The physician and the home health nurses would monitor closely her level of pain and overall physical function. Eventually my role would change from assisting Crystal's active mobility to teaching Clarence to most effectively lift and transfer her in and out of bed. The time would come when Crystal would enter the final stage of dying. Care would be planned so that Clarence would know what to expect and how to adapt to each situation. The stage would eventually be reached when active treatment was over and there was little to do but sit at the bedside and wait. This is a very delicate and difficult moment in care. It may be prolonged for days. Each succeeding hour may have to be explained to the family.

In caring for dying clients, the home health practitioner must understand the general pattern of events preceding death. Clients become more somnolent and diaphoretic. They must be patted dry, cleaned, and powdered more frequently. One cardinal rule understood by experienced hospice team members involves eating and drinking behaviors. If clients stop eating, death may be a week or so away. If clients stop drinking fluids, death may be a few days away. Reduction of pain medication is in response to the client's request; physical pain generally lessens at the end of life. Clients respond less to family members and their environment. Their eyes turn up and roll back. There is no urine output or a minimal quantity of very dark urine. Their fingers and toes become colder and cyanotic. It is now that family members, as well as medical caregivers, must say their goodbyes.

The fact of the actual dying process should be communicated honestly and appropriately to the family members. The actual death of most hospice clients is quiet and peaceful. Family members in attendance may actually wait for a time before informing the hospice program of the death and calling the funeral home.

DISCUSSION

Honest communication is essential to hospice care. Communication is probably the most important clinical skill in the care of the dying. The clinician must be guided by practical rules of effective communication in meeting many of the client's and family's nonphysical needs. The terminally ill client may care very little about what the clinician is thinking, and one need not offer an opinion unless asked. What is important is what the client is feeling and thinking. Effective workers never push for communication with the terminally ill, but are there if the client needs to talk. The practitioner should look as little like a physician or nurse as possible. Most clients have been through enough formal medicine. They need something different. The plan of intervention either works or does not work. This is high pressure for the clinician. There is no time for the strategy of trial and error, as the hospice worker must proceed with solving specific problems. If the solution to a physical problem is available, one arrives at what is physically possible or acknowledges and accepts the contrary. Saunders writes:

> It is far better to have a cup of tea on your last day than drips and tubes in every direction. I think this cup of tea comes best from someone who has compassion, understanding, and practicality—someone who adds heart to skill, and who has a sense of meaning and assurance in another dimension in life. We should never impose our own beliefs, or own feelings of meaning, onto another person, but I am quite sure we could help produce a climate in which the patients can find their own meanings, and can find the quietness and dignity of death as it can be when it is a person, not the apparatus around, that is the centre of attention (ref. 20, p. 31).

Studies comparing hospice care with conventional care for the terminally ill have been equivocal at best.[3,5,20-22] There is little consistency of dimensions studied and subjects vary to some extent. Generally, the studies indicate that the families of hospice clients were more satisfied with the care and support received, and were considered to make a better adjustment following the death, than families of clients receiving conventional care.[18,19]

A Personal Note

This chapter is personal as well as didactic. The mode of treatment described is less formal but not less competent. There continues to be a lack of objective literature regarding the overall efficacy of the hospice concept of care. Toot writes

> Those who believe that hospice should be a care alternative have the responsibility to satisfy the demand for objective rationales while retaining the unique humaneness of the hospice concept (ref. 23, p. 670).

The issue of effectively intervening with terminally ill clients is complicated further in home health care when hospice care is not available. The tenets of hospice care can be used in home care when a hospice program has not been established. The home health clinician does indeed need new tools to be effective in the care of the dying client. These tools constitute a different set of facts to work with, as in any other medical specialty. This does not preclude the practitioner from using old skills for new situations. The hospice concept of care provides the framework and facts for these situations.

SUMMARY

The whole hospice team is essential in the care of the dying client at home. To have been a vital part of a dynamic hospice team and to know that within the rules there truly are no rules, only guidelines to effectively lessen human suffering, has been gratifying. To serve terminally ill home health clients in communities without established hospice programs is a challenge to any health care worker. With a proper education in the psychological implications of dying, the process of grief, and the hospice philosophy of care, the home health clinician is well equipped to provide valuable assistance to the terminally ill client in conjunction with other members of the health care team.

REFERENCES

1. Kubler-Ross, E: On Death and Dying. Macmillan, New York, 1969.
2. Saunders, C, Summers, DH, and Teller, N (eds): Hospice: The Living Idea. WB Saunders, Philadelphia, 1980.
3. Mor, V and Masterson-Allen, S: Hospice Care Systems: Structure, Process, Costs and Outcome. Springer-Verlag, New York, 1987.
4. Paradis, LF: Hospice Handbook: A Guide for Managers and Planners. Aspen, Rockville, 1985.
5. Zimmerman, JM: Hospice: Complete Care for the Terminally Ill. Urban & Schwarzenberg, Baltimore, Munich, 1986.
6. Lamerton, RJ: Lecture, University of Cincinnati, Cincinnati, 1975.
7. McCann, BA: The Hospice Project Report. Chicago: Joint Commission on Accreditation of Hospitals, 1985.
8. National Hospice Organization: President's letter. Author, McLean, 1982.
9. Rhymes, J: Hospice care in America. JAMA 264:369, 1990.
10. Datzman, RC: Unpublished material, 1978.
11. Dobratz, MC: Hospice nursing: Present perspectives and future directives. Cancer Nurs 14:55, 1991.
12. Reuss, R: Hospice, one PT's personal account. Clinical Management in Physical Therapy 4:28, 1984.
13. Davis, CM: Hospice care: physical therapy has a role to play. Clinical Management in Physical Therapy 2:7, 1982.
14. Reuss, R and Last, S: Care of the terminally ill: Hospice, home and extended care facilities. In McGarvey, CL (ed): Physical Therapy for the Cancer Patient. Churchill Livingstone, New York, 1989.
15. Reuss, R: The use of TENS in the management of cancer pain. Clinical Management in Physical Therapy 5:16, 1985.
16. Folts, D, et al: Occupational therapy in hospice home care: A student tutorial. Am J Occup Ther 40:623, 1986.
17. Picard, HB, Magno, JB: The role of occupational therapy in hospice care. American Journal of Occupational and Physical Therapy 36:597, 1982.
18. Tigges, KN: The treatment of the hospice patient: From occupational history to occupational role. Am J Occup Ther 37:235, 1983.
19. Von Roenn, JH: Results of a physician's attitude toward cancer pain management survey by ECOG. Proceedings of the American Society of Clinical Oncology Annual Meeting 10:326, 1991.
20. Saunders, C: A death in the family: A professional view. BMJ 1:31, 1973.
21. Dawson, NJ: Need satisfaction in terminal care settings. Soc Sci Med 32:83, 1991.
22. Seale, C: A comparison of hospice and conventional care. Soc Sci Med 32:147, 1991.
23. Toot, J: Physical therapy and hospice: Concept and practice. Phys Ther 64:665, 1984

BIBLIOGRAPHY

Kopp, RL: Encounter With Terminal Illness. Zondervan Publishing, Grand Rapids, 1980.

Mor, V, Greer, DS, and Kastenbaum, R: The Hospice Experiment. John Hopkins University Press, Baltimore, 1988.

National Hospice Organization: The 1989 Guide to the Nation's Hospices. National Hospice Press, Arlington, 1989.

Purtilo, R: Similarities in patient response to chronic and terminal illness. Phys Ther 56:279–284, 1976.

Rando, T: Loss and Anticipatory Grief. Lexington Books, Lexington, MA, 1986.

Appendix 16–1

Datz's Observations*

GENERAL CONCEPTS

1. 9 in 10 clients (98%) die easily.
2. 8 in 10 have no appetite and no thirst when near death (a few are very thirsty).
3. Death is a natural weakening unless prolonged by hospital procedures—often painful.
4. When a client is near death (1–2 days), give only supportive treatment for decubitus.
5. New clients are described briefly at staff meetings; volunteers often ask for a certain client.

MEDICATIONS AND PAIN CONTROL

6. Get rid of pain and other symptoms, then live each day to the utmost.
7. Never give pain medication without offering a stool softener and a laxative.
8. Oral medication should be swished in the mouth a few seconds before swallowing, if possible. Give oral medication in any flavor of juice, milk, or soft drink.
9. During the first 4 days, give oral medication every 4 hours (15-minute leeway) around the clock.
10. Pain can be brought under control in 4 to 7 days if the client is seen twice daily.
11. Suspect oversedation or too many drugs if the client sleeps more and then does not respond and the respiration rate is less than 10 respirations per minute.
12. Specify old-fashioned easy-open caps for weaker clients (unless there are children in the family).
13. Ask the pharmacist for a measuring spoon or cup, or both, with the first oral medication.
14. Ask that all medicines be clearly labeled: name, what for, how much, how often.

FOODS AND FLUIDS

15. Sitting upright or lying on the right side after eating promotes stomach emptying.
16. Lying supine or on the left side encourages vomiting.
17. Vomiting (severe) still leaves 30 percent of stomach contents in the stomach.
18. Pinching the dorsum of the hand is the best way to determine adequate fluids (if it is slow to return to normal configuration, give more fluids).
19. Cold liquids promote stomach and intestinal contractions and emptying.
20. Client should decide on the temperature of liquids.
21. Cooking odors may change a client's desire for a food to revulsion.
22. Cancer clients may change previous food likes and dislikes.
23. Cancer clients may be more sensitive to seasoning. They usually give up sweets and prefer sour or tart items.

*Adapted from Datzman.[10]

24. Sucking pineapple chunks for dry mouth is often suggested but has not been very successful.

GENERAL CARE

25. Do a rectal examination once a week; it reduces the number of impactions.
26. Erythema on a pressure area should precipitate all preventive measures by family and client—skin breakdown is often disastrous.
27. Do not tire a client while assessing. Usually the client is too interested to stop, but ask frequently. It is better to discontinue and return.
28. Never turn down help from the family.
29. Foot and ankle edema is often resolved by elevation above the heart as little as 4 hours a day. Watch daily. Add Lasix for severe cases.
30. For mouth care; give water in a straw or soaked washcloth, Chapstick, Vaseline on lips, moistened Q-tips (clients do not like these, but effects are good), lemon and glycerine swabs.
31. Give physical examinations to hospice team members. Be lenient. There are many things they can do—give them a chance.
32. For terminal cases, give the "straw test": near the end, when it is difficult to swallow, the client may take water from a straw (use finger over straw end to offer an inch or two of water). Initially, the client may take 2 in of liquid without coughing; a little later, 1 in, and finally, ½ in. At this point, death is near.

PSYCHOLOGICAL CONSIDERATIONS

33. Always sit when visiting a client; never hurry; listen; do not try to help the client finish the sentence.
34. Sit at eye level or slightly below. Never look down on a client (this provokes a helpless feeling). Look the client in the eye.
35. Learn all family names by putting the names, ages, spouses, residences, and occupations in the assessment.
36. Go to every wake and funeral service.
37. A child that is old enough to understand death of a bird, pet, or relative should be spoken to honestly (not shielded).
38. Funeral home: Children (close) should go for viewing with a close adult before the regular visiting time.
39. Honesty of emotions should be encouraged. If the whole family is honest, there will be more crying together; it is better to vent than to have a knot in your stomach or lump in your throat.
40. Crying before death shortens bereavement time later.
41. Cool, strong composure raises doubts in client's mind about the health provider's level of care.
42. Touching, even if the family did not do it before, is worth learning.
43. Sex history, when appropriate, can work wonders for both spouses.
44. Given a choice of denial, anger, depression, or acceptance, a client who wants to live each day well will take acceptance.
45. Some clients will only confide in a health professional, but most clients will talk, or perhaps only confide, to volunteer when the volunteer takes time to listen.
46. It helps if the volunteer can identify with the client or a client-family situation. Confidences then are more easily shared.
47. Near the end of life, the client may say "I want to die" emphatically. I reassure them that I neither prolong nor shorten life. I can help clients sleep more by using a sedative, which they may choose.
48. Am I dying? This is a common question. I tell the client from the beginning to ask any time. Often the response comes with a change in symptoms or the development of a new condition.

INDEX

An "f" following a page number indicates a figure; a "t" following a page number indicates a table.